FIRST ON THE SCENE

THE COMPLETE GUIDE TO FIRST AID AND CPR

SECOND EDITION

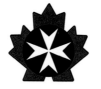

St. John Ambulance
OTTAWA, CANADA

Second Edition — 1996
First Impression — 15,000
Second Impression — 15,000

Canadian Cataloguing in Publication Data

First on the scene : the complete guide to first
aid and CPR

2nd ed.
Includes index.
ISBN 0-929006-89-5

1. First aid in illness and injury. 2. CPR (First
aid) I. St. John Ambulance.

RC86.8.F59 1996   616.02'52   C96-900770-1

First on the Scene: The Complete Guide to First Aid and CPR
is also printed as *The St. John Ambulance Guide to First Aid and CPR*
for distribution by Random House Press. The two books of the
second edition and first impression are identical.

EpiPen® Auto-Injector is a registered trademark of the EM Industries, Inc.
Ana-Kit® is a registered trademark of Miles Allergy Products Ltd.
HEROES™ is a registered trademark of SMARTRISK Foundation.
Tylenol® is a registered trademark of McNeil Consumer Products.
Tempra® is a registered trademark of Mead Johnson Canada.
Water-Jel® is a registered trademark of Water-Jel Technologies Inc.

St. John Ambulance
312 Laurier Avenue East
Ottawa, Ontario, K1N 6P6
Canada
613-236-7461

Printed in Canada
Stock No. 6504

St. John Ambulance

Since the days of the Crusades, St. John Ambulance has grown into a worldwide non-profit, non-denominational, multicultural, charitable organization committed to the service of others. Today, St. John Ambulance is one of two foundations of the *Most Venerable Order of the Hospital of St. John of Jerusalem.* The other foundation is the *St. John Ophthalmic Hospital* in Jerusalem, which specializes in the research and treatment of eye diseases, and which St. John Ambulance in Canada supports.

In Canada, St. John Ambulance is a national, voluntary agency founded over 110 years ago. Our mission is to enable Canadians to improve their health, safety and quality of life by providing training and community service. The work of St. John Ambulance in Canada is carried out by two distinct yet mutually dependent groups:

◆ the Brigade—uniformed volunteers who provide first aid coverage at public events and deliver community health promotion services

◆ the Association—a network of medical professionals, program development specialists, and instructors who provide first aid and health promotion courses to Canadians

Our mission is to enable Canadians to improve their health, safety and quality of life by providing training and community service.

We are

◆ 11,400 uniformed Brigade volunteers, including 2,500 youth

◆ 8,900 nationally certified instructors

◆ over 350 permanent staff members across Canada

◆ a Canadian Order headed by the Governor General as Prior, and the Queen as Sovereign Head

◆ throughout Canada, with Councils in each province, the Northwest Territories and in the National Capital Region (Federal District)

Acknowledgements

Book design:	Geoff Valentine, Beth Haliburton
Writer:	Geoff Valentine
Cover design:	Beth Haliburton
Cover photograph:	Richard Desmarais – photographer David Craib – art director
Illustrations:	Stanley Berneche – illustrator Marie-Hélène Baillot – assistant
NHQ Development Team:	Paula Dutz, Valerie Blais, Roger Lépine, Ileana Mavrodin, Josephine Hall

St. John Ambulance wishes to acknowledge and thank all the people who took time to answer questions, read pages and offer advice — you know who you are!

Special thanks to:

◆ The St. John Ambulance Professional Advisory Committee.

◆ Peter Johns, M.D., for his candid reviews of many portions of this book.

◆ The following St. John Ambulance Councils: Manitoba, Federal District, New Brunswick, Newfoundland, Prince Edward Island.

Contacting St. John Ambulance

St. John Ambulance welcomes your comments and suggestions for this manual. Please write, fax or e-mail us at the following address:

Training Department
St. John Ambulance National Headquarters
312 Laurier Avenue East
Ottawa, Ontario, K1N 6P6
Canada

fax: (613) 236-2425
e-mail: trainsja@nhq.sja.ca

Visit the St. John Ambulance World Wide Web site on the Internet at:
http://www.sja.ca

I am pleased to introduce *First on the Scene: The Complete Guide to First Aid and CPR*. Every Canadian should know basic first aid techniques and cardiopulmonary resuscitation. These easy-to-learn skills prepare an individual to provide immediate care when an injury happens. In a crisis situation, a person properly trained in first aid can make the difference between life and death.

First on the Scene: The Complete Guide to First Aid and CPR is a thorough reference manual and a valuable guide for those learning how to respond to a medical emergency. This book, which has been created under the counsel of medical professionals, presents the latest first aid and CPR techniques in a clear, informative manner that all Canadians will find useful. The manual's strong focus on managing an emergency scene offers first aid trainees the confidence and knowledge that will enhance their ability to provide safe and correct medical assistance.

The Order of St. John and the St. John Ambulance have a proud tradition of helping people in need and of training volunteers to help others. *First on the Scene: The Complete Guide to First Aid and CPR* is an important addition to this tradition and a laudable contribution to the well-being of Canadians. I commend all those involved with St. John Ambulance for their commitment to this organization's ideals and, as this book illustrates, for the exceptional quality of their work.

Ramon John Hnatyshyn

Governor General of Canada
Rideau Hall, Ottawa
October 1994

Prior of the Most Venerable Order
of the Hospital of St. John of
Jerusalem Priory of Canada

CONTENTS

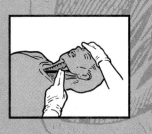

1 Introduction to first aid

2 Emergency scene management (ESM)

3 First aid for choking

4 Breathing emergencies and artificial respiration

5 Cardiovascular disease and CPR

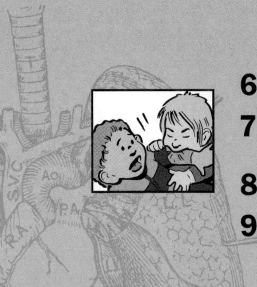

6 Wounds and bleeding

7 Injuries to bones, joints and muscles

8 Poisons, bites and stings

9 Burns

10 Environmental illnesses and injuries

11 Medical conditions

12 Emergency childbirth and miscarriage

13 Psychological emergencies

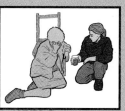

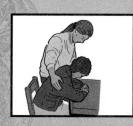

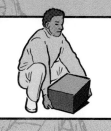

14 Lifting techniques and transportation

15 Be safe, be prepared

16 The body and how it works

Glossary

Index

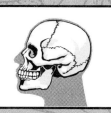

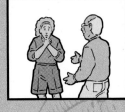

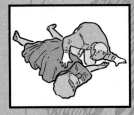

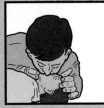

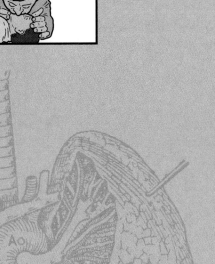

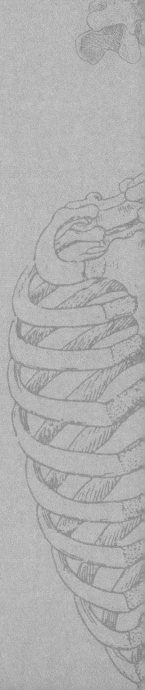

1

INTRODUCTION

TO FIRST AID

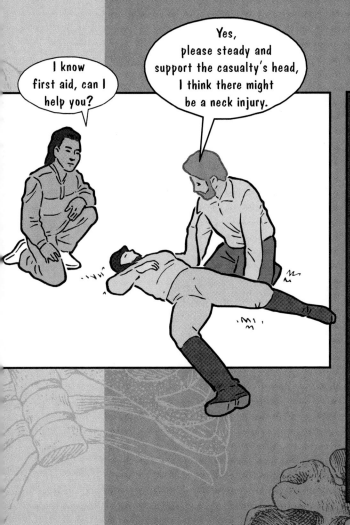

- ◆ *What is first aid?*
- ◆ *First aid and the law*
- ◆ *Safety and first aid*
- ◆ *Help at an emergency scene*
- ◆ *Getting medical help when you're alone*
- ◆ *History, symptoms and signs*
- ◆ *Shock*
- ◆ *Head and spinal injuries*
- ◆ *Levels of consciousness*
- ◆ *Recovery position*

1

This introductory chapter contains background information, definitions and other material related to giving first aid. There is first aid information at the end of the chapter on shock, head and spinal injuries and levels of consciousness, all of which you need to understand to act effectively at an emergency scene. Chapter 2 explains emergency scene management. Chapters 3 to 14 cover individual first aid topics. Chapter 15 has safety information to help you prevent injuries. Chapter 16 explains the parts of the body as related to first aid. This is followed by a complete glossary and index.

What is first aid?

First aid is emergency help given to an injured or suddenly ill person using readily available materials. It can be simple, like removing a sliver from a child's finger and putting on a bandage. Or, it can be complicated, like giving care to many casualties in a motor vehicle collision and handing them over to medical help. But no matter what the situation, the objectives of first aid are always the same. First aid tries to:

◆ preserve life

◆ prevent the illness or injury from becoming worse

◆ promote recovery

First aid is made up of both knowledge and skills. Most of the knowledge you will find in this book, and it can be learned by studying it. The skills are different. The best way to acquire first aid skills is to take a recognized first aid course from a qualified instructor. In an emergency where there are injuries, your ability to act calmly, assess the situation and give appropriate first aid will depend on your first aid skills. At St. John Ambulance, we strongly recommend you take a first aid course to learn the skills of first aid.

a **first aider** is someone who takes charge of an emergency scene and gives first aid

the injured or ill person is called a **casualty**

Who is a first aider?

Anyone can be a first aider. Often the first aider at an emergency scene is someone who was just passing by and wanted to help. A parent can be a first aider to her child, a firefighter can be a first aider to an injured pedestrian, or an employee can be trained as a first aider for her place of work. A first aider is simply someone who takes charge of an emergency scene and gives first aid.

First aiders don't *diagnose* or *treat* injuries and illnesses (except, perhaps, when they are very minor)—this is what medical doctors do. A first aider *suspects* injuries and illnesses and gives *first aid*.

What can a first aider do?

A first aider gives first aid, but she can also do much more. In an emergency, where there is confusion and fear, the actions of a calm and effective first aider reassure everyone, and make the whole experience less traumatic.

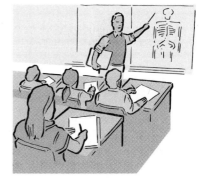

Besides giving first aid, she can:

- protect the casualty's belongings

- keep unnecessary people away

- reassure family or friends of the casualty

call the St. John Ambulance office nearest you to register for a first aid course—check your telephone book

- clean up the emergency scene and work to correct any unsafe conditions that may have caused the injuries in the first place

A casualty's age in first aid and CPR

In first aid and cardiopulmonary resuscitation (CPR):

- an **infant** casualty is under one year old

- a **child** casualty is from one to eight years old

- an **adult** casualty is eight years old and older

These ages are guidelines only; the casualty's size must also be considered.

Where does the term "first aid" come from?

"The term 'first aid' was officially adopted in England for the first time in 1879 by the St. John Ambulance Association, and the phrase 'first aid to the injured' appeared in its Annual Report for 1880."

Excerpted from *First Aid*, First Canadian Edition, 1959. Published under authority by The Priory of Canada of The Most Venerable Order of the Hospital of St. John of Jerusalem.

First aid and the law

Can a first aider be sued for giving first aid? Fear of being sued is one of the main reasons why people don't help when help is needed most. As a first aider, there are two "legal" situations in which you might give first aid. First, you may give first aid as part of your job—for instance, as a lifeguard or first aid attendant. Second, you might simply be a passer-by who sees an emergency situation and wishes to help an injured or ill person.

Note that St. John Ambulance is not giving legal advice here. This manual is not intended to replace advice given by a lawyer.

Giving first aid as part of your job

When giving first aid is part of your job, you have a legal duty to respond to an emergency situation at your workplace. You have a duty to use reasonable skill and care based on your level of training. This might include more than first aid—you may be trained in rescue, driving an emergency vehicle, etc. If you are a designated first aider at work, make sure your certification is always up-to-date. If you can, get a level of training higher than the minimum—you will be a more confident and effective first aider.

Giving first aid as a passer-by

In Canada (except Quebec) and most of the United States, you do not have a legal duty to help a person in need—if you do not help an injured person, you are not at fault. But our governments want to encourage people to help others, so they recognize the **Good Samaritan Principles**. These principles protect you if you choose to help someone in need. Once you begin to give assistance, you are obligated to use reasonable skill and care based on your level of training.

Giving first aid in Quebec

The *Quebec Charter of Human Rights and Freedoms* declares that any person whose life is in danger has the right to be helped. This means that you are required to help a person whose life is at risk, provided you do not put your own life, or anyone else's, in danger.

Principles of the Good Samaritan

You are a Good Samaritan if you help a person when you have no legal duty to do so. As a Good Samaritan, you give your help without being paid, and you give it in good faith (meaning you're helping because you care about the person and not for some other reason). Whenever you help a person in an emergency situation, you should abide by the following principles, each of which is discussed further below:

◆ you identify yourself as a first aider and get permission to help the injured or ill person before you touch her—this is called **consent**

◆ you use **reasonable skill and care** in accordance with the level of knowledge and skill that you have

◆ you are not **negligent** in what you do

◆ you do not **abandon** the person

Consent. The law says everyone has the right not to be touched by others. As a first aider, you must respect this right. Always identify yourself to a casualty and ask for permission to help before touching her. When you arrive at an emergency scene, identify yourself as a first aider to the casualty. If you are a police officer, nurse, first aider, etc., say so. Ask if you can help. If the casualty says, "yes," you have consent to go ahead and help. If the casualty doesn't answer you, or doesn't object to your help, you have what is called **implied consent,** and you can go ahead and help. There are some special situations:

◆ If the casualty is unresponsive and relatives are present, ask for consent from the casualty's spouse or another member of the casualty's immediate family.

Although it might not seem to make sense that you would identity yourself to an unresponsive person and ask for consent to help her, this is what you must do. Always ask for consent before touching a casualty. If there is no response, you have implied consent to carry on and give first aid.

◆ If the casualty is an infant or a young child, you must get consent from the child's parent or guardian. If there is no parent or guardian at the scene, the law assumes the casualty would give consent if she could, so you have implied consent to help.

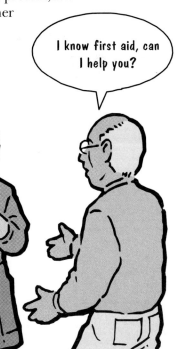

I know first aid, can I help you?

1

> I know first aid, can I help your baby?

A person has the right to refuse your offer of help and not give you consent. In this case, do not force first aid on a conscious casualty. Even if you do not have consent to touch the person and give first aid, there may be other actions you can take, like controlling the scene, calling for medical help, etc.

Reasonable skill and care.   As a Good Samaritan, when you give first aid you are expected to use reasonable skill and care according to your level of knowledge and skills. When in question, care that is given will be measured against what the reasonable person with the same level of knowledge and skill would do. Give first aid with caution so that you don't aggravate or increase an injury. Make sure you only try to do what you know you can do, and that all your actions help the casualty in some way.

Negligence.   The Good Samaritan principles say that, if you help someone who needs emergency medical care, you will not generally be considered negligent for what you do or don't do as long as you use reasonable skill and care according to your level of knowledge. When you give first aid, use common sense and make sure your actions are in the casualty's best interest. Simply put, give the care that you would like to receive if you were in the casualty's position.

Abandonment.   Never abandon a casualty in your care. Once the casualty accepts your offer of help, do not leave her. Stay with her until:

◆ you hand her over to medical help

◆ you hand her over to another first aider

◆ she no longer wants your help—this is usually because the problem is no longer an emergency and further care is not needed

In summary, there is no reason not to help a person in need. By following the guidelines above, you will minimize the risk of being held negligent for your actions.

Safety and first aid

1

The number one rule in giving first aid is, "Give first aid safely."
Emergency scenes can be dangerous and you have to make sure
your actions don't put you or anyone else in danger. Take the time
to look for hazards and assess the risks of any actions you take. You
don't want to become a casualty too!

There are three basic types of risks to be aware of:

◆ **the energy source that caused the original injury**—is the
energy still active and could anyone be injured by it? For
example, where an injury has been caused by machinery, is
the machinery still running?

◆ **the hazards from secondary or external factors**—are other
conditions present that could be a hazard? For example, at
the scene of a car crash, could there be an explosion or
perhaps injuries caused by passing vehicles?

◆ **the hazards of the rescue or first aid procedures**—is there
risk of someone being injured by the rescue and first aid
actions? For example, if the casualty is much larger than you
are, and you have to move that person, can you do so without
injuring your self?

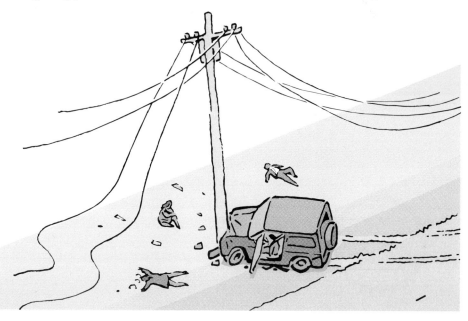

1

Preventing infection

A first aider and casualty are in very close contact with each other when first aid is given. This close contact means that an infection could pass from one person to the other. This risk of infection is a safety hazard a first aider always has to be aware of.

There is more risk of serious infection when blood and other bodily fluids are involved, as the viruses that cause AIDS (acquired immunodeficiency syndrome), hepatitis B and other illnesses may be present. If you don't know if someone is infected with an illness, you should use safety measures called **the universal precautions** to minimize the risk of transmission.

the risk of infection works both ways

The universal precautions are used in the health care professions to reduce the risk of infection for both the caregiver and the casualty. The universal precautions that apply to first aiders are: hand washing, wearing gloves, minimizing mouth-to-mouth contact during artificial respiration and the careful handling of sharp objects.

Gloves. Gloves prevent direct hand contact between the first aider and the casualty. Wear gloves when you might touch blood, bodily fluids, tissue or anything that has come in contact with one of these. Put on your gloves as you approach an emergency scene. Vinyl or latex gloves are equally effective, although latex irritates some peoples skin. Keep your gloves in a place you can get to easily, where they are not exposed to really hot or really cold temperatures. It's a good idea to keep a few pairs of gloves in your first aid kit. See page 1-10 for the correct method of removing and disposing of used gloves.

How big is the risk of getting AIDS?

· · · · · · · · · · · ·

If a casualty has AIDS, it is highly unlikely you would get AIDS by giving AR or CPR without a mask. The risk is very low — it has never actually happened.

Hand washing. Hand contact is one of the main ways infections are transferred from one person to another. Wash your hands with soap and running water immediately after any contact with a casualty. It is also a good idea to wash your hands often when you are around people who are sick with a cold, the flu, etc.

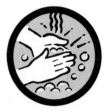

1

Minimizing mouth-to-mouth contact. There is a slight risk that an infection could be passed from one person to another during artificial respiration (AR). Use a special face mask or shield designed to prevent disease transmission during AR. Many brands and types of masks are available. Choose a disposable mask or one with a disposable one-way valve. Keep it in an accessible place where you can get it quickly. Follow the directions that come with the mask to use it properly.

Sharp objects. If a sharp object touches infected blood and then pricks or cuts you, you could become infected. Although first aiders do not routinely use sharp objects like scalpels and needles, there may be a need to use a knife or perhaps clean up broken glass that has been in contact with blood. In these cases, wear gloves and handle sharp objects with extreme care because one could cut through your gloves and skin and infect you.

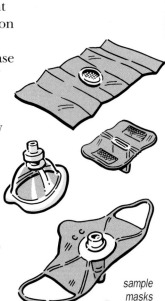

sample masks

The universal precautions are safety measures for protecting both the first aider and the casualty. Although it may seem like you are wasting precious time by pulling on gloves or getting your face mask ready, this is not the case. Safety is the most important concern while giving first aid. Use the universal precautions to ensure the safety of everyone at the scene.

Safety in a violent situation

Violent situations are not uncommon. Often there are injuries and your skills as a first aider can be valuable. In any emergency scene be on the lookout for violence. If there is violence, or the potential for violence, **be careful**. Your first priority is to protect your own safety—don't put yourself at risk. You are more valuable as a first aider than as a casualty!

Whenever injuries occur through violence, a crime has been committed. If you think a crime has been committed, call police to the scene. While waiting for

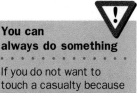

You can always do something

If you do not want to touch a casualty because of the risk of infection—is there anything you can do? Yes, there is plenty of first aid you can give. For instance, you can:

◆ take charge
◆ call bystanders and ask for help
◆ make the area safe
◆ send/get medical help
◆ give reassurance
◆ give information to ambulance officers

The risk of infection to a first aider is extremely small. In a situation where you think the risk is high, there are still many potentially life-saving actions you can take.

1

How to remove gloves

Once gloves have been used, they are contaminated and are a possible source of infection. Take them off without touching their outer surface following the steps below.

1 *grasp the outside of the glove*

Grasp the cuff of one glove.

2

Pull the cuff towards the fingers, turning the glove inside out.

3

As the glove comes off, hold it in the palm of your other hand.

4 *do not touch the outside of the glove*
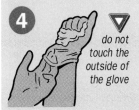

Slide your fingers under the cuff of the other glove.

5
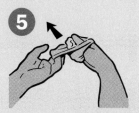

Pull the cuff towards the fingers over the first glove.

6 *first glove is inside the second*
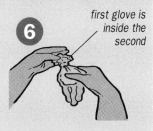

Tie a knot in the top of the outer glove and dispose of properly—see below.

7

Wash hands with soap and running water as soon as possible.

Torn gloves

If you tear your gloves while giving first aid, take them off right away. Wash your hands if possible, and put on a new pair of gloves.

Proper disposal

Seal the used gloves in a plastic bag and put them in your household garbage.

Check with a health professional or your first aid instructor for specific regulations in your area.

1

the police, do the following:

◆ protect your safety, and the safety of others if you can

◆ give first aid for any injuries, and be sensitive to the casualty's emotional state—see psychological first aid for assault, page 13-5

◆ keep onlookers away as much as possible—do what you can to ensure the privacy of any casualties

◆ leave everything at the scene as is—you may disturb evidence that could help police in their investigation

As a first aider, you may have additional information the police will find helpful. Remain at the scene until the police say you can leave. Answer all questions the police ask of you.

Child abuse

When giving first aid to a child with injuries, be on the alert for signs of child abuse. Child abuse is any form of physical harm, emotional deprivation, neglect or sexual maltreatment which can result in injury or psychological damage to a child. To detect possible child abuse, look for signs such as:

◆ injuries inconsistent with what a child could do

◆ unusually shaped bruises or burns

◆ the child's apparent fear of the parent or caregiver

If you suspect child abuse, do not accuse anyone. Insist that the child receive medical help for her injuries; this will permit a full medical assessment. If you don't think the child will be taken to a doctor, call an ambulance and the police to the scene—this will ensure a doctor sees the child.

If medical care for the child is refused and calling for an ambulance and/or the police is impossible, call a child welfare agency (often the Children's Aid Society) and report your suspicions. When you make such a call, you don't have to give your name if you don't want to.

1

Help at an emergency scene

As a first aider, the first thing you do when you arrive at an emergency scene is take charge of the situation. You stay in charge until you hand control of the scene over to more qualified people. While in charge, many other people may offer to help.

Other first aiders

If another first aider arrives on the scene, she should tell you, the first aider in charge, that she is trained in first aid and ask if she can help. If someone arrives on the scene and jumps right in, tell that person you are in charge, and ask if she wants to help you.

If you feel another first aider at the scene is more qualified to handle the situation, ask that person to take control. On the other hand, the most qualified person does not need to be in control. The first first aider at the scene takes charge and stays in charge until she decides to hand over control.

Bystanders

Emergency scenes attract a lot of attention and there may be many people standing around watching. To give the casualty the safest care possible, only the people really needed should be at the scene.

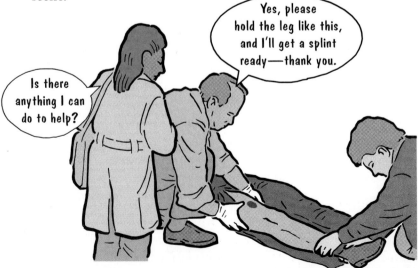

These include:

◆ relatives and close friends of the casualty

◆ any bystanders you ask to stay on the scene to help you

Everyone else should be asked to leave the scene. If needed, have a bystander control the crowd.

First responders—ambulance officers, police officers, fire fighters

Ambulance officers, police officers and fire fighters are known as first responders. It is their job to respond to an emergency. They are highly trained and will take charge of the scene as soon as they arrive. You can expect them to ask direct questions about the scene, the casualty and your involvement. Tell them you are a first aider, give the history of the scene and the condition of the casualty.

Depending on the scene, you may hand the care of the casualty over to the first responders immediately, especially if they are ambulance officers. Or, you may still be the best person to continue caring for the casualty at that time. Make sure that whatever happens is best for the casualty.

Other authorities—hydro, telephone, municipal personnel, etc.

Other authorities may be called to the scene. For example, if there are downed power lines, electrical utility personnel will be called. In these situations, the other authorities have a defined role that is not necessarily to give care to any casualties. Here, identify yourself, give the history of the scene and ensure the casualty's care is maintained.

Other authorities may arrive by chance. Here, use these people and their equipment to help manage the scene. They may have a radio or portable telephone to call for help. They can direct traffic,

---

Ten ways a bystander can help

1. Make the area safe.
2. Find all the casualties.
3. Find a first aid kit.
4. Control the crowd.
5. Call for medical help.
6. Help give first aid, under your direction.
7. Gather and protect the casualty's belongings.
8. Take notes.
9. Reassure the casualty's relatives.
10. Lead the ambulance attendants to the scene of the emergency.

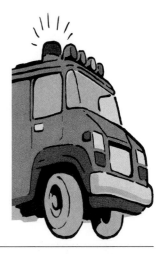

1

control any crowd or help give first aid. Commercial vehicles are often equipped with a first aid kit—this is a good source of first aid supplies if you do not have yours with you.

Off-duty doctors, nurses and other health professionals

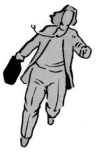

Health professionals are a valuable source of help at an emergency scene. If someone identifies herself as a health professional and asks whether she can help, tell her you are a first aider and that you are in charge of the situation. If the health professional has training and experience in managing the type of illness or injury present, ask for her opinion and advice (do this where the casualty cannot hear you). Make sure that whatever care is given makes sense to you and is best for the casualty.

Handing over control of a scene

When you are in charge of an emergency, you are responsible for the care of the casualty. At some point, you will hand control of the scene over to either another first aider, medical help or to the casualty herself. When deciding to hand over control of the scene, be sure that this is the best course of action for the casualty. You hand control of the scene to the casualty when the situation is minor and the casualty can manage without further help.

Tell whoever is taking charge of the scene the complete history of the incident including:

◆ your name

◆ the time you arrived

◆ the history of the illness or injury

◆ what first aid has been given

◆ any changes in the casualty's condition since you took charge

Also pass along any notes you have taken.

Medical Help

As a first aider, you cannot diagnose the exact nature and extent of an injury or illness; only a medical doctor has the legal right to do this. As a rule, always make sure the casualty receives medical care following first aid. Only for the most minor injuries is this not necessary. In first aid, medical care is called **medical help**.

Medical help is either given by a medical doctor or given under the supervision of a medical doctor. Ambulance officers (civilian only) and paramedics give medical help because they work under the supervision of medical doctors. Medical help is given in hospitals but it can also be given at the emergency scene or on the way to a medical facility, like a hospital.

Sometimes the need for medical help is urgent—here, calling for medical help right away is necessary to save the casualty's life. An example is a car collision where the driver hit the steering wheel and has severe bleeding inside her chest. Only getting her to a hospital where doctors can operate to stop the bleeding will save the casualty.

The Golden Hour

When there are severe, life-threatening injuries, doctors, ambulance officers and first aiders refer to the **golden hour**. The golden hour is the first hour after the casualty was injured. This time is "golden" because if she makes it to a hospital operating room within this hour, her chances of survival are "pretty good." After one hour, her chances for survival drop very quickly.

If you consider all the things that have to happen to get an injured person to an operating table, you'll see that there is no time to spare. For example, following a car crash:

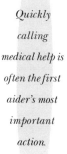

Quickly calling medical help is often the first aider's most important action.

◆ the crash scene has to be "discovered" by a passer-by

◆ the passer-by has to realize that medical help is needed

◆ the passer-by has to find a way to call medical help—this may mean using a car phone, sending another bystander, leaving the scene to call, or something else

◆ the ambulance has to be dispatched and travel to the scene

- the injured person may have to be freed from the car wreck

- the casualty needs to be loaded onto a stretcher and into the ambulance

- the ambulance has to reach the hospital and the stretcher has to be unloaded and wheeled to the waiting medical team

- once the casualty arrives at the hospital, time is needed for the medical team to make a careful assessment, take x-rays, do other required tests, prepare an operating room, etc.

In an emergency there is no time to spare. The faster the first aider calls for medical help, the better the chances are that the casualty will survive.

Call an ambulance or drive the casualty to the hospital?

Always call an ambulance if you can. Only transport the casualty to medical help yourself if that is the only possible way to get medical help. First, an ambulance or other rescue vehicle is well-equipped and the casualty can begin receiving medical help as soon as it arrives. Second, the Good Samaritan principles only protect you while giving care at the scene of the emergency, or, while transporting the casualty if transporting the casualty is needed to save the casualty's life, or is the only way to get the casualty to medical help. Choosing to transport the casualty yourself, when you could have called an ambulance, means your actions may not fall within the Good Samaritan principles.

The hospital versus the doctor's office

If you call an ambulance to an emergency scene, the ambulance officers will decide where to take the casualty. But if you or someone else is going to take the casualty to medical help, should you go to a hospital or a doctor's office?

If possible, always go to the emergency department of a hospital. Only go to a doctor's office if the situation is not urgent or there is no hospital nearby. As a rule, a doctor's office is not equipped to manage an emergency situation and often, the casualty will need the services of a hospital anyway.

1

How to get medical help

Medical help is organized under a community's **Emergency Medical Services** (EMS) system. The EMS system is made up of many parts, including ambulance services, hospital emergency departments, doctors, ambulance officers, paramedics and fire fighters. As a first aider, you are also an important part of the community EMS system. It is your role to recognize an emergency, give first aid and call for help. Without first aiders and bystanders, the other parts of the EMS system would not be able to respond quickly to emergencies.

To be an effective first aider, you have to know how to get medical help quickly. Know the EMS telephone number for your community (often 911). If you are outside of your community, the EMS phone number(s) is listed in the first few pages of the telephone book. When you call, follow the dispatcher's instructions. Don't hang up until you are told to, or the dispatcher hangs up first.

9-1-1

911 is the emergency phone number in many communities

Sending a bystander for medical help

• • • • • • • • • • • • • • • • • • •

If there is a bystander at the scene, it's best to send her to call for medical help. This lets you stay at the scene and give first aid.

Tell the bystander:

◆ to call an ambulance–give her the phone number

◆ what's wrong with the casualty–give the worst possible situation to make sure the casualty gets the urgent care she may need

◆ where you are

◆ to report back to you–this way you know the call for medical help has been made

If possible, always send someone out to meet the ambulance. Leading the ambulance officers to the emergency scene saves a lot of time.

Call an ambulance. Dial 911 and tell them an infant is unresponsive. The address is 321 Oak Street. Hang up when they tell you to and then come back here.

1

Getting medical help when you're alone

An emergency situation is immediately more complicated if you and the casualty are alone. You'll have to decide whether to stay with the casualty or leave to get help. The best course of action depends on the particular situation. Some typical situations are discussed below.

An unresponsive casualty

If a casualty is unresponsive, medical help is needed. You have to decide if, and when, you should leave to get medical help. To make this decision, first decide if help is "nearby."

What is "nearby"?

Help is nearby if you can get to a phone (or to a person), make the call and return within three minutes. If so, then go for medical help. Exactly when you go depends on the age of the casualty.

Adult casualty

With an adult casualty, go right away to call for medical help. When you return, start first aid with the primary survey*.

Child or infant casualty

You may be able to carry the infant or child to the phone and give first aid on the way. If so, do this, even if the phone is farther than "nearby."

If you cannot bring the child or infant to the phone, give first aid for one minute. You give first aid for one minute because in children and infants, unresponsiveness often follows a period of severe breathing difficulty. This means that the casualty's body is probably very low in oxygen and brain damage is likely to happen more quickly. By giving first aid for the ABCs right away, you may reduce the chance of brain damage or death by getting oxygen into the casualty's body.

Once you have given first aid for one minute, check the pulse:

◆ if the casualty is not breathing but has a

pulse and an open airway, stay and keep giving AR until medical help takes over
◆ if there is a pulse and breathing, or, if there is no pulse and no breathing, turn the casualty into the recovery position and go call for medical help. When you return, resume first aid with the primary survey*.

If a phone is not "nearby"

Complete the primary survey* and give life-saving first aid. Once this is done, consider the following in deciding whether to stay with the casualty or to go for medical help:

◆ how long might it be before someone finds us?
◆ how long will a return trip to the nearest phone or person take?
◆ if I leave, will the casualty survive until I return?
◆ if I stay, how long will the casualty survive?

These are the main considerations. If the casualty's life seems not to be in danger, and there is a good chance you will be found relatively soon, then you should probably stay with the casualty. If the casualty's only hope is medical help and you don't have to go too far to call and won't otherwise be found by anyone, then consider going to call.

You need to judge the situation, weigh the odds and do your best given your training and experience. Don't make any decision too quickly—and in making a decision, also consider your own safety. Whatever you do, keep the risk to yourself as low as possible. For example, if you are not outfitted to travel through the forest at night, then don't. The absolute worst decision you can make is one that results in you becoming a casualty too.

---

* "Primary survey" and "ABC's" are explained in chapter 2.

Deciding to leave an unresponsive casualty to call medical help

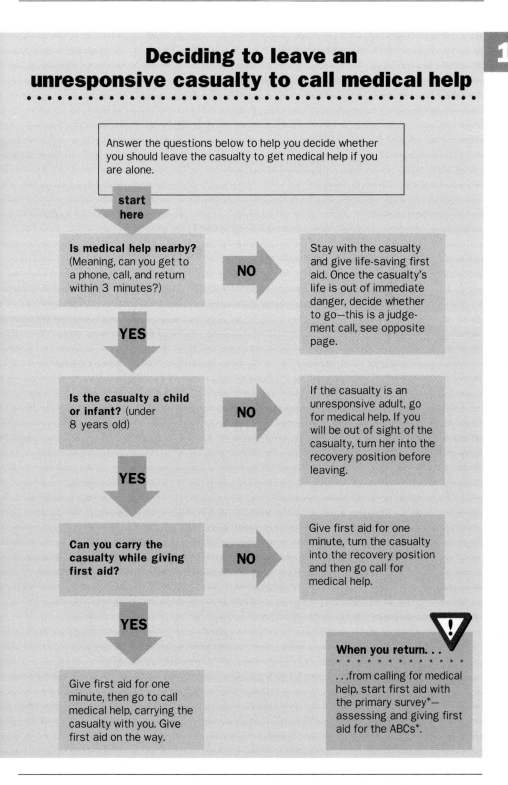

Answer the questions below to help you decide whether you should leave the casualty to get medical help if you are alone.

start here

Is medical help nearby? (Meaning, can you get to a phone, call, and return within 3 minutes?)

NO → Stay with the casualty and give life-saving first aid. Once the casualty's life is out of immediate danger, decide whether to go—this is a judgement call, see opposite page.

YES ↓

Is the casualty a child or infant? (under 8 years old)

NO → If the casualty is an unresponsive adult, go for medical help. If you will be out of sight of the casualty, turn her into the recovery position before leaving.

YES ↓

Can you carry the casualty while giving first aid?

NO → Give first aid for one minute, turn the casualty into the recovery position and then go call for medical help.

YES ↓

Give first aid for one minute, then go to call medical help, carrying the casualty with you. Give first aid on the way.

When you return. . .

. . .from calling for medical help, start first aid with the primary survey*— assessing and giving first aid for the ABCs*.

1

Background on injuries

When something from outside the body damages tissues, the damaged area is called an injury. How serious an injury is depends on:

- what tissues are injured—an injury to a vital organ, or tissues of a vital system, like the nervous system, is serious

- how bad the injury is—for instance, a bone broken in half may not be as serious as the same bone shattered into many pieces

- how much tissue is injured—a burned hand may be more serious than a burned finger

The closer an injury is to vital organs, the more serious the injury is. A broken rib can be more serious than a broken arm because the broken rib could injure the lung and affect breathing.

Injuries and energy

Injuries result from too much energy being applied to the body. For instance:

- a thermal burn is an injury caused by too much heat energy

- an acid burn is an injury caused by too much chemical energy

- snowblindness is an injury caused by too much light energy

- a broken bone is an injury caused by too much mechanical energy

- a stopped heart from an electric shock is an injury caused by too much electrical energy

The body can take a certain amount of energy without being injured. But too much of any sort of energy will cause injury. Three factors determine whether an injury will occur. They are:

- how intense the energy was

- how long the energy applied

- what part of the body the energy was applied to

Most injuries are caused either by something hitting the body or the body hitting something—this is mechanical energy. When something moves, it has mechanical energy. How much mechanical energy something has depends on how fast it is moving and how much it weighs.

Something moving slowly, like a person walking, has less mechanical energy than something the same weight that is moving fast, like a person skiing down a hill. Also, the heavier something is, the more energy it has when it is moving at a certain speed. Getting hit by a baseball hurts more than getting hit by a small stone—the baseball is heavier and has more energy—that's why it hurts more.

Mechanism of injury

Every injury has an exact cause. For example, in a car crash, the exact cause is not the driver falling asleep or the car skidding off the road, but the driver's head hitting the steering wheel. From the moment you arrive at an emergency scene, look for the causes of any injuries. Try to answer these questions:

◆ what happened to the casualty's body to cause the injury?

◆ how much force was involved?

◆ what parts of the body are involved?

The answers to these questions lead to the **mechanism of injury**, which is one of the first aider's most valuable tools. If you understand the mechanism of injury in an emergency situation, you are able to predict what injuries may be present, and what injuries are not likely. If you see that a lot of force or energy was involved, you know right away the person needs an ambulance. Doctors have a list of mechanisms of injury that automatically call for urgent medical help—these are listed in the sidebar. Remember the items in this list. If you recognize one of these mechanisms of injury, you will know that the casualty needs urgent medical help—call an ambulance right away.

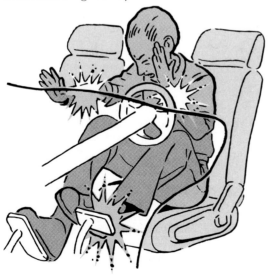

Mechanisms of injury that require an ambulance right away

◆ a free fall from more than 6.5 metres (20 feet)

◆ a vehicle collision that shows signs of a severe impact (such as major vehicle damage)

◆ severe damage to the inside of the vehicle that looks as if it was caused by impact with the casualty, like a bent steering wheel or a broken windshield

◆ casualty was thrown from the vehicle

◆ at least one casualty is dead

◆ the vehicle rolled over

◆ casualty was struck by a vehicle moving at 30 km/h or more

◆ severe crush injuries

When any of these mechanisms of injury are apparent, call an ambulance as soon as you can; you don't need any more information to make your decision.

1

Background on illness

We often think of first aid in the context of injuries only. But when someone becomes very sick, the result can be a medical emergency in which first aid can save a life.

Some illnesses, like heart attacks or strokes come on very fast. One minute the person seems to be in good health, and the next, they are seriously ill and you recognize a medical emergency. Other illnesses progress more slowly. Here, you may know the person is ill, and see that the condition is getting worse, but it can be hard to decide exactly when you have a medical problem that calls for a doctor's attention. The points below will help you decide when to get medical help for an ill person.

Get medical help when any of the following is present:

◆ sudden severe pain in any part of the body

◆ sudden changes in vision, headache or dizziness

◆ severe or persistent diarrhea or vomiting

◆ persistent high temperature

◆ changes in level of consciousness

◆ skin rash of unknown origin

◆ repeated fainting

◆ obvious depression, suicide threats or attempts

◆ whenever you are very worried about yourself or someone in your care

If the casualty is an infant (under one year old), the following are also reasons to get medical help (in addition to the reasons above):

◆ the baby has had a seizure

◆ the baby is blue or very pale

◆ you think the baby is having trouble breathing

◆ the baby cries a lot, or won't stop crying

History, signs and symptoms

Before you can give first aid, you need to assess the casualty to find out what is wrong. All your first aid actions are the result of what you find out in your assessments. History, symptoms and signs are the three ways you get information about a casualty.

History

History is all the information about the emergency situation and the condition of the casualty. You get this information by looking at the scene, talking to witnesses and to the casualty. The history answers the question, "What happened?" There is more about learning the history of the scene on page 2-12.

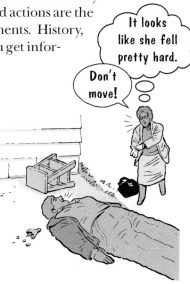

Signs

Signs are conditions of the casualty you can see, hear, feel and smell. You may see the signs of injury or illness immediately, or you may discover them while examining the casualty.

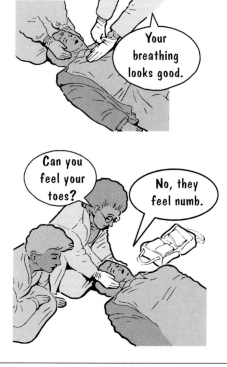

Symptoms

Symptoms are things the casualty feels and may be able to describe. You cannot discover symptoms on your own—the casualty must somehow communicate them to you.

1

Using history, signs and symptoms

As soon as you arrive on the scene, you are looking for signs and symptoms, and gathering information about the history of the incident. The table below gives examples of the things you may find at an emergency scene that can help you assess the casualty.

Chapter 2 describes how to look for signs, symptoms and the history in an orderly way using the **scene survey**, **primary survey** and **secondary survey**. Using your first aid knowledge, and the signs, symptoms and history at the scene, you decide what actions to take.

Examples of history, signs and symptoms	
things that can be part of the **history**	the condition of a vehicle, what bystanders tell you, what the casualty tells you about what happened, objects and substances at the scene, the time of day
signs you can **see**	blood, deformity, bruising, unequal pupils, painful expression, sweating, wounds, unusual chest movement, skin colour, swelling, foreign bodies, vomit, incontinence
signs you can **hear**	noisy or distressed breathing, groans, sucking wounds (chest injury), bones scraping together, quality of speech
signs you can **feel**	dampness, skin temperature, swelling, deformity
signs you can **smell**	casualty's breath (fruity breath or alcohol), vomit, incontinence, gas fumes, burning, solvents or glue
symptoms the casualty may **tell** you about	pain, fear, heat, cold, loss of normal movement, loss of sensation, abnormal sensation, thirst, nausea, tingling, faintness, stiffness, feeling faint, weakness, memory loss, dizziness, sensation of a broken bone

Vital signs

The casualty's temperature, pulse, respiration and level of consciousness are called vital signs. These signs show the basic condition of the casualty—if these signs are normal, the casualty is in pretty good shape. If any of these signs are abnormal, you should be concerned and look further for the reason. The vital signs are discussed in more detail in chapter 2, starting on page 2-13.

Shock

Any injury or illness can be accompanied by shock. Shock is a circulation problem where the body's tissues don't get enough blood. This is medical shock—don't confuse it with an electric shock or "being shocked" as in scared or surprised. Medical shock is life threatening because the brain and other organs cannot function properly. If shock gets bad enough, it leads to unconsciousness and even death. Because there is often shock in an emergency situation, and because it can progress very quickly, always check for shock and assess whether it is getting bad enough to be a medical emergency by itself. Like safety, shock is one of those things you always have to be thinking about.

Common causes of severe shock	
Cause of shock	**How it causes a circulation problem**
severe bleeding - internal or external (includes major fractures)	not enough blood to fill blood vessels
severe burns	loss of blood plasma (fluid) into tissues—not enough blood to fill blood vessels
crush injuries	loss of blood and blood plasma into tissues—not enough blood to fill blood vessels
heart attack	heart is not strong enough to pump blood properly
spinal cord or nerve injuries	brain can't control the size of the blood vessels and the blood can't get to the tissues properly
severe allergic reactions	many things can be affected—breathing, heart function, etc.

The table above gives some causes of shock. Severe shock can also result from medical emergencies such as diabetes, epilepsy, infection, poisoning or a drug overdose. Pain, anxiety and fear don't cause shock, but they can help make it worse, or make it progress faster. This is why reassuring a casualty and making her comfortable is so important.

Signs and symptoms of shock

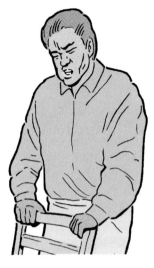

Signs	Symptoms
pale skin at first, turns bluish-grey	*restless*
bluish-purple lips, tongue, earlobes, fingernails	*anxious*
	disoriented
	confused
cold and clammy skin	*afraid*
breathing shallow & irregular, fast or gasping for air	*dizzy*
	*thirsty, maybe **very** thirsty*
changes in level of consciousness	
weak, rapid pulse— radial pulse may be absent	

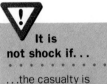

It is not shock if. . .

. . .the casualty is warm, the skin is dry with full colour and the person is fully conscious.

Minimizing shock

The following actions will minimize shock:

1 Give first aid for the injury or illness that caused the shock.

2 Reassure the casualty often.

3 Minimize pain by handling the casualty gently.

4 Loosen tight clothing at the neck, chest and waist.

5 Keep the casualty warm, but do not overheat—use jackets, coats, or blankets if you have them.

6 Moisten the lips if the casualty complains of thirst—don't give anything to eat or drink. If medical help is delayed many hours, give water or clear fluids to drink—make a note of what was given and when.

7 Place the casualty in the best position for her condition— see the positions on the next page.

8 Continue ongoing casualty care until hand over.

The above first aid for shock also prevents shock from getting worse. Whenever possible, add these steps to any first aid you give—this will minimize shock.

Positioning a casualty in shock

Putting the casualty in the right position can slow the progress of shock and make the casualty more comfortable. The position you use depends on the casualty's condition. The casualty should be as comfortable as possible in the position you use.

No suspected head/spinal injury; fully conscious

Place the casualty on his back with feet and legs raised—this position is often called the **shock position**. Once the casualty is positioned, cover him to preserve body heat, but do not overheat.

raise and support the feet and legs about 30 cm

No suspected head/spinal injury; less than fully conscious

Place the casualty in the recovery position—see page 1-32 and 1-33. When there is a decreased level of consciousness, airway and breathing are the priority—the recovery position ensures an open airway.

the recovery position—check the ABCs often

Suspected head/spinal injury

If there might be a head or spinal injury, steady and support the casualty in the position found and monitor the ABCs closely. This protects the head and spine from further injury.

As injuries permit

A casualty's injuries may not permit you to put her into the best position. For instance, raising the legs of a person with a fractured pelvis can cause more pain and aggravate the injury. Keep this person lying flat on her back. If possible, put her on a stretcher, or a backboard, and raise the foot of the stretcher. Always think of the casualty's comfort when choosing a position.

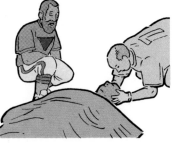

1

Head and spinal injuries

Injuries to the head and spine (especially the neck) are a special concern because they can be life threatening and/or cause life-long disability. Whenever you suspect a head injury, also suspect a neck injury, and whenever you suspect a neck injury, also suspect a head injury. Because the head and neck are so close to each other, often, when one is injured, so is the other.

Head/spinal injuries should be suspected when a casualty:

◆ has fallen from a height or down stairs

◆ has been in a motor vehicle collision

◆ has received a blow to the head, spine or pelvis

◆ has blood or straw-coloured fluid coming from the mouth, nose or ears

◆ is found unconscious and the history is not known

In every emergency situation, ask yourself if there is any way there could be a head or neck injury. Do this by looking at:

◆ the mechanism of injury

◆ the position of the casualty

◆ the history of the incident, including:

❖ what you are told

❖ what you can figure out from looking around the scene

sometimes it is easy to see that the casualty could have injured her head, neck or spine—but you have to assess the potential for a head or spinal injury in every situation

when you suspect a head or spinal injury, your job is to protect the head and spine from further injury by preventing unnecessary movement

Level of consciousness (LOC)

Consciousness means how aware a person is of herself and her surroundings. There is a full range of levels of consciousness, from completely conscious to completely unconscious. Many injuries and illnesses can cause changes in a casualty's level of consciousness. Some examples are:

- a breathing emergency
- a head injury
- shock
- a medical condition (epilepsy, diabetes, etc.)

- a heart attack
- poisoning
- alcohol or drug abuse

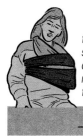

fully awake
speaks coherently
controls muscular activity
responds to speech or pain
fully aware of surroundings

no response to speech
no response to pain
not aware of surroundings

Decreasing consciousness

completely conscious

semi-conscious

completely unconscious

Unconsciousness may be a breathing emergency

Semi-consciousness and unconsciousness are breathing emergencies because, when an unconscious person is on her back, the tongue may fall to the back of the throat and block the airway. Also, saliva and other fluids can pool at the back of the throat. Since an unconscious person loses the reflex to cough up fluids in the throat, they block the airway and choke the person.

A progressive loss of consciousness means the casualty's condition is getting worse. Always monitor a casualty's level of consciousness and note any changes.

on his back, an unconscious casualty's airway may be blocked by either the tongue or fluids

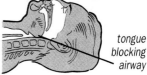

tongue blocking airway

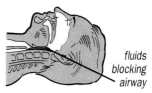

fluids blocking airway

Assessing level of consciousness

A first aider uses the **Modified Glasgow Coma Scale** to assess and describe levels of consciousness. The scale is based on the casualty's ability:

◆ to open the eyes—this is the **eye opening response**

◆ to speak—this is the **verbal response**

◆ to move muscles—this is the **motor response**

Use the information below to determine whether the casualty is conscious, semi-conscious or unconscious.

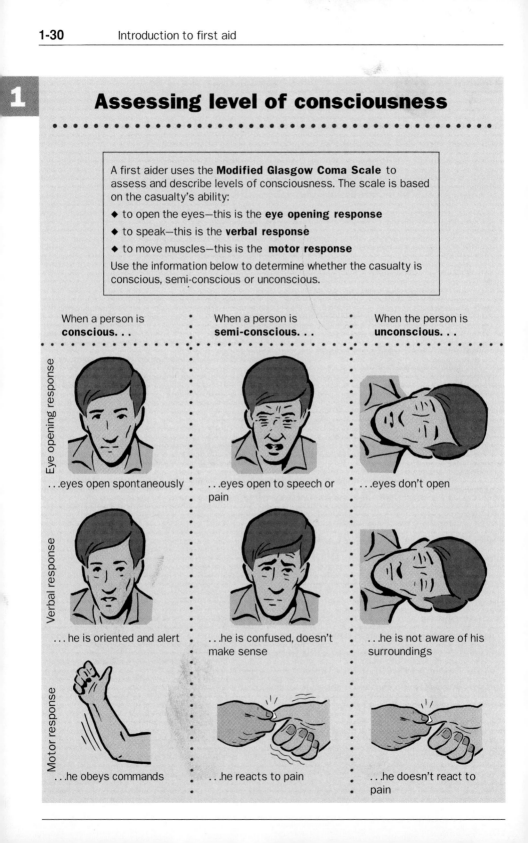

When a person is **conscious...**	When a person is **semi-conscious...**	When the person is **unconscious...**
Eye opening response ...eyes open spontaneously	...eyes open to speech or pain	...eyes don't open
Verbal response ...he is oriented and alert	...he is confused, doesn't make sense	...he is not aware of his surroundings
Motor response ...he obeys commands	...he reacts to pain	...he doesn't react to pain

First aid for semi-consciousness and unconsciousness

1   Start ESM—do a scene survey (see page 2-3). Have a by-stander call for medical help as soon as unresponsiveness is recognized. See page 1-19 for what to do if you are alone.

2   Do a primary survey and give life-saving first aid (see page 2-5).

3   Do a secondary survey if necessary and give first aid (see page 2-11).

4   Turn the casualty into the recovery position, if injuries permit. If injuries make it better for the casualty to be face up, monitor breathing continuously. If necessary, hold the airway open using the jaw-thrust without head-tilt (see page 4-22, step 3).

the recovery position

5   Loosen tight clothing at the neck, chest and waist, and continue ongoing casualty care until hand over. Record any changes in level of consciousness and when they happen.

Always ensure an open airway. If the casualty's injuries permit, put him into the recovery position. Otherwise, closely monitor breathing. Sometimes you cannot monitor the casualty's breathing. For instance, if:

◆ you have to leave to get medical help

◆ you have to give first aid to other casualties

Here, turn the casualty into the recovery position (see pages 1-32 and 1-33), being as careful as you can if there are any injuries. Although there is a risk of causing more injury, keeping the airway open is more important and must be your first concern.

Urgent medical help required

Decreased consciousness is always an urgent situation. The person can quickly become unconscious, and this is a breathing emergency. When you recognize decreased consciousness, get medical help as fast as possible.

1

How to put a casualty into the recovery position—method 1

The recovery position keeps an unconscious person's airway open. Always put a semi-conscious or unconscious person into the recovery position if you cannot constantly monitor the person's breathing. The method below is the preferred one.

1

place the near arm straight out

place the far arm with the back of the hand over the near cheek

Position the arms.

2

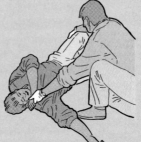

Bend and grab the far knee.

3

protect the casualty's head during the roll

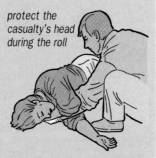

Roll the casualty towards you by pulling the far knee towards you and to the ground.

4

adjust the hand under the head so the neck is extended

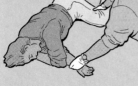

Adjust the position of the arms and leg so the casualty is in a stable position.

5

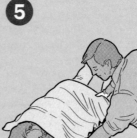

Continue ongoing casualty care.

Infant recovery position

support the head and neck

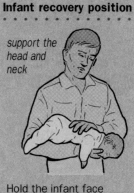

Hold the infant face down with the mouth and nose clear.

How to put a casualty into the recovery position—method 2

1

Use this method only if the casualty is much larger than you and too heavy to roll using method 1.

1

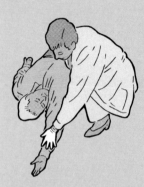

Position the arm closest to you.

2

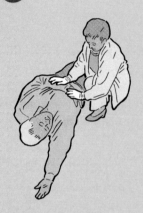

Position the arm furthest from you.

3

this will cause the casualty to roll over

Pick up the far lower leg and walk it around and over the casualty's near leg.

4

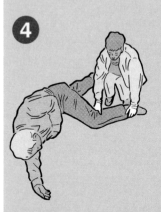

Position this leg with the knee bent.

5

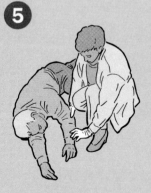

Position the arms to keep the neck extended.

6

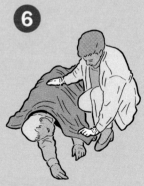

Continue ongoing casualty care.

1

Fainting

Fainting is a loss of consciousness that lasts a very short time—no more than a few minutes. It is caused by a temporary shortage of oxygenated blood to the brain. Some common reasons people faint are:

- fear or anxiety
- lack of fresh air
- severe pain, injury or illness
- the sight of blood
- underlying medical problem
- fatigue or hunger
- long periods of standing or sitting

A person losing consciousness is always a serious medical emergency. Do not assume a person has "just fainted" until there is a quick, full recovery and the reason for the fainting is known. If you think there might be a serious reason a person feels faint, or has fainted, get medical help.

Feels faint or "impending faint"

Sometimes when a person is about to faint, there are warning signs. The person:

- is pale
- is sweating
- feels sick, nauseous, dizzy and unsteady

When a person is about to faint, act quickly.

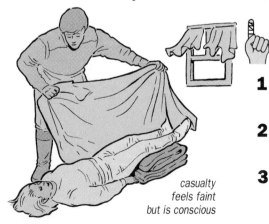

casualty feels faint but is conscious

First aid for an impending faint

1   Lay the casualty down with the feet raised about 30 cm (12 in).

2   Ensure a supply of fresh air—open windows or doors.

3   Loosen tight clothing at the neck, chest and waist.

4   Stay with the casualty until fully recovered.

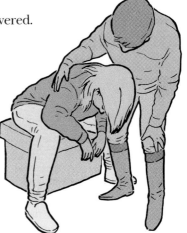

if you cannot lay the person down, (e.g. on an airplane or in a bus), have the person sit with her head lower than her shoulders

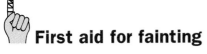

First aid for fainting

A person who has fainted is unconscious. The first aid for faint-ing is the same as the first aid for unconsciousness.

1   Start ESM—do a scene survey (see page 2-3). Have a bystander call for medical help as soon as unresponsiveness is recognized. See page 1-19 for what to do if you are alone.

2   Check the ABCs—make sure the casualty's airway is clear, that she is breathing and has a pulse, and check for shock.

3   Do a secondary survey if necessary and give first aid (see page 2-11).

4   Turn the casualty into the recovery position, if injuries permit (see pages 1-32 and 1-33).

5   Ensure a supply of fresh air and loosen tight clothing at the neck, chest and waist. Continue ongoing casu-alty care until hand over.

6   Make the casualty comfort-able as consciousness returns and keep her lying down for 10 to 15 minutes.

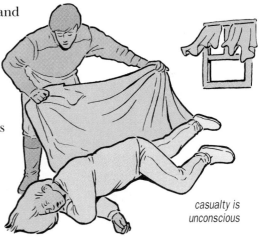

casualty is unconscious

Recovery from a faint should be quick and complete. If this is not the case, stay with the casualty until medical help takes over.

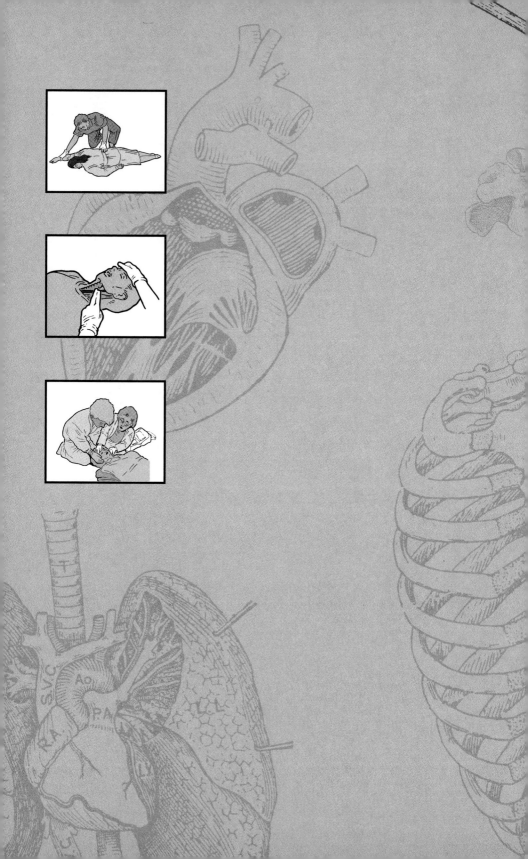

EMERGENCY SCENE MANAGEMENT (ESM)

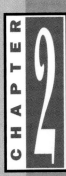

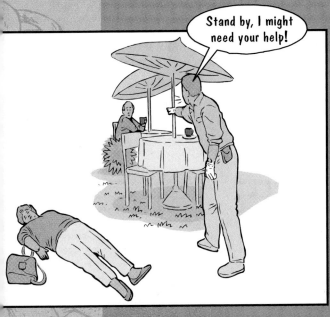

Stand by, I might need your help!

◆ *Introduction*

◆ *Scene survey*

◆ *Primary survey*

◆ *How to turn a casualty face up*

◆ *Secondary survey*

◆ *Taking the vital signs*

◆ *Head-to-toe examination*

◆ *Medical alert information*

◆ *Ongoing casualty care*

◆ *After the handover*

◆ *Multiple casualty management (triage)*

Introduction

Imagine a busy restaurant at lunchtime—people eating quickly and servers hurrying to get them on their way as fast as possible. Suddenly there is a commotion, and you see a woman lying on the ground… what happens now?

Emergency scenes like this usually begin with a lot of confusion as people realize there is an emergency unfolding in front of them— no one knows what to do first, who should be in charge or how they can help. In this situation, the first aider needs to follow a sequence of actions that ensure safe and appropriate first aid is given and everyone's safety is protected. St. John Ambulance first aiders use **emergency scene management** (called ESM for short) to do this.

Emergency scene management is the sequence of actions you should follow to ensure safe and appropriate first aid is given.

ESM has four steps:

◆ *scene survey*—here you take control of the scene, get an idea of what has happened and what is going on, and get things organized so you can start helping any casualties

◆ *primary survey*—here you assess each casualty for life-threatening injuries or illnesses and give the needed life-saving first aid

◆ *secondary survey*—here you assess the casualty for injuries or illnesses that are not life threatening and give appropriate first aid—sometimes you don't have to do this step

◆ *ongoing casualty care*—here you stay with the casualty until medical help arrives and takes over

These steps are always done in the order above, though sometimes you don't do the secondary survey. The pages that follow take you through the steps of ESM in detail. There is a four-page summary of ESM at the end of the chapter, on pages 2-30 to 2-33.

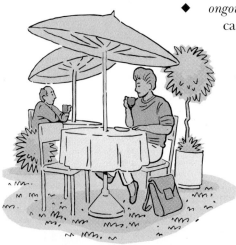

Scene survey

Every emergency scene is different, so the order of the steps of the scene survey will change depending on the situation. As much as possible, however, try to follow the order below.

1   Take charge of the situation

There won't be a head or spinal injury.

If you're the first first aider on the scene, take charge. If someone is already in charge, ask if you can help. If there is any chance the casualty could have a head or spinal injury, say, "Don't move!"

stay calm

collect your thoughts and decide to get involved

follow your common sense in deciding the best approach

2   Call out for help to attract bystanders

Stand by, I might need your help!

You can always use some help in an emergency situation—call out to attract the attention of any bystanders. Do this at any time if you need more help. See page 1-13 for a list of ten things a bystander can help with.

3   Assess hazards and make the area safe

An emergency scene can be a dangerous place. Look for anything that might be hazardous to the casualty, bystanders or yourself. If there are any hazards, do what you must to make the area safe—bystanders can help you with this. There is more about hazards at an emergency scene on page 1-7.

2

4 Find out the history of the scene, how many casualties there are and the mechanism(s) of injury

By looking at the scene, try to piece together what happened to cause the emergency situation. Look around for all possible casualties and count how many there are. For each casualty, note the mechanism of injury and consider whether there could be a head or spinal injury. See page 1-21 for more on mechanism of injury.

> If you suspect a head or spinal injury, you have to protect the casualty from unnecessary movement. See pages 2-6 and 2-7 for how ESM changes when there is a suspected head or neck injury.
>
> If there is more than one casualty, you have to decide who to assess first. See page 2-26 for more detail.

5 Identify yourself as a first aider and offer to help

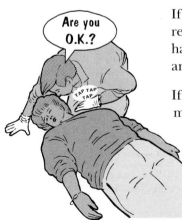

I know first aid, can I help you?

don't touch without consent

You can only touch someone if you have consent to do so. Before touching the casualty, ask for consent to help. If there is no response, you have implied consent to help. There is more about consent on page 1-5.

6 Assess responsiveness

Are you O.K.?

TAP TAP TAP

If the casualty is conscious, you know she is responsive. If she is not obviously conscious, you have to check responsiveness. Ask, "Are you O.K.?" and gently tap or shake her shoulders.

If she responds in any way, continue with the primary survey.

If she does not respond, send or go for medical help—see step 7.

7 Send or go for medical help

Send or go for medical help as soon as you know you will need it. In this case, the adult casualty is unresponsive so medical help is needed.

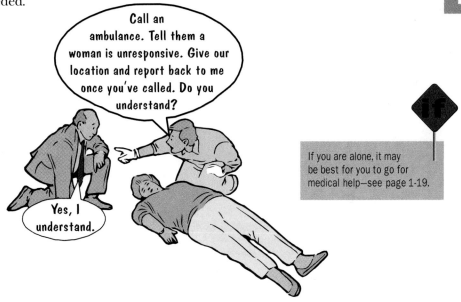

If you are alone, it may be best for you to go for medical help—see page 1-19.

. . . .

Next, start the primary survey

By the end of the scene survey, you have begun controlling the scene, have permission to give first aid to the casualty, and know whether the casualty is responsive. Next, focus your full attention on the casualty and do the primary survey.

. . . .

Primary survey

Airway, Breathing and Circulation are the ABCs.

With the primary survey you find out if the casualty has any life-threatening conditions and you give life-saving first aid. The primary survey focuses on the ABCs—airway, breathing and circulation. The exact techniques you use depend on the condition of the casualty. For instance, if the casualty is conscious and talking, you know she has an open airway and is breathing. If you suspect a neck injury, you must open the airway a special way to prevent movement of the head and neck.

continued on page 2-9

How ESM changes when a head or spinal injury is suspected

When there could be a head or spinal injury, protect the head and neck from any movement. Head or neck movement could result in life-long disability or death. Adjust your first aid to this situation as shown below.

1 *Don't move!*

I know first aid, can I help you?

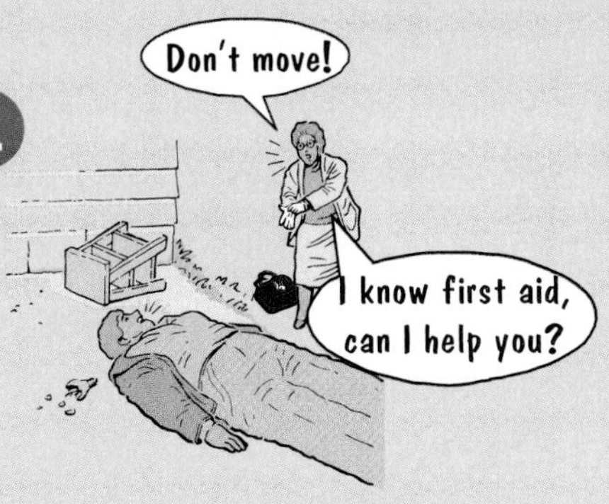

As soon as you see there might be a head or spinal injury, tell the casualty not to move.

2 *Are you O.K.?*

My head hurts.

firmly support the head in the position found

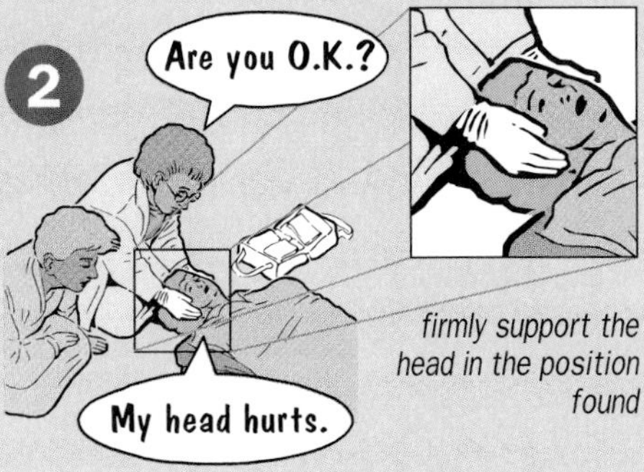

Once you have consent to help the casualty, steady and support the head and neck. Then, assess responsiveness.

3 *Don't let her head move at all, and if your arms get tired, tell me.*

keep elbows firmly supported on thighs or ground

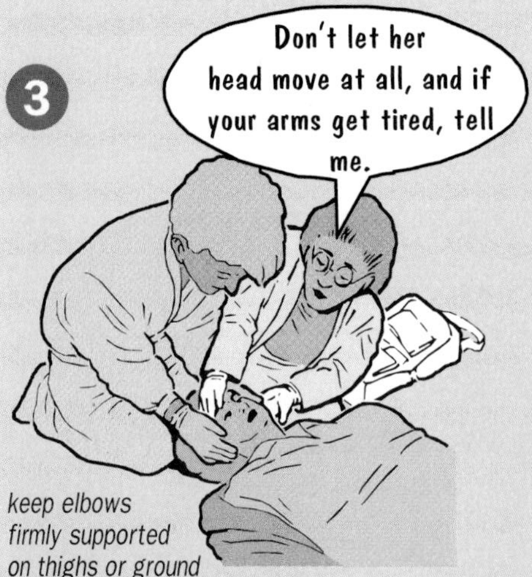

If there is a bystander to help, show her how to support the head and neck so you can continue your assessment.

4

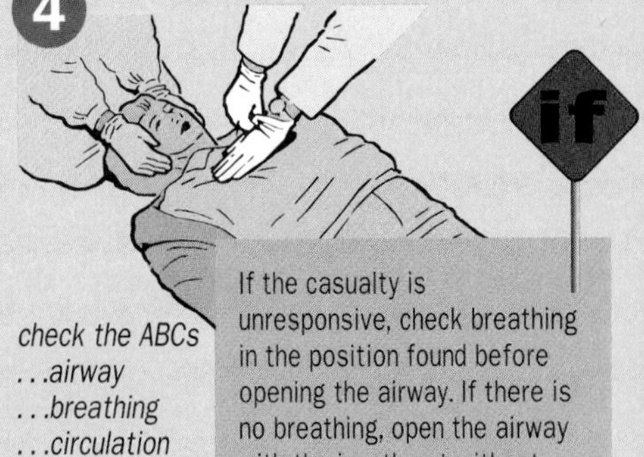

*check the ABCs
...airway
...breathing
...circulation*

if If the casualty is unresponsive, check breathing in the position found before opening the airway. If there is no breathing, open the airway with the jaw-thrust without head-tilt and check breathing again—see page 4-22.

Continue your assessment—check the ABCs.

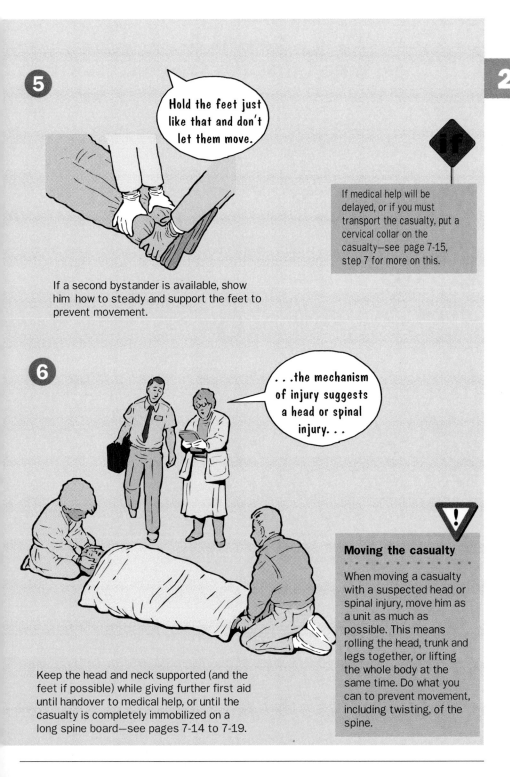

5

Hold the feet just like that and don't let them move.

If a second bystander is available, show him how to steady and support the feet to prevent movement.

If medical help will be delayed, or if you must transport the casualty, put a cervical collar on the casualty—see page 7-15, step 7 for more on this.

6

. . .the mechanism of injury suggests a head or spinal injury. . .

Keep the head and neck supported (and the feet if possible) while giving further first aid until handover to medical help, or until the casualty is completely immobilized on a long spine board—see pages 7-14 to 7-19.

Moving the casualty

When moving a casualty with a suspected head or spinal injury, move him as a unit as much as possible. This means rolling the head, trunk and legs together, or lifting the whole body at the same time. Do what you can to prevent movement, including twisting, of the spine.

2

How to
turn a casualty face up

You should give first aid in the position in which the casualty is found as much as possible. But sometimes you have to turn a casualty over to assess for life-threatening injuries or to give life-saving first aid. Two ways to do this are shown below.

**Turning a casualty face up—
no suspected head or spinal injury**

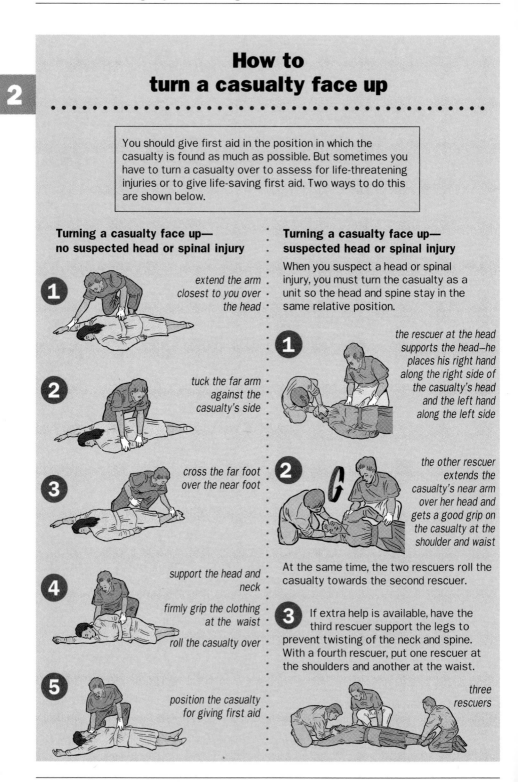

1 *extend the arm closest to you over the head*

2 *tuck the far arm against the casualty's side*

3 *cross the far foot over the near foot*

4 *support the head and neck*
firmly grip the clothing at the waist
roll the casualty over

5 *position the casualty for giving first aid*

**Turning a casualty face up—
suspected head or spinal injury**

When you suspect a head or spinal injury, you must turn the casualty as a unit so the head and spine stay in the same relative position.

1 *the rescuer at the head supports the head–he places his right hand along the right side of the casualty's head and the left hand along the left side*

2 *the other rescuer extends the casualty's near arm over her head and gets a good grip on the casualty at the shoulder and waist*

At the same time, the two rescuers roll the casualty towards the second rescuer.

3 If extra help is available, have the third rescuer support the legs to prevent twisting of the neck and spine. With a fourth rescuer, put one rescuer at the shoulders and another at the waist.

three rescuers

continued from page 2-5

The primary survey picks up from where the scene survey ends.

2

1 Check the airway

If the casualty is responsive, check the airway by asking a question and seeing how well the casualty can answer. If the casualty is unresponsive the airway may not be open. If there is no suspected head or neck injury, use the head-tilt chin-lift to open the airway.

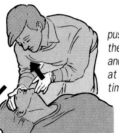

push back on
the forehead
and lift the jaw
at the same
time

one hand on
the forehead

fingers under
the bony part
of the jaw

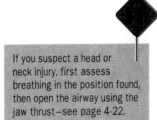

If you suspect a head or neck injury, first assess breathing in the position found, then open the airway using the jaw thrust—see page 4-22.

2 Check for breathing

Keep the airway open and check for breathing for 3 to 5 seconds.

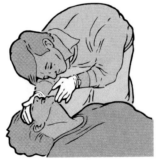

keep the head
tilted

with your ear
close to the
casualty's
mouth and
nose, check
for breathing

look... for
chest
movement

listen... for
sounds of
breathing

feel... for
breath on your
cheek

If the casualty is unresponsive, or appears to have difficulty breathing, assess to find out if breathing is **effective** or **ineffective**.

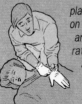

place a hand
on the chest
and assess
rate, rhythm
and depth

If there is no breathing, give two slow breaths and check for a carotid pulse for 5 to 10 seconds. If there is a pulse, give artificial respiration—see page 4-24, step 8. If there is no pulse, give CPR—see page 5-13, step 8.

If there is breathing but it is ineffective, give first aid that will help breathing and send for medical help. Assist the casualty's breathing—see page 4-33.

If breathing is effective, go to step 3, next page.

Signs of ineffective breathing:

♦ too slow* and shallow

♦ too fast* and shallow

♦ gasping for air

♦ bluish skin

* see page 4-3, *Breathing rates*

3 Check circulation

you may have to pull back your glove to feel the skin temperature

First, if there is any obvious, severe bleeding, give first aid to control it—see page 6-15. Bleeding is severe when blood spurts or flows freely from a wound. Second, check for shock by assessing skin condition and temperature. If there are signs of shock, send for medical help right away.

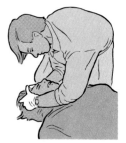

assess skin temperature using the back of your hand on the forehead, cheek or neck

check skin colour for paleness or blueness

look for sweating

Third, if you suspect other injuries, do a **rapid body survey** to check for hidden, severe, external bleeding and for signs of severe, internal bleeding. Quickly run the flats of your hands over the body looking for blood that is hidden from view and for obvious deformity that may indicate serious injury. Expose painful areas to look for signs of internal bleeding. The rapid body survey should take 30 seconds or less.

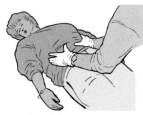

check the head and neck...

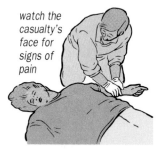

watch the casualty's face for signs of pain

... the shoulders, arms and hands...

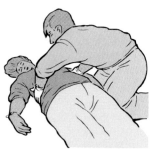

... the chest and under...

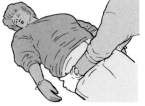

...the abdomen and under...

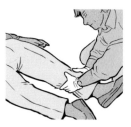

... the pelvis and buttocks...

... the legs and feet

If you find blood, expose the wound and control the bleeding if it is severe. Send for medical help. Support an obviously deformed limb with your hands.

Evaluate the situation
and decide whether to do a secondary survey

Whether you do a secondary survey depends on the situation.
Do a secondary survey if:

◆ the casualty has more than one injury

◆ medical help will be delayed more than 20 minutes

◆ medical help is not coming to the scene and you have to
  transport the casualty

If you do not do a secondary survey, steady and support any
injuries and give ongoing casualty care—see page 2-24.

Secondary survey

Do a secondary survey if there is more than one injury, medical help will be delayed, or you have to transport the casualty.

The secondary survey follows the primary survey and any life-saving
first aid you had to give. It is a step-by-step way of gathering information to form a complete picture of the condition of the casualty. You
are looking for injuries or illnesses that were not revealed in the
primary survey, but could benefit from first aid. Only do a secondary
survey if there is more than one injury, medical help will be delayed
more than about 20 minutes, or you have to transport the casualty.

The secondary survey has four steps:

1. the history of the casualty

2. the vital signs

3. the head-to-toe examination

4. first aid for injuries and illnesses found

Do not examine for unlikely injuries. For instance, if the casualty
cut his hand with a knife while preparing food, there is no need to
examine for injuries to the legs. Use the history of the situation
and the signs and symptoms of the casualty to decide how much of
the head-to-toe examination you need to do. When it is obvious
only one part of the body is affected, and the person has no other
complaints, a complete head-to-toe examination is not needed.

2

History of the casualty

When taking a complete history of the casualty, you are trying to find out everything that could be important about the casualty and the situation. This information can help you give the best first aid possible, and passing this information on may be helpful to others who care for the casualty.

If the casualty is fully conscious, ask him questions directly. If the casualty is semi-conscious or unconscious, ask friends, relatives and bystanders about her and the situation.

A simple way to take a complete history of the casualty is to re-member the word **SAMPLE**. Each letter stands for a part of the history, as follows:

S   =   *symptoms.* Symptoms are sensations the casualty feels such as pain, nausea, etc. If the casualty is conscious, ask him what he feels. If he is unconscious, ask bystanders if he complained of any symptoms before losing conscious-ness.

A   =   *allergies.* If the casualty is conscious, ask him if she has any allergies. Particularly important here are allergies to drugs.

M   =   *medications.* Ask if the casualty has taken any medication in the past 24 hours.

P   =   *past medical history.* Ask about the casualty's past medical history and whether there is anything that could be related to the current injury or illness. Check for a medical alert device (pendant or bracelet).

L   =   *last meal.* Find out when the casualty ate his last meal. This may be important information for medical help.

E   =   *events leading to the incident.* Ask how the incident happened. Get exact information about how the casual-ty's body was affected—this will help you find all injuries.

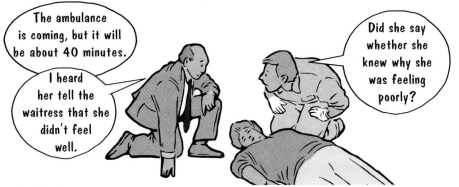

Vital signs

The **four vital signs** show the basic condition of the casualty.
These are:

- level of consciousness
- breathing
- pulse
- skin condition and temperature

Any change in a casualty's vital signs can indicate a serious change
in condition. Once you have assessed (or "taken") the vital signs,
monitor them closely— every few minutes, or whenever you think
the casualty's condition may have changed.

Taking the vital signs

1 Assess level of consciousness.

use the Modified
Glasgow Coma
Scale to assess
LOC—see
page 1-30

2 Assess breathing.

assess
breathing for
rate, rhythm
and depth—see
page 2-15

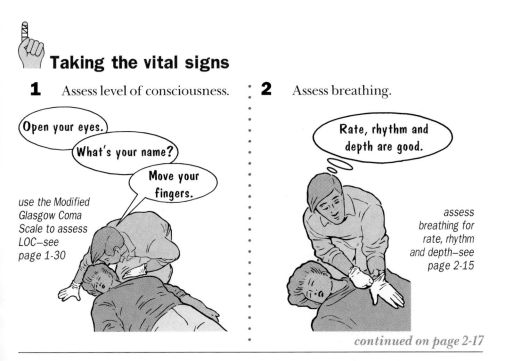

continued on page 2-17

Vital signs – How to assess level of consciousness (LOC)

1 *Open your eyes.*

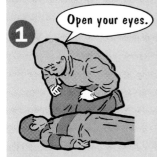

2 *What is your name?*

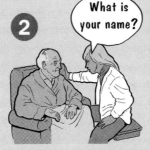

3 *Move your fingers.*

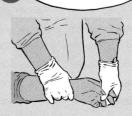

Check eye opening response. If the casualty's eyes are open, he is conscious. If the casualty's eyes are not open, say, "Open your eyes." If the casualty's eyes still don't open, pinch the skin on the forearm to see if mild pain causes the eyes to open.

Check verbal response. Ask questions and listen to how well the casualty can speak. Is the casualty:

♦ oriented and alert?

♦ confused and not making sense?

♦ not able to speak?

Check motor response. How well can the casualty move? Ask him to move part of his body. If there is no response, squeeze the thumbnail to cause mild pain and see if that causes the casualty to move.

Record the LOC

1. Eye opening response
   - ☐ eyes open
   - ☑ eyes open to speech or pain
   - ☐ eyes don't open

2. Verbal response
   - ☐ oriented and alert
   - ☐ confused, doesn't make sense
   - ☑ no speech

3. Motor response
   - ☑ obeys commands
   - ☐ moves to pain
   - ☐ no movement

This casualty's LOC would be described as, "Eyes open to speech, no verbal response, moves fingers on command."

This method of assessing LOC is called the **Modified Glasgow Coma Scale.**

Causing pain

You could cause the unconscious casualty pain during the primary and secondary surveys when you find and expose injuries. Note any pain reactions and use these to assess LOC.

Obstacles to casualty's response

Some conditions affect how well the casualty can respond. For instance:

♦ an eye injury or swelling around the eyes will affect eye opening response

♦ a throat injury, speech disability or a language barrier may affect verbal response

♦ paralysis will affect motor response— if you suspect paralysis, check motor response by asking the casualty to blink his eyes

Vital signs –
How to assess breathing

During the primary survey you checked whether or not the casualty was breathing, and, if the casualty was breathing, whether breathing was effective or ineffective.

In the secondary survey, you assess breathing rate, rhythm and depth, as they are important indictors of a person's state of health. These signs give early warning of physical changes and of life-threatening conditions. Breathing:

◆ **rate** refers to how many breaths the person takes in one minute—it is assessed as "breaths per minute."

◆ **rhythm** refers to how regular the intervals between breaths are—rhythm is assessed as either "regular" or "irregular."

◆ **depth** refers to how deeply the person is breathing—depth is assessed as "shallow," "normal" or "deep." There is more on breathing rate, rhythm and depth starting on page 4-3.

If the casualty is conscious

Look at the casualty's chest and abdomen and ask about her breathing. Listen not only to what the casualty says, but also, to how well she is able to say it. If she has difficulty responding, or cannot respond, place a hand on her chest and assess breathing rate, rhythm and depth.

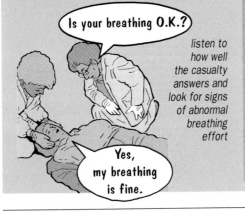

Is your breathing O.K.?

listen to how well the casualty answers and look for signs of abnormal breathing effort

Yes, my breathing is fine.

If the casualty is unconscious

Place a hand on the chest and assess breathing rate, rhythm and depth. Look for other signs of severe breathing difficulties also—see page 4-5.

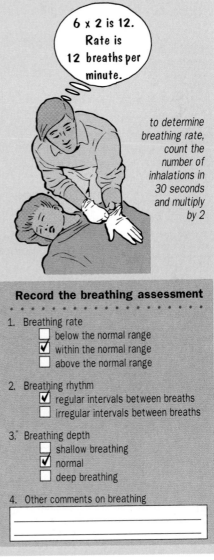

6 x 2 is 12. Rate is 12 breaths per minute.

to determine breathing rate, count the number of inhalations in 30 seconds and multiply by 2

Record the breathing assessment

1. Breathing rate
   - ☐ below the normal range
   - ☑ within the normal range
   - ☐ above the normal range

2. Breathing rhythm
   - ☑ regular intervals between breaths
   - ☐ irregular intervals between breaths

3. Breathing depth
   - ☐ shallow breathing
   - ☑ normal
   - ☐ deep breathing

4. Other comments on breathing
   _____
   _____

Vital signs –
How to take the pulse

For an adult or child casualty, take the pulse at the wrist and/or neck. For an infant casualty, take the pulse on the upper arm.

Taking an adult's or child's pulse

The pulse at the wrist, called the **radial pulse**, is commonly used for an adult or child casualty.

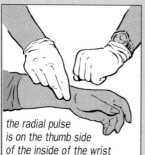

the radial pulse is on the thumb side of the inside of the wrist

use light pressure

count the number of heartbeats in 30 seconds and multiply by 2.

The neck pulse, or **carotid** pulse, is best when the casualty's blood pressure might be low. Use this pulse when shock might be present. There is a carotid pulse on either side of the neck—feel for a pulse on the side closest to you. **Do not feel or compress both sides at the same time.**

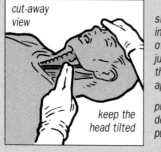

cut-away view

keep the head tilted

slide 2 fingers into the groove of the neck just down from the Adam's apple

press gently to detect the pulse

Taking an infant's pulse

The best place to take the pulse of an infant is on the upper arm. This pulse is called the **brachial** pulse. You find it halfway down the inside of the upper arm, between the large muscle of the arm and the bone.

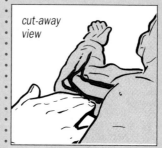

cut-away view

press gently to feel the pulse

count the number of heartbeats in 30 seconds and multiply by 2.

⚠ Never use your thumb to take the pulse of an adult, child or infant—it has a pulse of its own, and you will feel your own pulse instead of the casualty's.

Normal pulse rates, by age

age	rate (heartbeats per min.)
adult (8 and over)	50 to 100
child (1 to 8)	80 to 100
infant (< 1 yr.)	100 to 140

Vital signs – How to assess skin condition and temperature

> The condition and temperature of the skin change when there is shock. By assessing the skin, you are checking for shock. The signs and symptoms of shock are listed on page 1-26.

To assess skin condition, look for:

◆ the skin colour
  – is the skin pale, reddish or bluish?
◆ the presence of sweating
  – is the skin wet or clammy?

To assess skin temperature, use the back of your hand on the skin.

place the back of the hand on the forehead, neck or cheek

pull back your glove if you have to

continued from page 2-13

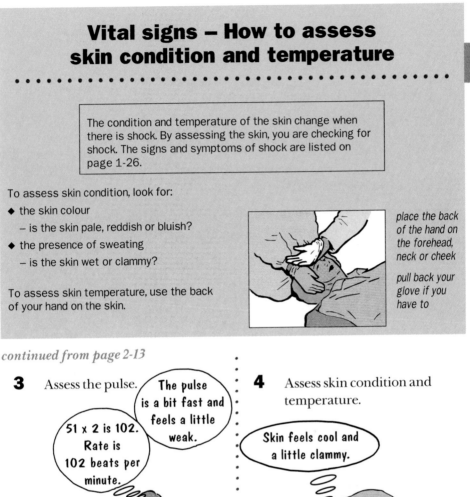

3   Assess the pulse.

The pulse is a bit fast and feels a little weak.

51 x 2 is 102. Rate is 102 beats per minute.

assess for rate, rhythm and strength–see page 2-16

4   Assess skin condition and temperature.

Skin feels cool and a little clammy.

assess the skin for colour, whether it is dry or wet and whether it is hot or cool– see above

Reassess the vital signs every few minutes or when you think the casualty's condition has changed. Write down what you find using a form like the one shown on page 2-29, if you have one. Once you have taken the vital signs, do a head-to-toe examination of the casualty.

Head-to-toe examination

Use the head-to-toe examination to find and examine other injuries and illnesses that may be helped with first aid.

Fully conscious casualty

If the casualty is fully conscious:

◆ ask him where it hurts and examine that area first. If he tells you there are two or more areas that hurt, ask, "Which one is bothering you most?"

◆ ask if anything else is wrong and make sure there are no injuries that are masked by pain, numbness or drugs

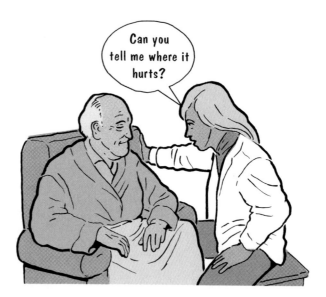

General guidelines

Remember the following when doing a head-to-toe examination:

◆ don't move the casualty unless there is danger

◆ protect yourself—if you have gloves, wear them

◆ if you can, stay on one side of the casualty. If you must get to the other side, walk around the casualty—never step over a casualty

◆ use gentle but firm pressure to examine the casualty and:

   ❖ if possible, compare the part of the body you are examining with the same part on the other side. Look for differences between the two

   ❖ check your hands often for blood and other body fluids

   ❖ check every part of the body for deformity, swelling, bruising—any sign of injury

   ❖ watch the casualty's face, including the unconscious casualty, for any sign of pain

   ❖ listen to the casualty's speech or for sounds that may indicate pain or some other symptom

◆ the exact order you follow in the head-to-toe examination doesn't matter as long as you examine the entire body

If you must get to the other side, walk around the casualty— never step over a casualty.

As you do the head-to-toe examination, talk to the casualty even if he is unconscious. Although an unconscious casualty cannot respond to you, he may still be able to hear you. By telling the casualty what you are doing, he will be reassured whether he is fully conscious or just barely able to understand you. Ask the conscious casualty his name and use it when speaking to him.

Don't comment on "how bad" an injury is and don't tell the casualty what you think the problem might be—only a medical doctor can properly diagnose an illness or injury. Instead, tell the casualty what you are going to do, what you are doing, and why you are doing it. If the casualty asks you specific questions about his injuries, tell him what you see and that a doctor will determine the extent of the injury or illness.

Is my wrist broken?

I don't know. There is bruising and a bump on the front. The doctor will tell you exactly what is wrong.

Doing the head-to-toe examination

2

1 Examine the head.

I'm checking your head for injuries.

check the skull and scalp...
...look for bruising, blood and swelling
...feel for bumps, depressions or anything abnormal

check the face...
...compare one side to the other

check the eyes—look for any bruising

gently open both eyes and compare the pupils— are they both the same size?

Both pupils are the same size.

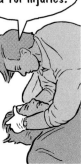

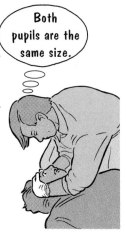

check the lips and mouth—are the lips burned, bleeding or discoloured? Is there an odour on the breath?

open the mouth with the tongue-jaw lift and look in—is there anything in the mouth the casualty could choke on, like candy, gum, loose dentures or loose teeth? Remove any loose objects

check the ears for blood or clear fluid that may indicate a head injury

check the nose for swelling, blood or clear fluid

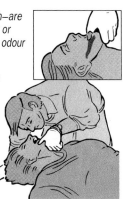

2 Check the neck.

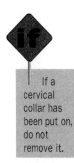

If a cervical collar has been put on, do not remove it.

look and gently feel for deformities

check for a medical alert necklace

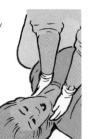

3 Check both collarbones at the same time.

gently run your fingers along the full length of the collarbones, feeling for deformities

look for signs of injury

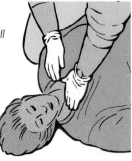

2

4   Check the shoulders, arms and hands. Check one side first,
then check the other side. If you can't safely reach over the
casualty, walk around to the other side.

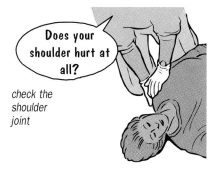

Does your shoulder hurt at all?

check the
shoulder
joint

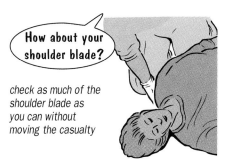

How about your shoulder blade?

check as much of the
shoulder blade as
you can without
moving the casualty

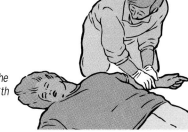

check the
full length
of the
arm

squeeze the hand and check each
of the fingers

check the colour of the
fingernails—are they bluish?

ask the
conscious
casualty if she
has feeling in
her arm, hand
and fingers,
and if she can
move them

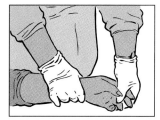

Medical alert information

People who have ongoing medical conditions that need specific treatment often wear or carry medical information in the form of a bracelet, necklace or pocket card. Sometimes this information is kept in a specially marked container on the top shelf in the person's refrigerator.

These medical alert devices state the condition and perhaps the treatment required. Sometimes there is a phone number to call for further information.

When examining an unconscious casualty, look for medical alert information. It could help in your assessment and might warn of allergies or health problems that would make certain first aid or medical procedures dangerous. Tell whoever you hand the casualty over to about the medical alert information.

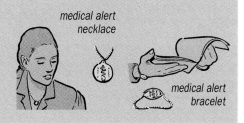

medical alert
necklace

medical alert
bracelet

5   Check the chest and under.

watch and feel the chest move—does it expand easily, evenly and equally on both sides?

feel for wounds and other injuries

ask the conscious casualty to take a deep breath to see if this causes any pain

6   Check the abdomen and under.

gently press on the abdomen–does this cause pain? Is the abdomen tender? Does it feel rigid?

ask the conscious casualty to pull in and push out the abdomen —does this cause any pain?

check as much of the back as possible without moving the casualty

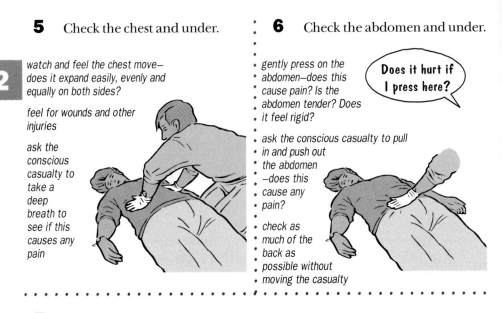

7   Check the pelvis and buttocks.

find the tops of the hips

push the tops of the hips towards each other and check whether this causes pain

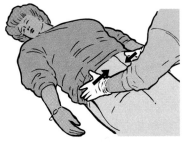

8   Check the legs, ankles and feet.

look at the legs—is there any obvious deformity? Is one foot turned in or out in an unnatural way? Is one leg shorter than the other?

feel for injuries one leg at a time. With firm pressure, check the upper leg, all around the knee, the front and back of the lower leg and all around the ankle

squeeze the foot and each toe

ask the conscious casualty if she has feeling in the leg, foot and toes and whether she can move them

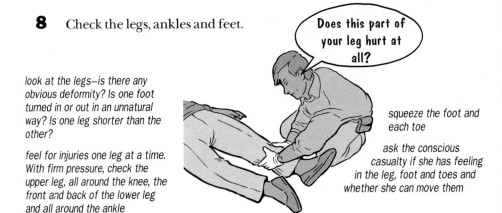

2

Finding injuries during the head-to-toe examination

When a casualty tells you where an injury is, or when you find an injury during the head-to-toe examination, don't stop your examination. Instead, examine the injury just enough to determine the type and severity, then complete the head-to-toe examination. By stopping at one injury, you can forget to examine the rest of the casualty.

Giving first aid for injuries and illnesses found

To give appropriate first aid, each injury must be carefully examined. You need to have a good look to find out the nature and extent of the tissue damage. The most important part of examining an injury is exposing it. If clothing is in the way, it is best to cut it—trying to take it off may cause you to move the injured part in the process. If clothing is stuck to the injury, don't pull it off—this could cause further tissue damage. Always tell the casualty what item of clothing you are removing and why. And always respect a casualty's privacy when removing clothing.

The most important part of examining an injury is exposing it.

When you have finished the head-to-toe examination, give the appropriate first aid for any injury or illness you have found or suspect. If there is more than one injury or illness, use the priorities for casualties with more than one injury (see page 2-27) to decide which injury to attend to first.

Deciding what first aid to give depends on whether medical help will be coming to the scene, how long it will take to arrive if it is coming, and the first aid the casualty needs. For instance, if medical help will arrive in 30 minutes, and it will take 35 minutes to immobilize the person on a spine board, it may be best to simply support the casualty in the position found until medical help arrives. The best first aid depends on the details of the situation.

There is no obvious injury—maybe the condition on the medical alert bracelet is the problem. It's best to give ongoing casualty care until medical help takes over.

Ongoing casualty care

2

Once first aid for injuries and illnesses that are not life threatening has been given, one of three things happens:

◆ you hand over control of the scene to the casualty, or someone else, and end your involvement in the emergency. For more on this see page 1-14, or

◆ you stay in control of the scene and wait for medical help to take over, or

◆ you stay in control of the scene and transport the casualty to medical help—see page 1-16 on when to do this

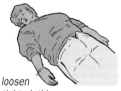

*loosen
tight clothing*

When you stay in control of the scene, you should continue giving first aid to keep the casualty in the best possible condition. This first aid is called **ongoing casualty care**. It includes:

◆ showing a bystander how to maintain manual support of any injuries, if needed

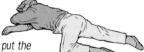

*put the
casualty in
the best position for her
condition*

◆ giving first aid for shock, which includes:

❖ reassuring the casualty

❖ loosening tight clothing

❖ placing the casualty in the best position for her injuries or illnesses

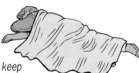

*keep
the casualty warm*

❖ covering the casualty to preserve body heat

There is more on minimizing shock on page 1-26.

◆ monitoring the casualty's condition, especially the ABCs

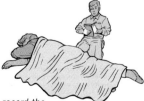

*record the
casualty's condition*

◆ giving nothing by mouth—if the casualty complains of thirst, moisten her lips with a wet cloth

◆ recording the casualty's condition, any changes that occur, and the first aid given. Use a form like the one on page 2-29

◆ protecting the casualty's personal belongings

◆ handing the casualty over to medical help and
   reporting on the incident, the casualty's
   condition and the first aid given

Do not leave the casualty until you hand control
of the scene to someone else.

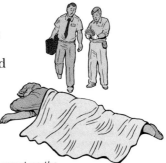

*report on the
incident to whoever takes over*

After the handover

In first aid, we prepare ourselves to care for an injured or ill
person. We don't often think about what happens after the
casualty has left our care. Immediately following the handover of
the casualty, to medical help or whoever, you may have a number
of practical details to attend to. These can include cleaning up
after the emergency, correcting any unsafe conditions that caused
the injury, or, in your workplace, making a report on the incident
and your involvement.

Once these practical matters are out of the way, we expect things to
"return to normal." However, you will likely find yourself thinking
about the situation and the details of what happened while you
were involved—the more serious the injury or illness, the more you
will think about it. Following a stressful event, many people
review the details and try to evaluate what they did and how they
could have done it better.

This reviewing of the events is completely normal and you can
expect it to happen. But if thoughts of the incident continue for
many weeks, or if they affect your day-to-day life, you may be
experiencing the negative effects of **critical incident stress** (CIS).

Critical incident stress is a common reaction to a stressful emergency situation. The effects of CIS can interfere with your daily
life—your job, your relationships, your peace of mind. If this
happens to you, you need to do something about it, and help is
readily available. Start by talking to your family doctor, or a
doctor at a walk-in clinic. He or she will understand what you are
going through, and will suggest a course of action for dealing with
the effects of critical incident stress.

The effects of critical incident stress can appear many weeks, months or years after the event.

Multiple casualty management (triage)

You are travelling alone and arrive at the scene of a car crash—there are at least four casualties. Who do you go to first?

When there are more casualties than first aiders, you need a system to ensure that the casualties get the best treatment without time being wasted on unnecessary things. You need an approach that will help you save as many lives as possible.

The process of making these decisions during an emergency scene where people are injured is called **triage**. In triage, First aiders quickly examine all casualties and place them in order of greatest need for first aid and for transportation. The idea is to do the most good for the greatest number of casualties.

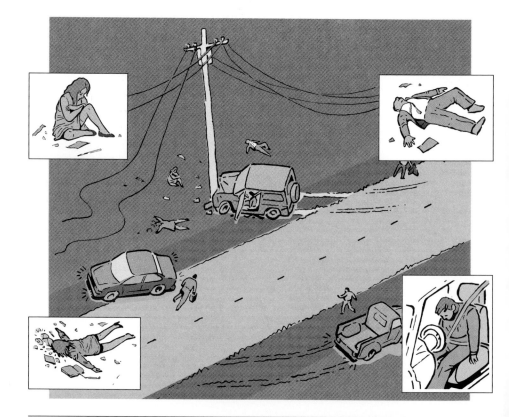

2

Three levels of priority

The table below shows the priorities for different injuries and conditions. There are three levels of priority:

◆ **highest priority**—casualties who need immediate first aid and transportation to medical help

◆ **second priority**—casualties who probably can wait one hour for medical help without risk to their lives

◆ **lowest priority**—casualties who can wait and receive first aid and transportation last, or casualties who are obviously dead

		The first aid priorities for injuries	
	Priority	**Condition**	**Examples**
high priority	**1st – Airway**	foreign body blocking airway	choking on food
		tongue or fluids blocking airway	unconscious, lying on back
		swollen airway	allergic reaction, airway infection
	2nd – Breathing	injured chest and/or lungs	chest injury, broken ribs
		brain not controlling breathing properly	poisoning, drug overdose, stroke, electric shock
		not enough oxygen reaching blood	not enough oxygen in air, carbon monoxide poisoning
	3rd – Circulation	severe bleeding	external bleeding or internal bleeding
		severe shock	bleeding, serious illness, poisoning
medium priority	**Injuries that may affect ABCs or have potential for life-long disability**	fractures that could affect breathing	broken ribs, shoulder blade
		fractures—open, severe or multiple bones	broken upper leg, pelvis, crushed arm
		head/spinal injuries	fall from a 6-foot ladder
		critical burns	3rd degree burns to the hands
low priority	**Minor injuries or obviously dead**	minor fractures	broken lower leg, lower arm, hand, finger, etc.
		minor bleeding	bleeding not spurting or free-flowing
		non-critical burns	2nd degree burns to the forearms
		behavioural problems	grief or panic
		obviously dead	obvious massive injuries, no pulse* or other signs of life

* except for lightning injuries—see page 10-14

2

Triage sequence of actions

Often, the more casualties there are, the more confusion there is and the greater the chance people will panic. Triage is a decision-making process. The more cool-headed you are, the better your decisions will be. One person should be in charge of the triage process—this should be the most experienced first aider. Stay calm, continually assess the hazards of the situation, and don't take any risks to your own safety.

1 Begin ESM—start the scene survey. Try to determine how many casualties there are.

2 Go to the nearest casualty, provided it is safe to do so. Assess responsiveness and do a primary survey. Give first aid for life-threatening conditions—only do what you have to do to save the person's life. If the person is obviously dead, don't waste time. Go to the next nearest casualty.

3 Repeat step 2 for each casualty in turn, always going to the next nearest casualty.

4 Once you have done a primary survey on each casualty, decide which casualties have injuries of the highest priority, second priority and lowest priority—see table, page 2-27.

5 If there are injuries of the highest priority, and transportation to medical help is available, begin to transport those casualties.

6 Do a secondary survey of each casualty, starting with the casualties of the highest priority. Give appropriate first aid, considering the situation—if medical help is nearby, most injuries can simply be steadied and supported.

7 Give ongoing casualty care to each casualty.

If there are bystanders or other first aiders at the scene, tell them you are in charge and assessing the situation. Assign these people, and any equipment, to help the highest priority casualties.

In a multiple casualty situation, you must constantly assess the changing conditions of both the casualties and the situation itself. Make changes to the priorities you have assigned accordingly. When medical help arrives, tell the ambulance officers it is a triage situation and answer their questions.

Sample first aid report form

First Aid Report

Date _____

Location _____

First aider

Name _____

Address _____

City _____

Province _____ Postal code _____

Telephone number _____

Casualty

Name _____

Address _____

City _____

Province _____ Postal code _____

Telephone number _____

☐ Male   ☐ Female   Age (approx.) _____

Scene survey

Type of incident _____

Number of casualties _____
(use a separate form for each casualty)

Casualty responsiveness
   ☐ responsive   ☐ unresponsive

Primary survey

Airway
   ☐ clear
   ☐ partly blocked
   ☐ completely blocked

Breathing
   ☐ yes....☐ effective   ☐ ineffective
   ☐ no

Circulation
   Pulse   ☐ yes   ☐ no
   Severe bleeding   ☐ yes   ☐ no
   Shock   ☐ yes   ☐ no

Secondary survey

History
   Symptoms _____
   _____
   Allergies _____
   Medications _____
   Past medical history _____
   Last meal _____
   Events leading to incident _____
   _____

Vital signs
   Time taken   _____   _____   _____
   Level of consc.   _____   _____   _____
   Breathing rate   _____   _____   _____
   Breathing rhythm _____   _____   _____
   Breathing depth   _____   _____   _____
   Pulse rate   _____   _____   _____
   Skin cond./temp. _____   _____   _____

Head-to-toe examination
   Head _____
   Neck _____
   Collarbones _____
   Shoulders arms/hands _____
   Chest and under _____
   Abdomen and under _____
   Pelvis and buttocks _____
   Legs/feet _____

First aid given

_____
_____
_____
_____
_____

Hand over to medical help

_____
_____
_____

Emergency scene management summary

• •

Emergency scene management has many steps and can be quite complicated, but the initial scene survey, primary survey and the start of life-saving first aid usually happens very quickly—within one or two minutes. This summary shows all the steps on four pages and gives an idea of the flow of steps.

Scene survey

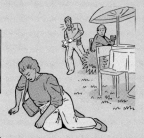

Take charge of the situation.

↓

Call out for help to attract bystanders. **Assess hazards** and make the area safe.

↓

Find out the **history of the scene, how many casualties** there are and the **mechanism(s) of injury**.

↓

Identify yourself as a first aider and offer to help.

↓

Assess responsiveness **Send, or go for medical help.**

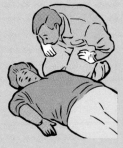

2

Primary survey

Don't move the casualty to do the primary survey unless you absolutely have to. Give first aid for life-threatening conditions as you find them while checking the ABCs.

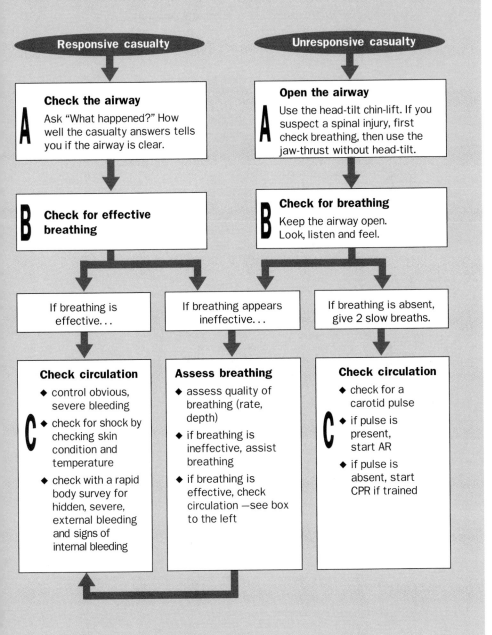

Responsive casualty

A **Check the airway**
Ask "What happened?" How well the casualty answers tells you if the airway is clear.

B **Check for effective breathing**

If breathing is effective...

If breathing appears ineffective...

C **Check circulation**
◆ control obvious, severe bleeding
◆ check for shock by checking skin condition and temperature
◆ check with a rapid body survey for hidden, severe, external bleeding and signs of internal bleeding

Assess breathing
◆ assess quality of breathing (rate, depth)
◆ if breathing is ineffective, assist breathing
◆ if breathing is effective, check circulation —see box to the left

Unresponsive casualty

A **Open the airway**
Use the head-tilt chin-lift. If you suspect a spinal injury, first check breathing, then use the jaw-thrust without head-tilt.

B **Check for breathing**
Keep the airway open. Look, listen and feel.

If breathing is absent, give 2 slow breaths.

C **Check circulation**
◆ check for a carotid pulse
◆ if pulse is present, start AR
◆ if pulse is absent, start CPR if trained

Secondary survey

After giving first aid for life-threatening injuries, do a secondary survey if medical help is delayed, you have to transport the casualty or the casualty has more than one injury.

1

History of the casualty

S symptoms
A allergies
M medications
P past and present medical history
L last meal
E events leading to the incident

2

Assess the vital signs

◆ level of consciousness
◆ breathing
◆ pulse
◆ skin temperature

Head-to-toe examination

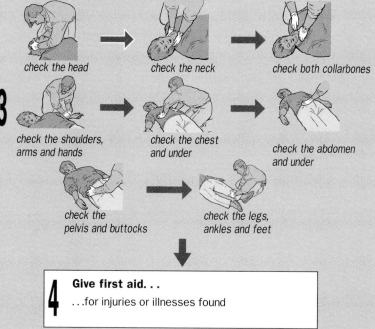

check the head   *check the neck*   *check both collarbones*

3

check the shoulders, arms and hands   *check the chest and under*   *check the abdomen and under*

check the pelvis and buttocks   *check the legs, ankles and feet*

4

Give first aid. . .

. . .for injuries or illnesses found

Ongoing Casualty Care

Instruct a bystander to maintain manual support of the head and neck, if head/spinal injuries are suspected.

Continue to steady and support any injuries manually, if needed.

1
Give first aid for shock
- ◆ reassure the casualty
- ◆ loosen tight clothing
- ◆ place the casualty in the best position for the condition
- ◆ cover the casualty to preserve body heat

2
Monitor the casualty's condition
- ◆ check the ABCs often
- ◆ give nothing by mouth

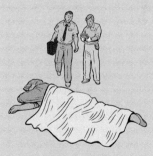

3
Record the events of the situation
- ◆ protect the casualty's belongings

4
Report on what happened
- ◆ tell whoever takes over what happened and what first aid has been given

Do not leave the casualty until you hand control of the scene over to someone else.

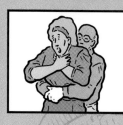

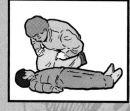

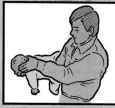

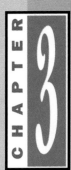

CHAPTER 3

FIRST AID FOR CHOKING

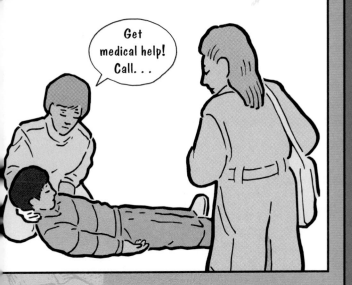

- ◆ *Introduction*

- ◆ *Air exchange*

- ◆ *Signs of choking*

- ◆ *First aid for choking*

- ◆ *Ongoing casualty care for choking*

- ◆ *Choking adult*

- ◆ *First aid for obese or pregnant choking casualties*

- ◆ *Self-help*

- ◆ *Choking child*

- ◆ *How the Heimlich manoeuvre works*

- ◆ *Choking infant*

- ◆ *How to prevent choking*

Introduction

open and clear airway

partly blocked airway

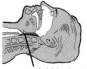

partial blockage

completely blocked airway

foreign object

A person chokes when the airway is partly or completely blocked and airflow to the lungs is reduced or cut off. The choking casualty either has trouble breathing or cannot breathe at all. A choking casualty may die if first aid for choking is not given right away. For information on other breathing emergencies, see page 4-2.

Air exchange – good, poor or none

A person's airway can be either partly or completely blocked. With a partially blocked airway, there is either **good air exchange** or **poor air exchange**. With good air exchange, the person can still cough forcefully, breathe and speak. With poor air exchange, the person cannot cough forcefully, has trouble breathing, or cannot speak. With a completely blocked airway, there is no air exchange—coughing, breathing and speaking are impossible.

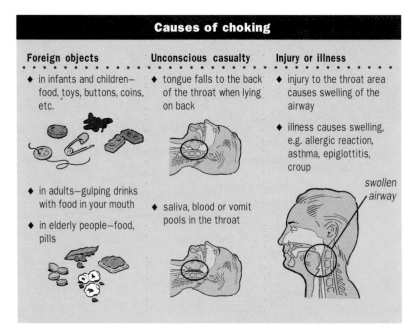

Causes of choking

Foreign objects

♦ in infants and children—food, toys, buttons, coins, etc.

♦ in adults—gulping drinks with food in your mouth

♦ in elderly people—food, pills

Unconscious casualty

♦ tongue falls to the back of the throat when lying on back

♦ saliva, blood or vomit pools in the throat

Injury or illness

♦ injury to the throat area causes swelling of the airway

♦ illness causes swelling, e.g. allergic reaction, asthma, epiglottitis, croup

swollen airway

What happens when a person chokes

Choking is a life-threatening emergency. When the air supply to the lungs is cut off, the person's face immediately becomes reddish. Shortly after, as the oxygen in the body is used up, the face becomes grey and the lips and ear lobes become bluish. This change in colour is called **cyanosis**. Soon, the person becomes unconscious and eventually the heart stops beating.

3

Signs of choking

The most obvious sign of choking is grabbing the throat. The other signs are given in the illustration below. Notice how they are different with good air exchange or poor/no air exchange.

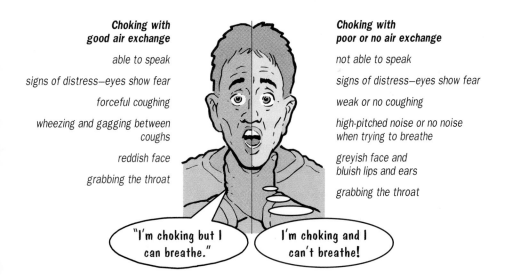

Choking with good air exchange

able to speak

signs of distress—eyes show fear

forceful coughing

wheezing and gagging between coughs

reddish face

grabbing the throat

"I'm choking but I can breathe."

Choking with poor or no air exchange

not able to speak

signs of distress—eyes show fear

weak or no coughing

high-pitched noise or no noise when trying to breathe

greyish face and bluish lips and ears

grabbing the throat

I'm choking and I can't breathe!

You need to know how to recognize whether a choking person has good air exchange or poor/no air exchange because the first aid is different for each.

First aid for choking

There are two choking situations you may have to deal with:

◆ a conscious choking person who may become unconscious while you are giving first aid

◆ an unconscious person who, you discover through your first aid actions, has a blocked airway

The first aid you give depends on the casualty's age. In first aid for choking, an adult is eight years old and over, a child is between one and eight years old and an infant is under one year old. These ages are guidelines only; the casualty's size must be also considered. There are variations in the techniques for a casualty who is pregnant, obese or in a wheelchair.

If choking is caused by swelling of the airway from an infection, injury or allergic reaction, the Heimlich manoeuvre won't work–get medical help quickly.

 ## Choking adult – conscious who may become unconscious

1   Begin ESM—do a scene survey (see page 2-3).

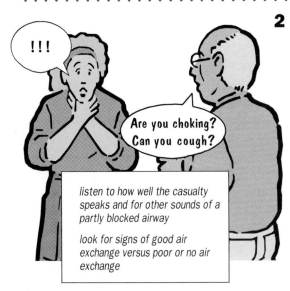

!!!

Are you choking?
Can you cough?

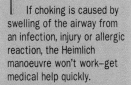

listen to how well the casualty speaks and for other sounds of a partly blocked airway

look for signs of good air exchange versus poor or no air exchange

2   If the casualty can cough forcefully, speak or breathe, don't touch her. Tell her to try to cough up the object. If a partial blockage lasts for a few minutes, get medical help.

If you think there might be poor or no air exchange, check by asking, "Can you cough?" If the casualty cannot cough forcefully, speak or breathe, use the Heimlich manoeuvre to try to remove the blockage—go to step 3.

3   Stand behind the casualty ready to support her if she becomes unconscious. Find the correct hand position and give abdominal thrusts to try to remove the airway blockage.

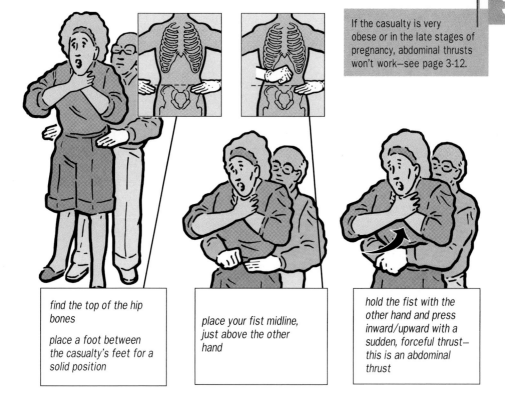

If the casualty is very obese or in the late stages of pregnancy, abdominal thrusts won't work—see page 3-12.

find the top of the hip bones

place a foot between the casualty's feet for a solid position

place your fist midline, just above the other hand

hold the fist with the other hand and press inward/upward with a sudden, forceful thrust— this is an abdominal thrust

Give each abdominal thrust with the intention of removing the object. Use only your fist—make sure you don't press against the ribs with your forearms.

4   Keep giving the Heimlich manoeuvre until either the object is removed or the casualty becomes unconscious. If the airway is cleared, give ongoing casualty care for choking as described on page 3-8.

If the casualty becomes unconscious, don't panic. Continue first aid with step 5 on the next page.

If the casualty is sitting, try to get her to stand up. If the casualty can't stand up, try reaching around from the back of the chair to give the Heimlich manoeuvre. See page 3-14 for what to do for a casualty in a wheelchair.

3

5   As the casualty collapses, lower her to the ground. Send someone to call for medical help.

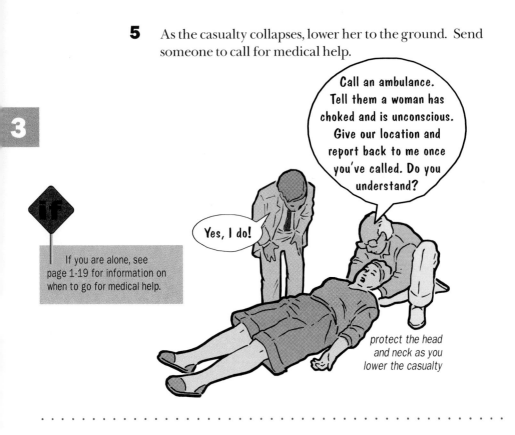

Call an ambulance. Tell them a woman has choked and is unconscious. Give our location and report back to me once you've called. Do you understand?

Yes, I do!

If you are alone, see page 1-19 for information on when to go for medical help.

protect the head and neck as you lower the casualty

6   Check the mouth. Open the mouth with the tongue-jaw lift. The forward movement of the tongue may loosen the blockage. Finger sweep to remove any matter.

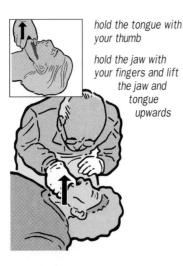

hold the tongue with your thumb

hold the jaw with your fingers and lift the jaw and tongue upwards

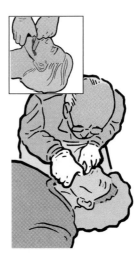

hold the jaw in position and slide a hooked finger down the far side of the mouth to the base of the tongue

hook any foreign matter and pull it up against the near cheek—be careful, the object may be sharp or slippery

7 Try to breathe into the casualty's mouth.

push back on the
forehead and lift
the jaw

seal your mouth
around the
casualty's mouth

pinch the nostrils

blow slowly—watch
for the chest to
rise

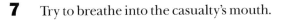

if the chest doesn't
rise, reposition the
head, check the seals
at the nose and mouth
and try again.

if the chest does rise,
give another breath
and go to page 4-24,
step 7

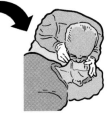

if the chest doesn't rise on your
second try, conclude the airway
is blocked—try to clear the
airway—go to step 8

8 Use the Heimlich manoeuvre to clear the airway. Find the
right hand position and give up to five abdominal thrusts.

keep the fingers raised, in line
with the centre of the body and
interlocked if you wish

kneel astride
the casualty

find the top
of the hips
with your
hands

place the
heel of one
hand midline
slightly
above the
other hand

give up to five
quick, inward and
upward thrusts—
give each with the
intention of
removing the
object

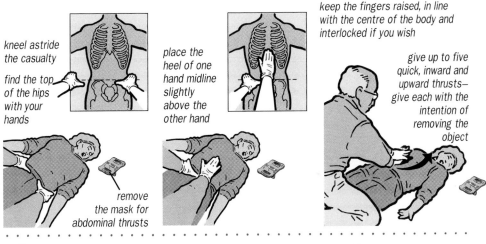

remove
the mask for
abdominal thrusts

9 Repeat steps 6, 7 and 8 until the chest rises when you blow
into the casualty's mouth or medical help takes over. If the
chest rises, go to step 10.

step 6: tongue-jaw lift and
finger sweep

step 7: tilt the head and try
to ventilate twice

step 8: give up to
five abdominal
thrusts

keep
repeating
steps 6, 7
& 8

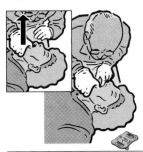

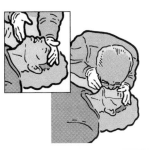

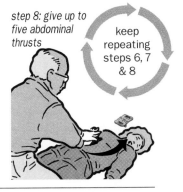

3

10 If you remove the blockage, or if the chest rises when you ventilate, give a total of two slow breaths, then, continue the primary survey—check breathing and pulse. If the casualty is breathing effectively, give ongoing casualty care for choking as described below.

Ongoing casualty care for choking

Your job as a first aider is not over when the airway blockage is removed. When a choking casualty's airway has been cleared, she may be conscious, semi-conscious or unconscious. Continue giving first aid as described below.

If the casualty is conscious	**If the casualty is semi-conscious**	**If the casualty is unconscious**
◆ monitor breathing often. Breathing difficulties can develop following a choking incident	◆ call for medical help if not called already	◆ monitor ABCs
	◆ give first aid for shock	◆ if the casualty is breathing, place her in the recovery position and give first aid for shock
◆ stay with the casualty until normal breathing returns	◆ monitor ABCs closely	
◆ urge the casualty to see a medical doctor— the Heimlich manoeuvre can cause internal injuries	◆ stay with the casualty until medical help takes over	

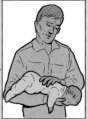

infant recovery position

We're going to the hospital to see if those chest thrusts hurt you.

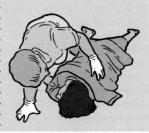

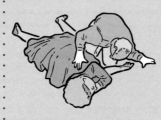

place a semi-conscious casualty into the recovery position

Choking adult – found unconscious

You arrive at a scene. . .there is an unconscious person lying on the floor. . .

1 Begin ESM—start the scene survey (see page 2-3).

3

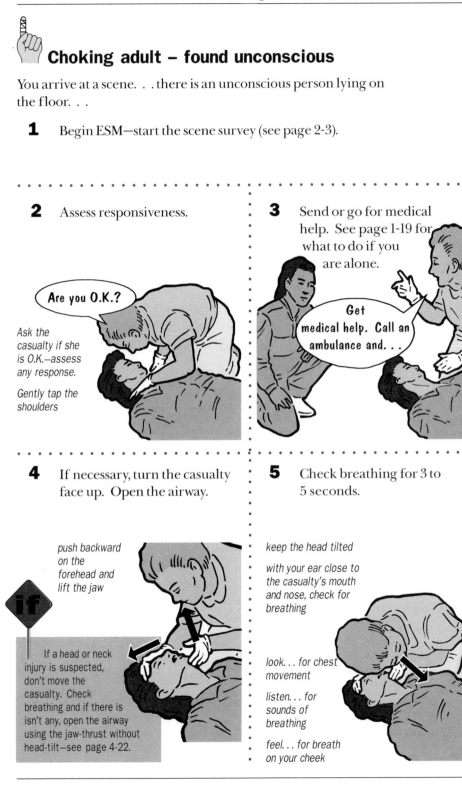

2 Assess responsiveness.

Are you O.K.?

Ask the casualty if she is O.K.–assess any response.

Gently tap the shoulders

3 Send or go for medical help. See page 1-19 for what to do if you are alone.

Get medical help. Call an ambulance and. . .

4 If necessary, turn the casualty face up. Open the airway.

push backward on the forehead and lift the jaw

if

If a head or neck injury is suspected, don't move the casualty. Check breathing and if there is isn't any, open the airway using the jaw-thrust without head-tilt—see page 4-22.

5 Check breathing for 3 to 5 seconds.

keep the head tilted

with your ear close to the casualty's mouth and nose, check for breathing

look. . . for chest movement

listen. . . for sounds of breathing

feel. . . for breath on your cheek

6   Try to breathe into the casualty's mouth.

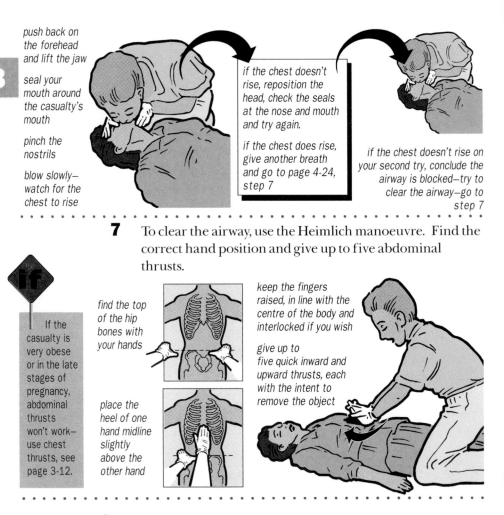

push back on
the forehead
and lift the jaw

seal your
mouth around
the casualty's
mouth

pinch the
nostrils

blow slowly—
watch for the
chest to rise

if the chest doesn't
rise, reposition the
head, check the seals
at the nose and mouth
and try again.

if the chest does rise,
give another breath
and go to page 4-24,
step 7

if the chest doesn't rise on
your second try, conclude the
airway is blocked—try to
clear the airway—go to
step 7

7   To clear the airway, use the Heimlich manoeuvre. Find the
correct hand position and give up to five abdominal
thrusts.

if

If the
casualty is
very obese
or in the late
stages of
pregnancy,
abdominal
thrusts
won't work—
use chest
thrusts, see
page 3-12.

find the top
of the hip
bones with
your hands

place the
heel of one
hand midline
slightly
above the
other hand

keep the fingers
raised, in line with the
centre of the body and
interlocked if you wish

give up to
five quick inward and
upward thrusts, each
with the intent to
remove the object

8   Open the mouth with the tongue-jaw lift. Finger sweep the
mouth to remove any matter.

hold the tongue with
your thumb

hold the jaw with your
fingers

lift the jaw and tongue
upwards

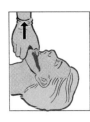

hold the jaw in position
and slide a hooked finger
down the far side of the
mouth to the base of the
tongue

hook any foreign matter
and pull it up against the
near cheek—be careful,
the object may be sharp
or slippery

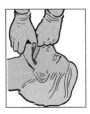

9   Try breathing into the casualty's mouth again—maybe the abdominal thrusts loosened the blockage enough for you to get some air into the lungs.

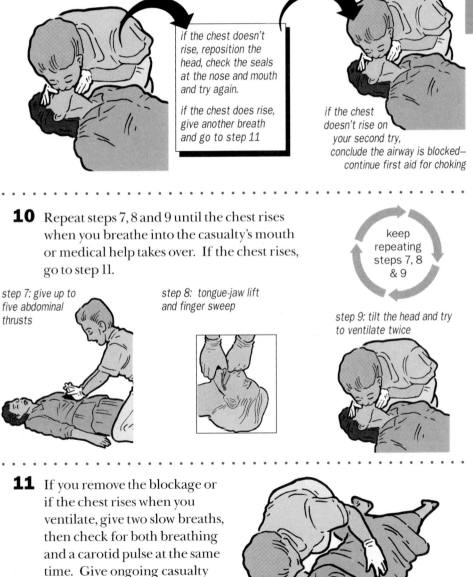

if the chest doesn't rise, reposition the head, check the seals at the nose and mouth and try again.

if the chest does rise, give another breath and go to step 11

if the chest doesn't rise on your second try, conclude the airway is blocked— continue first aid for choking

10   Repeat steps 7, 8 and 9 until the chest rises when you breathe into the casualty's mouth or medical help takes over. If the chest rises, go to step 11.

keep repeating steps 7, 8 & 9

step 7: give up to five abdominal thrusts

step 8: tongue-jaw lift and finger sweep

step 9: tilt the head and try to ventilate twice

11   If you remove the blockage or if the chest rises when you ventilate, give two slow breaths, then check for both breathing and a carotid pulse at the same time. Give ongoing casualty care described on page 3-8.

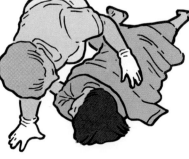

Choking adult – first aid for obese or pregnant choking casualties

If a choking casualty is very obese, abdominal thrusts won't be effective. If the casualty is in the late stages of pregnancy, abdominal thrusts may be dangerous to the baby. Instead of abdominal thrusts, use chest thrusts as described below.

Chest thrusts for a conscious choking casualty

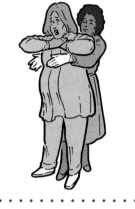

stand behind the casualty

wrap your arms around the chest

keep arms horizontal and snug up under the armpits

place your fist against the lower half of the breastbone, thumb-side in

hold the fist with your other hand

pull inward forcefully

give chest thrusts until either the object is removed or the casualty becomes unconscious

give each thrust with the intention of removing the blockage

Chest thrusts for an unconscious choking casualty

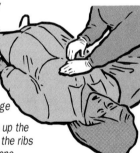

place the casualty face up on a firm, flat surface

with the hand closest to the feet, find the edge of the rib cage

move your fingers up the rib cage to where the ribs meet the breastbone

place the heel of the other hand midline on the lower part of the breastbone

raise the fingers off the chest

using a sudden, downward thrust to depress the breastbone 3.8 to 5 cm, give up to five chest thrusts

make each thrust distinct, given with the intention of removing the object

Actual size

0 cm

3.8 cm
(1½ in)

5 cm
(2 in)

Positioning a pregnant casualty

Whenever a pregnant casualty is positioned face up, place something like a jacket or a pillow, if you have one, under the right hip. This positions the baby off an important blood vessel in the mother.

baby is shifted to the left

rolled up jacket

Choking adult – self-help

If you begin to choke on an object, what should you do?

1   Don't panic, though that's not easy. If there are people around, get their attention—grab your throat to show them you are choking— this is the universal sign of choking. **Do not isolate yourself from others when you are choking**.

2   If you can cough forcefully, try to cough up the object. Don't let anyone slap you on the back, this could drive the object further down your airway.

3   If you can't cough forcefully, breathe or speak, and there is no one else to give you the Heimlich manoeuvre, do it to yourself as shown below. Use either your hands or a piece of furniture, whatever gives the best effect.

If you are alone and choking, you must get help quickly—you will be unconscious within minutes.

Do whatever is necessary to get someone's attention. If all else fails, and you have 911 emergency service in your area, call 911. In some areas, the 911 operator can see on her equipment the address of the phone the caller is using. If 911 gets your call, help will be sent even though you cannot tell them what's wrong.

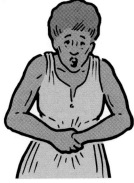

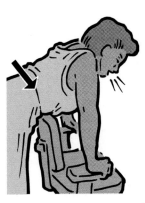

put a fist, thumb-side in, midline on your abdomen just above your hips

hold the fist with your other hand and pull inward/upward forcefully

give yourself abdominal thrusts until you can cough forcefully, breathe or speak

a second method is to use a solid object like the back of a chair, a table or the edge of a counter

position yourself so the object is just above your hips. Press forcefully to produce an abdominal thrust—keep giving yourself thrusts until you can cough forcefully, breathe or speak

If you are very obese or in the late stages of pregnancy, give yourself chest thrusts instead. Place a fist, thumb-side down, in the middle of your chest. With your head turned to the side, fall against a wall hard enough to produce a chest thrust.

Choking adult – first aid for a casualty in a wheelchair

The way you do the Heimlich manouvre for someone in a wheelchair depends largely on the type of wheelchair. If you can reach around from behind the wheelchair, use the Heimlich manouvre as you would for any conscious casualty of the same age. If you cannot reach around the wheelchair, use the technique shown below.

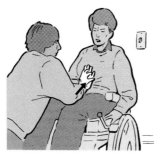

position the wheelchair against a wall

put the wheelchair brake on

put the heel of one hand, with the other on top, in the middle of the abdomen, well below the notch where the ribs meet

give sudden, inward/upward thrusts until the object is removed or the casualty becomes unconscious

· ·

If the casualty becomes unconscious, take her out of the wheelchair.

grip the casualty's clothing

pull the casualty forward supporting her with your arm and leg

lower yourself and the casualty to the ground using the strength in your legs and not your back as much as possible

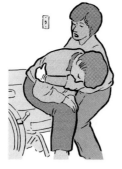

if

If a doctor, physiotherapist or other health professional has shown you a different way of giving the Heimlich manoeuvre to a person in your care, use the method that you prefer.

supporting the casualty, and protecting the head as much as possible, roll the casualty to the floor to a face-up position

when she is face up, give first aid for choking—go to step 6, page 3-6

Choking child – conscious who may become unconscious

1 Begin ESM—do a scene survey (see page 2-3), Identify yourself as a first aider to the parent or guardian and offer to help.

> If choking is caused by swelling of the airway from an infection, injury or allergic reaction, the Heimlich manoeuvre won't work–get medical help quickly.

3

· ·

2 Find out how badly the child is choking. Ask, "Are you choking?"

If he can speak, breathe or cough, don't touch him. Tell him to try to cough up the object. If this partial blockage lasts for more than a few minutes, get medical help.

If you think there might be poor or no air exchange, check by asking, "Can you cough?" If the casualty cannot cough, use the Heimlich manoeuvre to try to remove the blockage—go to step 3.

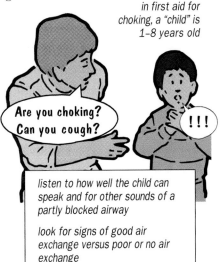

in first aid for choking, a "child" is 1-8 years old

Are you choking? Can you cough?

!!!

> listen to how well the child can speak and for other sounds of a partly blocked airway
>
> look for signs of good air exchange versus poor or no air exchange

How the Heimlich manoeuvre works

· ·

When you choke on something, your body tries to unblock your airway by coughing. The Heimlich manoeuvre tries to do the same thing with an artificial cough. The illustration below shows how an abdominal thrust creates a cough.

foreign object

diaphragm

an abdominal thrust pushes the diaphragm up towards the lungs very quickly—this forces air from the lungs up the airway and, hopefully, blows out the object

for the best effect, the fist has to be in the right place, your forearms off the abdomen and each thrust a strong and sudden movement

3   Stand or kneel behind the casualty ready to support him if he becomes unconscious. Find the correct hand position. Give abdominal thrusts to try to remove the airway blockage.

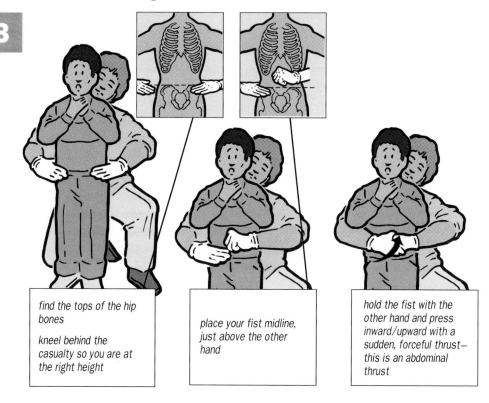

find the tops of the hip bones

kneel behind the casualty so you are at the right height

place your fist midline, just above the other hand

hold the fist with the other hand and press inward/upward with a sudden, forceful thrust— this is an abdominal thrust

Give each abdominal thrust with the intention of removing the object. Use only your fist—make sure you don't press against the ribs with your forearms.

4   Keep giving the Heimlich manoeuvre until either the airway is cleared or the child becomes unconscious.

If the object is removed, give ongoing casualty care for choking as described on page 3-8.

If the child becomes unconscious, don't panic. Continue first aid with step 5 on the next page.

5 As the child collapses, lower him to the ground. Send someone to call for medical help.

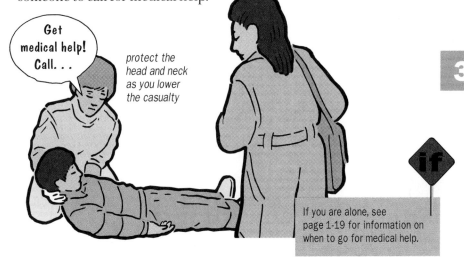

Get medical help! Call. . .

protect the head and neck as you lower the casualty

If you are alone, see page 1-19 for information on when to go for medical help.

6 Check the mouth. Open the mouth with the tongue-jaw lift and look for any foreign matter—remove any matter you see and reach with a hooked finger.

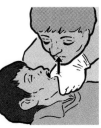

hold the tongue with your thumb

hold the jaw with your fingers

lift the jaw and tongue upwards

look for any foreign matter and remove what you see

Only. . .

. . .finger-sweep a child's mouth if you can see and reach the object, otherwise you could push the object further down the airway.

7 Try to breathe into the casualty's mouth. If the chest rises, go to step 10. If it doesn't, go to step 8.

push back on the forehead and lift the jaw

seal your mouth around the casualty's mouth

pinch the nostrils

blow slowly—watch for the chest to rise

if the chest doesn't rise, reposition the head, check the seals at the nose and mouth and try again.

if the chest does rise, give another breath and go to page 4-27, step 7

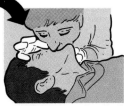

if the chest doesn't rise on your second try, conclude the airway is blocked—try to clear the airway— go to step 8

8 Use the Heimlich manoeuvre. Find the correct hand position and give up to five abdominal thrusts.

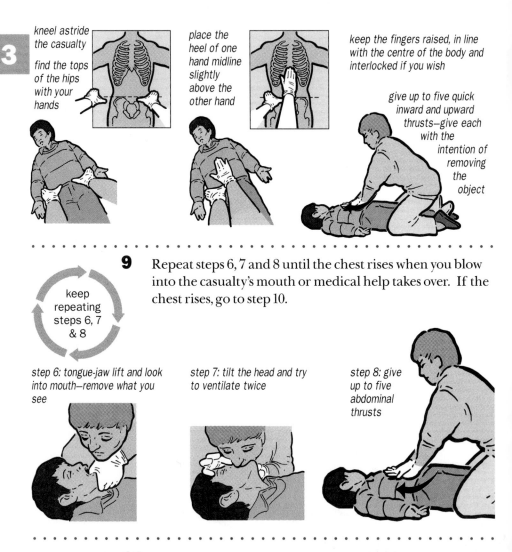

kneel astride the casualty

find the tops of the hips with your hands

place the heel of one hand midline slightly above the other hand

keep the fingers raised, in line with the centre of the body and interlocked if you wish

give up to five quick inward and upward thrusts–give each with the intention of removing the object

9 Repeat steps 6, 7 and 8 until the chest rises when you blow into the casualty's mouth or medical help takes over. If the chest rises, go to step 10.

keep repeating steps 6, 7 & 8

step 6: tongue-jaw lift and look into mouth–remove what you see

step 7: tilt the head and try to ventilate twice

step 8: give up to five abdominal thrusts

10 If you remove the blockage, or if the chest rises when you ventilate, give two slow breaths, then check for both breathing and a carotid pulse at the same time. Give the ongoing casualty care described on page 3-8.

Choking child – found unconscious

You arrive at a scene. . .there is a child lying on the floor. . .

1   Begin ESM—start the scene survey (see page 2-3). Identify
yourself as a first aider to the parent or guardian and offer
to help.

2   Assess responsiveness.

3   Send for medical help. If you
are alone, keep giving
first aid.

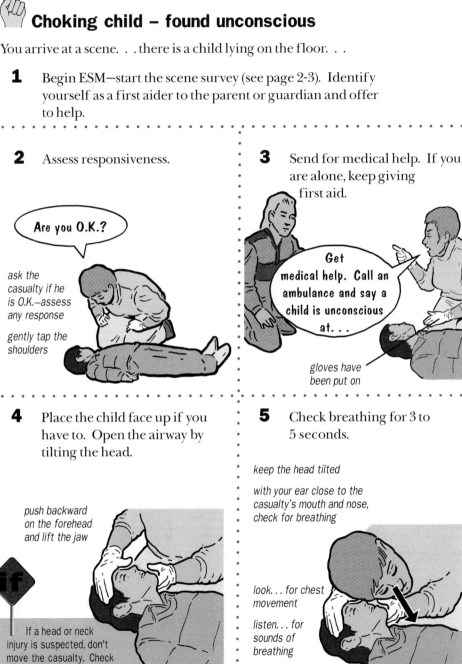

Are you O.K.?

*ask the
casualty if he
is O.K.–assess
any response*

*gently tap the
shoulders*

**Get
medical help. Call an
ambulance and say a
child is unconscious
at. . .**

*gloves have
been put on*

4   Place the child face up if you
have to. Open the airway by
tilting the head.

*push backward
on the forehead
and lift the jaw*

if

If a head or neck
injury is suspected, don't
move the casualty. Check
breathing and if there isn't any,
open the airway using the jaw
thrust without head-tilt—see
page 4-22.

5   Check breathing for 3 to
5 seconds.

keep the head tilted

*with your ear close to the
casualty's mouth and nose,
check for breathing*

*look. . . for chest
movement*

*listen. . . for
sounds of
breathing*

*feel. . . for breath
on your cheek*

6   Try to breathe into the casualty.

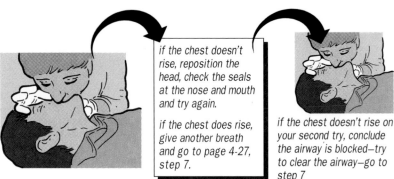

seal your
mouth around
the casualty's
mouth

pinch the
nostrils

blow slowly—
watch for the
chest to rise

if the chest doesn't
rise, reposition the
head, check the seals
at the nose and mouth
and try again.

if the chest does rise,
give another breath
and go to page 4-27,
step 7.

if the chest doesn't rise on
your second try, conclude
the airway is blocked—try
to clear the airway—go to
step 7

7   To clear the airway, use the Heimlich manoeuvre. Find the
correct hand position and give up to five abdominal thrusts.

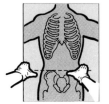

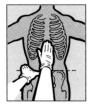

keep the fingers
raised, in line with the
centre of the body and
interlocked if you wish

give up to
five quick inward and
upward thrusts, each
with the intention of
removing the object

find the tops of
the hip bones with
your hands

place the heel of
one hand midline
slightly above the
other hand

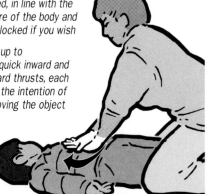

8   Open the mouth with the tongue-jaw lift and look for
foreign matter.

hold the tongue with your thumb
and the jaw with your fingers

lift the jaw and
tongue upwards

look for any
foreign
matter

if you see anything, hold the jaw
in position and slide a hooked
finger down the far side of the
mouth to the base of the tongue

hook any
foreign
matter and
pull it up
against the
near cheek

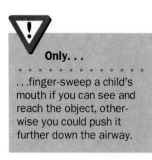

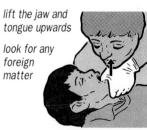

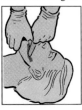

Only. . .

. . .finger-sweep a child's
mouth if you can see and
reach the object, other-
wise you could push it
further down the airway.

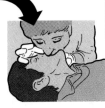

9 Try breathing into the casualty's mouth again—the abdominal thrusts may have loosened the blockage enough for you to get some air into the lungs.

push back on the forehead and lift the jaw

seal your mouth around the casualty's mouth

pinch the nostrils

blow slowly— watch for the chest to rise

if the chest doesn't rise, reposition the head, check the seals at the nose and mouth, and try again

if the chest does rise, go to step 11.

if the chest doesn't rise on your second try, conclude the airway is blocked— continue first aid for choking

10 Repeat steps 7, 8 and 9 until the chest rises when you try to breathe into the casualty's mouth or medical help takes over. If the chest rises, go to step 11.

keep repeating steps 7, 8 & 9

step 7: give up to five abdominal thrusts

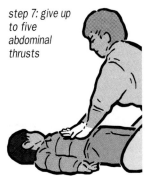

step 8: tongue-jaw lift and finger sweep

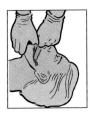

step 9: tilt the head and try to ventilate twice

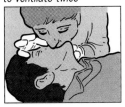

11 If you remove the blockage, or if the chest rises when you ventilate, give a total of two slow breaths, then check for both breathing and a carotid pulse at the same time. Give ongoing casualty care as described on page 3-8.

If you are alone, see page 1-19 for information on when to go for medical help.

Infant choking casualty

Suspect an infant is choking when she suddenly has trouble breathing, even if you haven't seen the baby actually put something into her mouth. Coughing, gagging, and high-pitched, noisy breathing all indicate breathing difficulty. Whenever you suspect an infant is choking, start first aid right away.

Choking infant – conscious who may become unconscious

if

If choking is caused by swelling of the airway from an infection, injury or allergic reaction, the Heimlich manoeuvre won't work–get medical help quickly.

1 Begin ESM—do the scene survey (see page 2-3). Identify yourself as a first aider to the parent or guardian and offer to help.

2 Assess the baby's breathing. If the baby can cough forcefully or breathe, stand by and don't interfere, let the baby try to cough up the object. If a partial blockage lasts for more than a few minutes, get medical help.

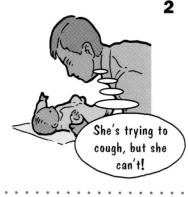

She's trying to cough, but she can't!

If the baby cannot cough forcefully, cannot breathe, makes a high-pitched noise when trying to breathe or starts to turn blue, give back blows and chest thrusts to try to relieve the blockage. Go to step 3.

3 Pick the baby up and turn her over. Support the head and neck throughout the movement.

arm between the legs

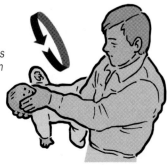

sandwich the baby between your forearms and turn her face down

head and neck supported

4   Give five back blows between the shoulder blades.

with the baby's head lower than the body, use the heel of your hand to give five forceful back blows

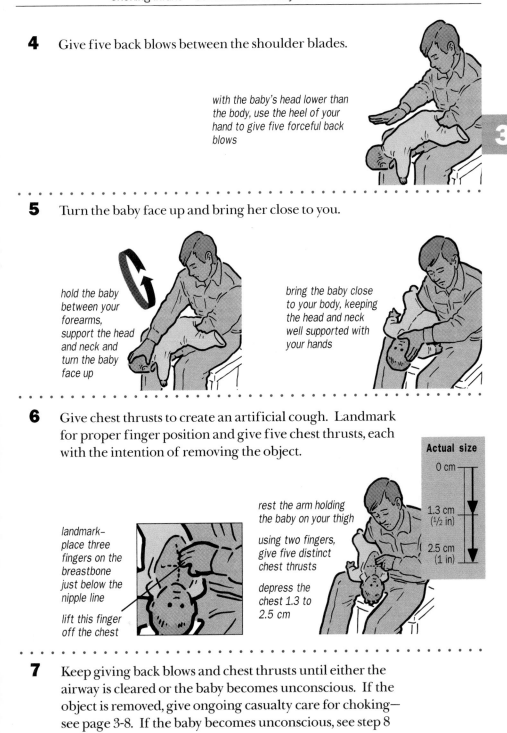

3

5   Turn the baby face up and bring her close to you.

hold the baby between your forearms, support the head and neck and turn the baby face up

bring the baby close to your body, keeping the head and neck well supported with your hands

6   Give chest thrusts to create an artificial cough. Landmark for proper finger position and give five chest thrusts, each with the intention of removing the object.

Actual size

0 cm

1.3 cm
(½ in)

2.5 cm
(1 in)

landmark– place three fingers on the breastbone just below the nipple line

lift this finger off the chest

rest the arm holding the baby on your thigh

using two fingers, give five distinct chest thrusts

depress the chest 1.3 to 2.5 cm

7   Keep giving back blows and chest thrusts until either the airway is cleared or the baby becomes unconscious. If the object is removed, give ongoing casualty care for choking— see page 3-8. If the baby becomes unconscious, see step 8 on the next page.

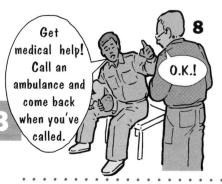

Get medical help! Call an ambulance and come back when you've called.

O.K.!

8 If the baby becomes unconscious, send a bystander, if there is one, to call for medical help.

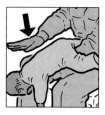

If you are alone, see page 1-19 for information on when to go for medical help.

Only. . .

. . .finger-sweep an infant's mouth if you can see and reach the object, otherwise you could push the object further down the airway.

9 Check the mouth. Open the mouth with the tongue-jaw lift and look for any foreign matter—remove anything you see with a hooked finger.

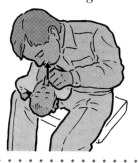

hold the tongue with your thumb and the jaw with your fingers

lift the jaw and tongue upwards and look for foreign matter

if you see an object you can reach, slide your little finger down the far side of the mouth to the base of the tongue

hook any foreign matter and pull it up against the near cheek

---

10 Tilt the baby's head back and try to breathe into the baby's mouth and nose. If the chest rises, give another breath and go to page 4-32, step 7.

tilt the head back

seal your mouth around the baby's mouth and nose

blow into the baby

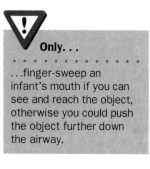

If the chest doesn't rise, reposition the head and try breathing into the infant again. If the chest still doesn't rise, give back blows and chest thrusts—go to step 11.

---

11 Turn the baby over and give up to five back blows.

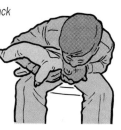

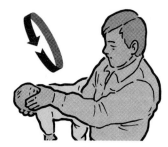

with the baby's head lower than the body, use the heel of your hand to give up to five forceful back blows

12 Turn the baby over, landmark and give up to five chest thrusts.

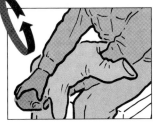

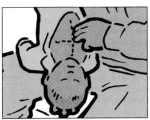

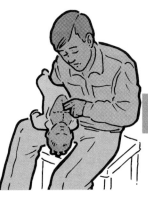

hold the baby between your forearms, support the head and neck and turn the baby face up

place three fingers on the breastbone just below the nipple line and lift the finger closest to the head off the chest

give up to five chest thrusts, making each one distinct

13 Check the mouth and try to breathe into the baby.

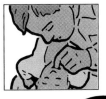

check the mouth using the tongue-jaw lift, remove any foreign matter you can see

push back on the forehead and lift the jaw

seal your mouth around the baby's mouth and nose

blow slowly—watch for the chest to rise

if the chest doesn't rise, reposition the head, check the seals at the nose and mouth and try again.

if the chest does rise, give another breath and go to page 4-32, step 7

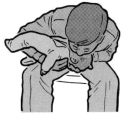

if the chest doesn't rise on your second try, conclude the airway is blocked—try to clear the airway—go to step 14

14 Repeat steps 11, 12 and 13 until the chest rises when you breathe into the baby's mouth or until medical help takes over.

keep repeating steps 11, 12 & 13

If medical help has not been called, after one minute of first aid, decide what to do—see page 1-19.

If you remove the blockage, or if the chest rises when you ventilate, give another breath and then check for both breathing and a brachial pulse at the same time. Give the ongoing casualty care described on page 3-8.

if

If you are alone, see page 1-19 for information on when to go for medical help.

Choking infant – found unconscious

When you find a baby unconscious, you don't know what has happened. By following the correct first aid sequence, you may discover the baby has choked.

1 Begin ESM—start the scene survey (see page 2-3). Identify yourself as a first aider to the parent or guardian and offer to help.

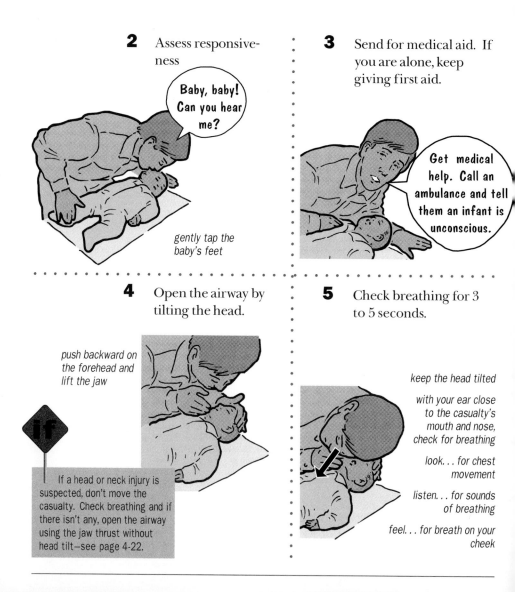

2 Assess responsive-ness

Baby, baby! Can you hear me?

gently tap the baby's feet

3 Send for medical aid. If you are alone, keep giving first aid.

Get medical help. Call an ambulance and tell them an infant is unconscious.

4 Open the airway by tilting the head.

push backward on the forehead and lift the jaw

If a head or neck injury is suspected, don't move the casualty. Check breathing and if there isn't any, open the airway using the jaw thrust without head tilt—see page 4-22.

5 Check breathing for 3 to 5 seconds.

keep the head tilted

with your ear close to the casualty's mouth and nose, check for breathing

look... for chest movement

listen... for sounds of breathing

feel... for breath on your cheek

6   Try to breathe into the casualty's mouth. If the chest rises, give another breath. If it doesn't, conclude the airway is blocked and give first aid for choking.

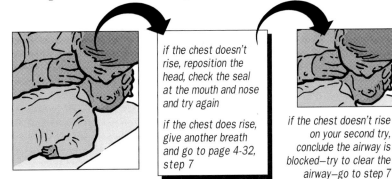

seal your mouth around the infant's mouth and nose

blow slowly– watch for the chest to rise

if the chest doesn't rise, reposition the head, check the seal at the mouth and nose and try again

if the chest does rise, give another breath and go to page 4-32, step 7

if the chest doesn't rise on your second try, conclude the airway is blocked–try to clear the airway–go to step 7

3

7   Pick the baby up, turn her over and give up to five back blows between the shoulder blades. Support the head and neck throughout the movements.

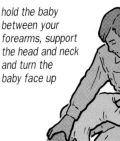

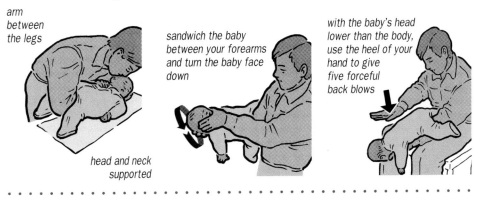

arm between the legs

head and neck supported

sandwich the baby between your forearms and turn the baby face down

with the baby's head lower than the body, use the heel of your hand to give five forceful back blows

8   Turn the baby face up and bring her close to you.

hold the baby between your forearms, support the head and neck and turn the baby face up

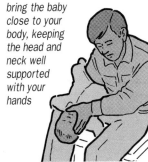

bring the baby close to your body, keeping the head and neck well supported with your hands

9 Give chest thrusts to create an artificial cough. Landmark for proper finger position and give five chest thrusts, each with the intent of removing the object.

Actual size

0 cm

1.3 cm
(½ in)

2.5 cm
(1 in)

*landmark–
place three
fingers on the
breastbone
just below the
nipple line*

*lift this finger
off the chest*

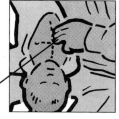

*rest the arm holding
the baby on your thigh*

*using two fingers,
give five distinct
chest thrusts*

*depress the chest
1.3 to 2.5 cm*

10 Check the mouth and try to breathe into the baby.

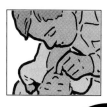

*check the mouth using the
tongue-jaw lift, remove any
foreign matter you can see*

*push back on the
forehead and lift the
jaw*

*seal your mouth
around the baby's
mouth and nose*

*blow slowly–watch for
the chest to rise*

*if the chest doesn't
rise, reposition the
head, check the seals
at the nose and mouth
and try again.*

*if the chest does rise,
give another breath
and go to page 4-32,
step 7*

*if the chest doesn't rise on your second
try, conclude the airway is blocked–try
to clear the airway–go to step 11*

11 Repeat steps 7, 8, 9 and 10 until the chest rises when you breathe into the baby's mouth or until medical help takes over.

*keep
repeating
steps 7, 8,
9 & 10*

If medical help has not been called, after one minute of first aid, decide what to do—see page 1-19.

if

If you relieve the blockage, or if air goes in when you ventilate, give another breath and then check for both breathing and a brachial pulse at the same time. Give the ongoing casualty care described on page 3-8.

If you are alone, see
page 1-19 for information on
when to go for medical help.

FOCUS ON SAFETY

How to prevent choking

• •

3

> The prevention tips below are based on the most common causes of choking. Use these tips to reduce the risk of choking.

Preventing choking in adults

◆ Cut food into small pieces or take small bites when not using a knife and fork.

◆ Drink alcohol in moderation. Alcohol causes you to lose the coordination of the muscles used in swallowing, and makes it easier to choke.

◆ Don't talk, laugh or gulp drinks with food in your mouth.

Preventing choking in children

◆ Supervise children when they are eating.

◆ Don't feed the following food items to children under four years of age:

– nuts	– popcorn
– round candies	– grapes
– hot dogs	– thickly-spread peanut butter

◆ Cut hot dogs in half lengthwise for older children.

◆ Teach children not to run or move about when eating.

◆ Balloons are a common cause of choking—always supervise children when they're playing with balloons.

◆ Check your house regularly for items that could cause choking, especialy under furniture and between the cushions on couches and chairs—coins are a common hazard.

Preventing choking in infants

◆ Inspect all toys for small parts that may come off—keep these toys away from infants.

◆ Only give infants small bite-sized pieces of food, especially when the infant has few teeth or is just learning to eat solids.

◆ Keep all toys out of the baby's crib.

◆ Check pacifiers for small parts or worn nipples. Throw these away immediately.

◆ Don't let infants play with balloons.

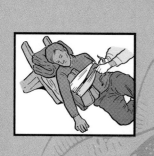

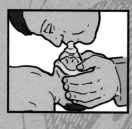

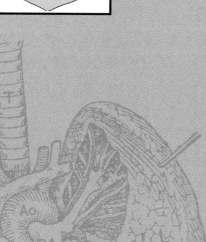

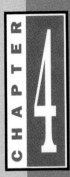

CHAPTER 4

BREATHING EMERGENCIES AND ARTIFICIAL RESPIRATION

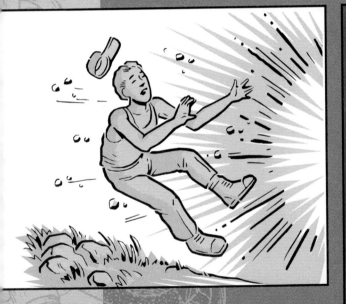

- ◆ *Requirements for effective breathing*

- ◆ *Ineffective breathing*

- ◆ *Breathing emergencies caused by injuries*

- ◆ *First aid for a penetrating chest wound*

- ◆ *First aid for a flail chest*

- ◆ *First aid for a severe asthma attack*

- ◆ *Artificial respiration*

- ◆ *How to prevent breathing emergencies*

Breathing emergencies

Continuous, effective breathing is vital for life. When a person's breathing is affected through injury or illness, his life can be in immediate danger. As a first aider, you have to be able to recognize a breathing emergency very quickly and know what first aid to give—the casualty's life may depend on it.

Hypoxia

A breathing emergency causes a lack of oxygen in the blood. This condition, called **hypoxia**, can damage vital tissues and eventually cause death, if not corrected. The causes of hypoxia are grouped under three headings:

◆ **lack of oxygen** —for example:

❖ an environment where the oxygen level is low, such as at a high altitude

❖ the oxygen is displaced by other gases, such as carbon monoxide, silo gas on a farm or hydrogen sulphide (H_2S) in an industrial setting

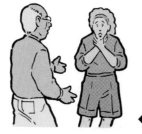

silo gas displaces oxygen

❖ the oxygen in a small space is used up—for instance, a young child trapped in an old refrigerator quickly uses up all the air

◆ **blocked airway**—for example:

❖ the casualty chokes on a foreign object, like food

❖ the casualty is face up while unconscious and the tongue blocks the airway

❖ the casualty's airway is swollen from an infection

◆ **abnormal heart and lung function**—the lungs and heart are not working properly, for example:

❖ an illness such as chronic obstructive pulmonary disease, pneumonia or congestive heart failure

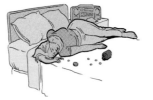

❖ an injury to the head, spine, chest, etc.

❖ a drug overdose or poisoning

Requirements for effective breathing

To breathe effectively, we need at least the following:

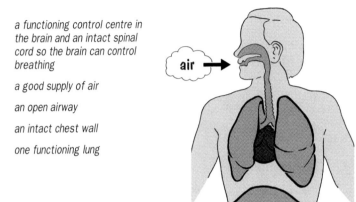

a functioning control centre in
the brain and an intact spinal
cord so the brain can control
breathing

a good supply of air

an open airway

an intact chest wall

one functioning lung

4

There is more detail about the parts and functioning of the body's
respiratory system on page 16-12.

Signs of normal, effective breathing

The rate, rhythm and depth of breathing are important signs for
the first aider to use to assess breathing.

Breathing **rate** is the number of breaths (inhalations and exhala-
tions) in one minute. The normal breathing rate varies for infants,
children and adults. The table below gives the range of normal
breathing rates for different ages. The table also gives the rates
that are too slow and too fast for each age group. A breathing rate
that is too slow or too fast is a sign of a breathing emergency.

Breathing rates – breaths per minute			
age group	range of normal rates	too slow	too fast
adult (over 8 yrs.)	10 to 20	below 10	above 30
child (1 to 8 yrs.)	20 to 30	below 15	above 40
infant (under 1 yr.)	30 to 50	below 25	above 60

Breathing **rhythm** refers to the interval between breaths. In normal breathing, the intervals are even and breathing is effort-less—this is regular breathing. In irregular breathing, the intervals between breaths are uneven. This usually indicates a respiratory disorder or distress.

Breathing **depth** refers to the amount of air moved in and out of the lungs with each breath. Learn to recognize the difference between normal breathing depth and shallow or deep breathing.

Other signs of normal breathing include:

◆ quiet and effortless breathing

◆ chest movement that is equal on both sides

◆ the person is alert and relaxed

◆ normal skin colour

◆ able to speak without taking a breath every few words

Signs of ineffective breathing

When a person is breathing normally, breathing is **effective**. This means the body is getting the oxygen it needs to function. As a person's breathing becomes more and more impaired, there is a point where the body needs more oxygen than it is getting. At this point, breathing becomes **ineffective**. There are different levels of ineffective breathing, as the illustration below shows. As a first aider, you need to be able to tell the difference between breathing that is "just a little" ineffective, where the casualty's life is not in immediate danger, and breathing that is very ineffective, where the casualty's life is in immediate danger. When breathing is very ineffective, the casualty has **severe breathing difficulties**.

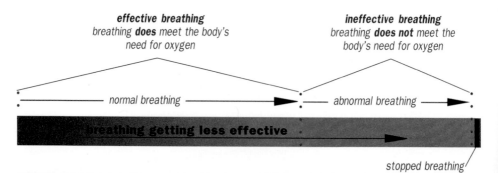

Signs and symptoms of severe breathing difficulties

Look for the signs and symptoms below. Notice whether the person's condition changes over time. For example, if a person with breathing difficulties who was fully conscious begins to get drowsy, you know the breathing difficulties are severe and medical help is urgently needed.

4

person may be anxious, afraid, terrified, etc. because of the breathing difficulty (dyspnea)

breathing is difficult—the casualty is struggling for breath or gasping for air

breathing rate may be too fast or too slow

breathing rhythm may be irregular

breathing depth may be too shallow or too deep

breathing may be noisy or raspy

person may say he's "getting tired" from trying to breathe

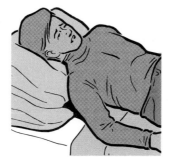

the casualty may be sweaty from working so hard at breathing

decreased level of consciousness

*the lips, ears and fingernail beds look bluish (this bluish tinge is called **cyanosis**)*

chest movement may be abnormal—the chest goes in and the abdomen puffs out during inhalation

there may be little or no chest movement or breathing effort

you may not be able to feel air moving in and out of the nose and mouth

First aid for ineffective breathing

Ineffective breathing is a life-threatening breathing emergency. Give first aid for ineffective breathing as soon as you see that breathing is ineffective, or when the situation suggests that breathing could become ineffective. The first aid for ineffective breathing has two parts:

1   First aid for the cause of the breathing emergency, such as:

◆ sealing a chest wound

◆ supporting an area of broken ribs

◆ positioning the casualty to make breathing easier

4

2 If the above first aid actions don't make the casualty's breathing effective, give the casualty assisted breathing. Assisted breathing is explained on page 4-33.

The table below lists some of the causes of breathing emergencies. To give first aid, first determine the cause of the breathing emergency, then decide on the best first aid actions.

Causes of breathing emergencies		
Injuries that can cause a breathing emergency	**Illnesses that can cause a breathing emergency**	**Poisoning that can cause a breathing emergency**
broken ribs	asthma	inhaled poison – e.g. carbon monoxide poisoning H_2S
near drowning	stroke	
knife or gunshot wound	allergic reaction	swallowed poison – medication like sleeping pills
burns to the face	pneumonia	
head injury	congestive heart failure	injected poison – e.g. bee sting
compression of the chest preventing chest expansion	emphysema	

Breathing emergencies caused by injuries

Poisoning and breathing emergencies

If poisoning caused the breathing emergency, give first aid as follows:

♦ do a scene survey and primary survey and give first aid for the ABCs

♦ send someone to call for medical help as soon you recognize a breathing emergency

♦ see chapter 8 for first aid for poisoning

If the breathing problem was caused by an injury, what part of the body was injured? If the head was injured, including the mouth and nose, something could be blocking the airway. Check the mouth for loose teeth, dentures, blood or other body fluids. With a head injury, there may also be a spinal injury, so protect the head and neck from movement the best you can while making sure the casualty has a clear airway.

A chest injury may be the cause of the breathing difficulty. Chest injuries can be open or closed. In an **open chest injury** the skin has been broken. The cause is either an external object or a broken rib that has been forced through the chest wall. In a **closed**

chest injury, the skin of the chest has not been broken and there may be no visible sign of injury, but there could be serious damage to the ribs, sternum, lungs, heart or the nerves that control breathing. This often happens in a car crash when the casualty is thrown against the steering wheel or dashboard.

If the mechanism of injury suggests a chest injury, and there is difficulty breathing, or if the casualty complains of pain in the chest carefully examine the area. Expose it and look for signs of broken ribs or a wound (try to ensure a female casualty's privacy). Look for bruises, deformity, blood and abnormal chest movement while breathing. Two serious complications of chest injuries are pneumothorax and flail chest.

Pneumothorax

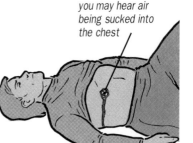

A **pneumothorax** (new-mow-thor-ax) is the result of an injury where air gets into the chest cavity—page 4-37 explains this in detail. Pneumothorax can cause one or both lungs to collapse, resulting in a life-threatening breathing emergency. If air is getting into the chest cavity through an open wound, the wound is called a **penetrating chest wound**. There may be bloodstained bubbles around the wound when the casualty exhales—these come from air being sucked into, and out of the wound as the casualty breathes (which is why these wounds are also called **sucking chest wounds**). First aid is needed right away.

you may hear air being sucked into the chest

First aid for a penetrating chest wound

1 Begin ESM—do a scene survey and primary survey. As soon as you identify a sucking chest wound, cover it by pressing the casualty's hand, a bystander's hand or your own hand over the wound. This stops air from flowing in and out of the chest cavity.

If the first aid makes the casualty worse

Sealing a sucking chest wound can make the casualty worse. See step 5 on page 4-9 for what to do if this happens.

2   Place the casualty in the position that makes breathing easiest—this is usually semisitting, leaning slightly towards the injured side. This position keeps the uninjured side of the chest upward so it can be used most effectively for breathing.

If you suspect a head or spinal injury, leave the casualty in the position found, supporting the head and neck.

If breathing is not effective, give assisted breathing (see page 4-33). If the casualty must be moved to do this, support the head and neck during movement.

use the casualty's hand on the uninjured side to cover the wound

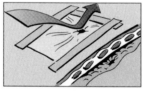

airtight materials that can be used to seal a sucking chest wound

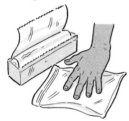

3   Seal the wound with an airtight dressing taped on three sides. The dressing should work as a flutter-type valve, letting air from the chest cavity out while preventing air from going into the wound. If there is an embedded object, tape dressings around the object and try to make a flutter-type valve.

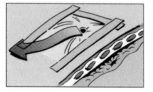

the flutter valve stops air from going into the wound by being sucked up tight against the wound when the casualty inhales

when the casualty exhales, the valve opens and allows air to exit from the chest

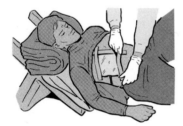

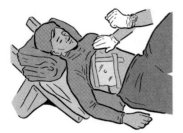

4   Assess breathing. If breathing is still ineffective, give assisted ventilations—see page 4-33. If breathing gets worse, see *tension pneumothorax* in step 5, next page. If breathing is effective, go to step 5.

5 Give ongoing casualty care, monitoring breathing often. If breathing becomes more difficult, a **tension pneumothorax** may be developing. First, unseal the wound for a few seconds—air may rush out. Then adjust the dressing to make sure it seals the wound as the casualty breathes in, and unseals the wound as the casualty breathes out. You have to check this kind of dressing often to make sure it is working properly.

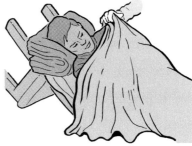

There is not always an open wound with a pneumothorax. A pneumothorax can be caused by broken ribs, or it can happen for no obvious reason. A pneumothorax always has the potential to be a life-threatening breathing emergency and medical help is needed as quickly as possible.

Flail chest

A flail chest results when several ribs in the same area are broken in more than one place. The injured part of the chest wall is called a **"flail"** or **"loose" segment**. The flail segment is no longer a rigid part of the chest wall, so it doesn't move normally during breathing. As the casualty inhales, the chest should expand, but the flail segment is pulled into the chest instead. As the casualty exhales, the chest should move inward, but the flail segment puffs outward. This abnormal chest movement is called **paradoxical chest movement**. This injury makes breathing very difficult because of the pain and the tissue damage.

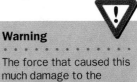

Warning

The force that caused this much damage to the chest may also have caused a head or spinal injury—see page 2-6.

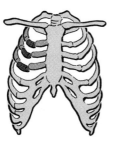

a flail segment results when a number of ribs in the same area are broken and the chest wall is no longer rigid

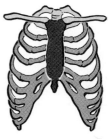

if many of the ribs that attach to the breastbone are broken, the whole breastbone can become a flail segment—this can happen if the chest hits the steering wheel during a motor vehicle collision

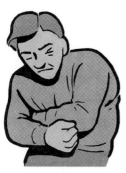

4

Signs and symptoms of a flail chest

◆ paradoxical chest movement (see page 4-9)—this is the sign that will tell you whether there is a flail chest

◆ breathing is very painful, and the casualty may be positioned to support the injured area

◆ bruising at the injury site

First aid for a flail chest

The aim of first aid for a flail chest is to give first aid for the ABCs, immobilize the casualty and get medical help.

1   Begin ESM—do a scene survey. As soon as you suspect major injuries, tell the casualty not to move.

2   Steady and support the head and neck.

3   Start the primary survey—check airway and breathing.

4   If the casualty complains of difficulty breathing and pain in the chest, expose and examine the injury.

5   Support the injured area with your hand—this may make breathing easier.

6   Give first aid for ineffective breathing if needed—See page 4-5.

7   Check circulation and give first aid if needed.

8   Give ongoing casualty care until medical help takes over. Monitor ABC's often.

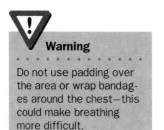

Warning

Do not use padding over the area or wrap bandages around the chest—this could make breathing more difficult.

Blast injury

Most people never see explosives in their lifetimes. But for some Canadians, working with explosives is a way of life. This is especially true in the mining and construction industries. There are three mechanisms of injury from an explosion, apart from being right in the blast:

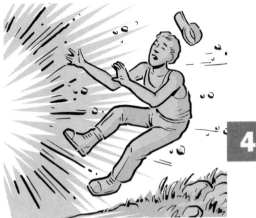

- ◆ injuries from being struck by material thrown by the blast

- ◆ injuries from being thrown by the blast

- ◆ injuries to hollow organs, including the lungs, caused by the shock wave from the blast—these can cause life-threatening breathing emergencies

The violent shock wave of an explosion can damage the lungs (and the stomach and intestines), even when there is no other visible sign of injury. The casualty may complain of chest pain and cough up frothy blood.

First aid for a blast injury that affects breathing

1 Begin ESM—do a scene survey (see page 2-3). If the casualty was thrown by the blast, suspect a head or spinal injury and prevent any unnecessary movement.

2 Do a primary survey (see page 2-5). Place the casualty at rest in a semisitting position if there is no suspected head or spinal injury—raise and support the head and shoulders. Send for medical help.

3 Monitor breathing closely. If it is ineffective, give assisted breathing—see page 4-33. If breathing stops, give AR.

4 Give first aid for shock.

5 Give ongoing casualty care until medical help arrives.

4

Inhalation injuries

Inhalation injuries happen when the casualty inhales:

- hot steam or hot (superheated) air

- smoke or poisonous chemicals

- carbon monoxide (the most common inhalation injury in a fire)

Inhalation injuries are the most common cause of death from a fire in a building—suspect an inhalation injury when a casualty has been in a fire. An inhalation injury is always considered a life-threatening breathing emergency. It can be many hours after inhaling the hot air or poisonous gas that breathing is seriously affected. For this reason, every casualty of an inhalation injury needs to be transported to medical help. Only a medical doctor can determine the extent of the injuries.

Signs and symptoms of inhalation injury

Signs of hypoxia:

- dizziness, restlessness, confusion, unconsciousness
- pallor or cyanosis

Signs of severe breathing difficulty:

- noisy breathing
- abnormal breathing rate or depth
- pain during breathing

Signs of being close to heat:

- burns on the face, especially the mouth and nose
- singed hair on the face or head

Signs of breathing smoke:

- sooty or smoky smell on breath
- sore throat, hoarseness, barking cough, difficulty swallowing

First aid for an inhalation injury

1 Begin ESM—do a scene survey (see page 2-3). Make sure you can give first aid safely without putting yourself in danger.

2 Do a primary survey (see page 2-5). Give first aid for the ABCs. Make sure the casualty has a supply of fresh air.

3 Make breathing easier for the casualty—place him in the semisitting position and loosen tight clothing at the neck, chest and waist.

4 Monitor breathing closely. If breathing is ineffective, give assisted breathing. If breathing stops, give AR.

5 Give first aid for shock.

6 Give ongoing casualty care until handover to medical help.

Breathing emergencies caused by illness

If the casualty has trouble breathing and there is no reason to suspect an injury or poisoning, the breathing difficulty is probably related to an illness. Illnesses that can lead to severe breathing difficulties include asthma, allergies, chronic obstructive pulmonary disease (e.g. emphysema), congestive heart failure, pneumonia, etc. The basic first aid for all these emergencies is the same.

 ## First aid for breathing emergencies caused by illness

1 Begin ESM—do a scene survey (see page 2-3) and primary survey see page 2-5).

2 Place the casualty in the most comfortable position—this is often semisitting. Send for medical help.

3 Find out the history of the situation using the **SAMPLE** method (see page 2-12). You may be able to discover the exact cause of the breathing difficulties.

4 Ask the casualty if he has any medication for this condition. See page 4-36 for information on helping with asthma medications, and pages 4-34 and 4-35 for information on medications for severe allergic reactions.

5 Stay with the casualty. Give ongoing casualty care until medical help arrives. If breathing becomes ineffective, give assisted breathing (see page 4-33). If the casualty becomes unconscious, place him in the recovery position and monitor his breathing closely.

There is more information below on the following breathing emergencies:

◆ asthma (bronchial asthma)—see page 4-15

◆ severe allergic reaction—see page 4-16

◆ hyperventilation—see page 4-17

4

Sudden Infant Death Syndrome (SIDS)

There is one breathing emergency that every new parent knows of and dreads—**sudden infant death syndrome**, or **SIDS**. Also called crib death, SIDS is the unexplained death of an apparently healthy infant. The infant dies suddenly and unexpectedly, usually while sleeping. One or two infants per 1,000 die of SIDS in Canada. This makes SIDS the leading cause of death for infants older than four months. SIDS is not likely to occur after one year of age.

First aid for SIDS

The first aid for SIDS is the same as for any unresponsive infant (see page 5-26). Your actions include:

◆ assess responsiveness

◆ open the airway

◆ assess breathing

  – if there is no breathing, give 2 breaths

◆ assess the pulse

  – if there is a pulse, continue AR—see page 4-33, step 8

  – if there is no pulse, give CPR—see page 5-28, step 8

◆ give first aid for one minute, then get medical help as quickly as possible, while continuing first aid—see page 1-19 for what to do if you are alone.

Reducing risk factors

Although the exact cause(s) of SIDS is unknown, you can help reduce the risk of SIDS by:*

◆ putting the baby to sleep on his back or side, on a firm, flat surface

◆ keeping the baby in a smoke-free environment

◆ not overheating the baby

◆ breast-feeding the baby, if possible

* source: The Canadian Foundation for the Study of Infant Deaths, Canadian Institute for Child Health, Canadian Pediatric Society, and Health Canada

More about SIDS

When a baby dies of SIDS, it is nobody's fault. Although we can reduce the risk factors for SIDS, we cannot prevent it. When even doctors cannot explain the cause, SIDS deaths seem very mysterious and many parents blame themselves or each other. They think it was something they did, or did not do. Sometimes the baby has seen the doctor just before dying, so the parents blame the doctor. But there is no way to tell if a baby is going to die of SIDS. Most babies who have died of SIDS were well fed, well cared for, and seemed to be in good health.

A baby who dies of SIDS does not suffer. The baby does not cry out or struggle in any way. SIDS is not caused by smothering. Occasionally a baby who died of SIDS is found face down and covered in blankets, which may suggest smothering, but this is rarely the case. Most SIDS deaths occur when there was no chance of smothering or strangulation.

**For more
information on SIDS**

Write or call:

Canadian Foundation
for the Study of Infant Deaths
P.O. Box 190, Station R
Toronto, Ontario
M4G 309

1-800-END-SIDS

Bronchial asthma

Bronchial asthma (often called "asthma") is a respiratory illness in which the person has repeated attacks (asthmatic attacks) of shortness of breath, often with wheezing and coughing. Between attacks, the person has no trouble breathing.

Signs and symptoms of a severe asthmatic attack

◆ shortness of breath with obvious trouble breathing

◆ coughing or wheezing (a whistling noise caused by air moving through narrowed airways)—may get louder or stop

◆ fast and shallow breathing

◆ casualty sitting upright trying to breathe

◆ bluish colour in the face (cyanosis)

◆ anxiety, tightness in the chest

◆ fast pulse rate, shock

◆ restlessness at first, and then fatigue—the casualty becomes tired from trying so hard to breathe

First aid for a severe asthma attack

1 Begin ESM—do a scene survey (see page 2-3) and a primary survey (see page 2-5). As soon as you identify a severe asthma attack, send for medical help.

2 Have the casualty stop any activity and place him in the most comfortable position for breathing. This is usually sitting upright with arms resting on a table.

3 Help the casualty take his prescribed medication—see sidebar.

4 Give ongoing casualty care. Stay with the casualty until medical help takes over. Give plenty of reassurance since fear and anxiety may cause the casualty to breathe faster, making the situation worse.

Asthma medications

There are a variety of asthma medications and the casualty may have more than one type of medication. See page 4-36 for information on inhaler-type medications. See pages 4-34 and 4-35 for information on injection-type medication.

4

Severe allergic reaction

A life-threatening breathing emergency can result from a severe allergic reaction called **anaphylaxis** (an-a-fi-lak-sis). This reaction usually happens when a substance to which the casualty is very sensitive enters the body. But anaphylaxis can also be caused by exercise or have no known cause. Anaphylaxis is a serious medical emergency that needs urgent medical attention.

Anaphylaxis can happen within seconds, minutes or hours of a substance entering the body. As a rule, the sooner the casualty's body reacts, the worse the reaction will be.

Common causes of anaphylaxis

· · · · · · · · · · · · · ·

Stings—by bees, hornets, wasps and fire ants

Medications—including antibiotics (esp. penicillin), seizure medications, ASA and muscle relaxants

Foods—like milk, eggs, nuts (incl. peanuts), shellfish, whitefish, food additives

Exercise

Signs and symptoms of anaphylaxis	
The early signs and symptoms of anaphylaxis may include:	**As anaphylaxis progresses, the signs and symptoms may include:**
itchy, flushed skin, raised skin rash (hives)	pale skin and/or cyanosis
sneezing, running nose and watery eyes	anxiety and perhaps a severe headache
swelling of the airway	wheezing, chest feels like it's being squeezed
a "lump" or "tickle" in the throat that won't go away	breathing difficulties, coughing
coughing	pulse is rapid and irregular
sense of impending doom	shock—wrist pulse may be hard to find
nausea and vomiting	swelling of the lips, tongue, throat, hands and feet
	unconsciousness, stopped breathing, stopped heart (cardiac arrest)

First aid for a severe allergic reaction

1   Begin ESM—do a scene survey (see page 2-3) and a primary survey (see page 2-5). As soon as you identify a severe allergic reaction, send for medical help.

2   Stop any activity and place the casualty in the most comfortable position for breathing—usually sitting upright.

3 Help the casualty take his prescribed medication. Some people with known allergies carry medication with them. Some times these medications are in the form of a prepared hypodermic syringe in an allergy kit. See pages 4-34 and 4-35 for information on helping give the type of medication.

4 Give ongoing casualty care. Stay with the casualty until medical help takes over. Give plenty of reassurance, as fear and anxiety will make the casualty's condition worse.

Hyperventilation

Hyperventilation is a condition of "overbreathing." It can be caused by acute anxiety or emotional stress, drug withdrawal or aspirin poisoning or for no obvious reason. A hyperventilation attack can be very dramatic—the casualty may be very frightened, and the people with the casualty may also become upset.

Signs and symptoms of hyperventilation

◆ breathing is faster and deeper, the casualty may say:

"I can feel my heart pounding!"

"I feel like I am smothering and can't get enough air!"

"I'm having trouble swallowing."

◆ pulse is rapid, skin colour is usually good

◆ headache, chest pains, dizziness, tingling, shaking

> **Don't use a brown paper bag**
>
> Do not have a hyperventilating casualty breathe into a bag and re-breathe his own air. This old technique does not work and it can be dangerous.

First aid for hyperventilation

The aim of first aid for hyperventilation is to calm the person and reassure him. In stress-related hyperventilation, quietly reassuring and encouraging the person to slow the rate of respiration will usually bring relief and ease the symptoms. Ask the person to match your normal rate and depth of breathing.

Casualties in hyperventilation should be taken to medical help for evaluation and further care. Some serious medical conditions look like hyperventilation and these need medical care.

First aid for stopped breathing – Artificial respiration (AR)

The vital organs of the body such as the brain and heart need a continuous supply of oxygen to stay alive. Artificial respiration (AR) is a way you can supply air to the lungs of a casualty who is breathing ineffectively or not breathing at all.

In the second step of the primary survey, you check for breathing. If there is no breathing, you start AR. If there is breathing, assess whether the casualty is having severe breathing difficulties. If so, give first aid to make breathing more effective. If there are still severe breathing difficulties, assist breathing using the techniques of AR.

The brain may be permanently damaged if it doesn't have oxygen for more than four minutes.

As you breathe, the air you exhale contains enough oxygen to keep a non-breathing person alive. Artificial respiration involves blowing this air into the casualty's lungs to deliver oxygen to the non-breathing person. The number of times you blow in one minute is called the **rate**—AR has to be given at the proper rate to make sure the casualty is getting enough oxygen.

There are a number of different techniques of AR and the one you use depends on the situation. These are:

◆ **mouth-to-mouth AR** — this is the most commonly used method of AR. The first aider pinches the casualty's nose closed and blows into his mouth

◆ **mouth-to-nose AR** — this method is used in situations where mouth-to-mouth is not appropriate, such as when your mouth won't cover the casualty's mouth. You hold the casualty's mouth closed and blow into his nose. There is more on mouth-to-nose AR on page 4-30

◆ **mouth-to-mouth-and-nose AR** — this method is used for infants and small children where your mouth easily fits over the casualty's mouth and nose

◆ **mouth-to-stoma AR** — this technique is for a casualty who has previously had a laryngectomy and breathes through a hole in his neck (called a stoma)

Artificial respiration can be given in a wide range of situations. In an emergency situation, keep the following in mind:

◆ you can start AR right away in any position (but it is best if the casualty is on his back on a firm, flat surface)

◆ you can continue AR while the casualty is being moved to safety by other rescuers

◆ you can give AR for a long time without getting too tired

◆ AR techniques can be used to help a casualty with severe breathing difficulties

Giving AR in some situations, may be more difficult than in others. When this happens, you have to do the best you can (based on your level of training) without putting yourself into danger. Sample situations are:

◆ when severe deforming injuries to the mouth and nose prevent a good seal around the mouth

◆ blood and/or other body fluids drain into the throat and block the airway when you try direct AR (do your best to drain the mouth)

◆ the casualty was poisoned by a toxic gas like hydrogen sulphide and coming in contact with the casualty may result in you being poisoned

◆ the casualty has a corrosive poison on the face or in the mouth, and you don't have a face mask

How to give artificial respiration

The following pages illustrate, in detail, how to give artificial respiration to adult, child or infant casualties. The methods are presented as rescue sequences and show all the actions you should take when you find a unresponsive casualty. These sequences follow the same steps as the scene survey and primary survey described in chapter 2, but here casualties are given first aid for stopped breathing.

Ages in AR

In AR, first aid for choking and CPR, the following age guidelines are used:

◆ adult = 8 years and up
◆ child = between 1 and 8 years old
◆ infant = under 1 year old

These ages are guidelines only; the casualty's size must also be considered. For example, you would give adult AR to a tall, husky seven-year-old.

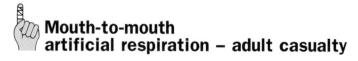

Mouth-to-mouth
artificial respiration – adult casualty

You arrive at a scene… an unconscious adult (someone eight years old or older) is lying on the floor…

if

If there could be a head or spinal injury, continue as shown on page 4-22 and 4-23.

4

1   Begin ESM—start the scene survey (see page 2-3).

. . . .

2   Assess responsiveness. If there is no response, go to step 3.

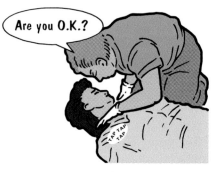

Are you O.K.?

ask the casualty if she is O.K. Assess any response.

gently tap the shoulders

. . . .

3   Send or go for medical help.

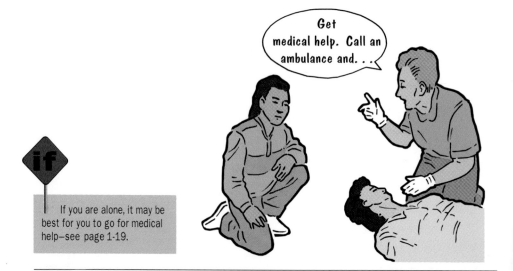

Get medical help. Call an ambulance and. . .

if

If you are alone, it may be best for you to go for medical help—see page 1-19.

4 Place the casualty face up, protecting the head and neck during any movement. Open the airway by tilting the head.

to open the airway push backward on the forehead and lift the jaw

If you suspect a head or spinal injury, don't move the casualty. See page 4-22 for how to open the airway and check for breathing.

4

airway closed   *airway open*

when the head is tilted back, the tongue is lifted off the back of the throat, opening the airway

5 Check for breathing for 3 to 5 seconds.

keep the head tilted

place your ear just above the casualty's nose and mouth

look... for chest movement

listen... for sounds of breathing

feel... for breath on your cheek

If there is no breathing, go to step 6.

6 Breathe into the casualty twice. For an adult casualty, blow for 1½ to 2 seconds. Use enough air to make the chest rise.

take a deep breath and seal your mouth around the casualty's mouth

pinch the nostrils

blow slowly and watch for the chest to rise

move your mouth away and release the nostrils to allow the air to escape

look for the chest to fall, listen for air sounds and feel for air being exhaled against your cheek

give another breath and go to step 7

If the chest doesn't rise when you blow:

♦ reopen the airway by tilting the head

♦ pinch the nose again

♦ make a better seal around the mouth

♦ try blowing again

If the chest still doesn't rise, give first aid for choking—see page 3-10, step 7.

continued on page 4-24

4

How to give AR when you suspect a head or spinal injury

The usual AR technique involves moving the head and neck to open the airway. If the casualty has a head or neck injury, this movement could cause paralysis or even death.

When you suspect a head or spinal injury, prevent head and neck movement and open the airway using the **jaw-thrust without head-tilt** as shown below.

1 *place your hands on either side of the casualty's head so the head and neck cannot move*

Tell the casualty not to move. Support the head and neck and assess responsiveness—instead of tapping, gently pinch the earlobes. Send for medical help if the casualty is unresponsive.

2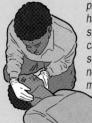

Check for breathing in the position found. Look, listen and feel for signs of breathing.

3 *open the airway— press on the chin to open the mouth and lift the jaw*

steady your hands on the cheek bones

grasp the angle of the jaw and lift to open the airway

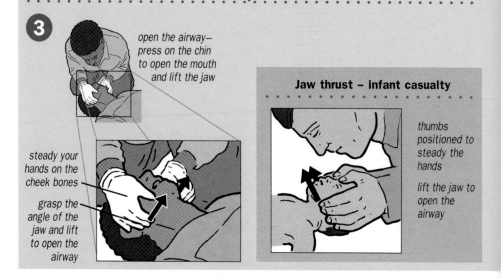

Jaw thrust – infant casualty

thumbs positioned to steady the hands

lift the jaw to open the airway

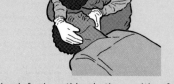

4

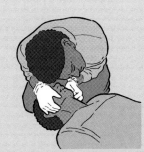

look... for chest movement

listen... for sounds of breathing

feel... for breath on your cheek

Check for signs of breathing for three to five seconds while holding the airway open with the jaw thrust.

If you must reposition the casualty to properly assess him or give AR, move or turn him as a unit as much as possible—see page 2-8.

4

5

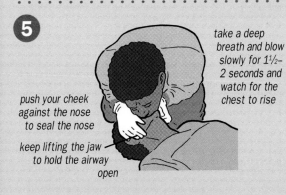

take a deep breath and blow slowly for 1½– 2 seconds and watch for the chest to rise

push your cheek against the nose to seal the nose

keep lifting the jaw to hold the airway open

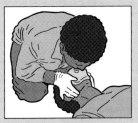

opening the airway with the jaw-thrust without head-tilt using a face mask

If there is no breathing, put your mouth over the casualty's mouth and press your cheek against the casualty's nose to seal it. Blow into the casualty's mouth and watch for the chest to rise.

If the chest rises, give another breath and continue AR. If the chest doesn't rise, try opening the airway again with the jaw thrust, but this time:

◆ apply gentle traction to the head and neck by pulling the head gently away from the body

◆ tilt the head slightly backwards—just enough to open the airway (although these actions move the neck, it is more important to get air into the casualty's lungs than to protect the neck)

◆ try to breathe into the casualty again.

If the chest still does not rise, conclude the airway is blocked by a foreign object and

start first aid for choking—see page 3-10, step 7.

Using the jaw thrust, continue giving AR as described on step 7, next page.

For an infant casualty

Cover both the mouth and nose with your mouth, or with a face mask if you are using one. Blow for 1 to 1½ seconds.

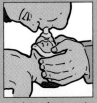

using a face mask

continued from page 4-21

7 Check for a pulse at the neck. There is a carotid pulse on either side of the neck—feel for a pulse on the side closest to you— **do not feel or compress both sides at the same time**

First aider's view of the pulse check

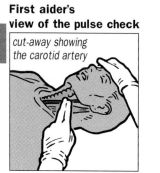

cut-away showing the carotid artery

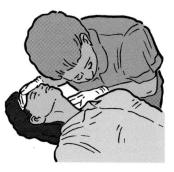

keep the head tilted

slide 2 fingers into the groove of the neck just down from the Adam's apple

press gently to detect the pulse, take 5 to 10 seconds

If there is no pulse, start CPR—see page 5-13, step 8.

If there is a pulse, continue AR—see step 8, below.

· ·

8 Breathe into the casualty once every five seconds (12 times a minute). After one minute of AR, recheck the pulse for five seconds, and at the same time, look, listen and feel for breathing:

◆ if there is no pulse, start CPR—see page 5-13, step 8

◆ if there is a pulse and breathing, continue the primary survey—see page 2-9, step 2

◆ if there is a pulse and still no breathing, continue AR. Recheck the pulse and breathing every few minutes. Keep giving AR until the casualty starts to breathe on her own, medical help takes over or you are too tired to continue

Don't blow too hard
· · · · · · · · · · · · ·
If you blow into a casualty too hard or too fast, the air may go into the stomach instead of the lungs. This can cause a few problems—see page 4-28 for more on this. Only blow hard enough to make the chest rise.

Mouth-to-mouth artificial respiration – child casualty

You arrive at a scene… an unconscious child (someone between one and eight years old) is lying on the floor…

1   Begin ESM—start the scene survey (see page 2-3). Ask a parent or guardian for consent to help, if present.

If there might be a head or spinal injury, continue as shown on page 4-22 and 4-23.

4

. . . .

2   Assess responsiveness.

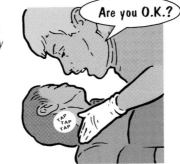

ask the casualty if he is O.K. and assess any response

gently tap the shoulders

Are you O.K.?

TAP TAP TAP

If there is no response, go to step 3.
. . . .

3   Send a bystander for medical help. If you are alone, keep giving first aid for one minute before considering getting medical help.

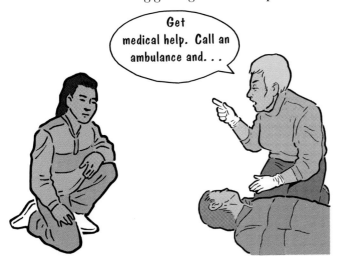

Get medical help. Call an ambulance and. . .

4 Place the casualty face up, protecting the head and neck during any movement. Open the airway by tilting the head.

airway closed

airway open

to open the airway push backward on the forehead and lift the jaw

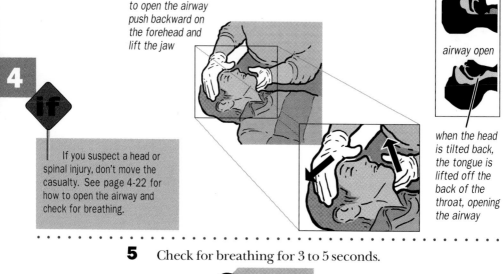

If you suspect a head or spinal injury, don't move the casualty. See page 4-22 for how to open the airway and check for breathing.

when the head is tilted back, the tongue is lifted off the back of the throat, opening the airway

- -

5 Check for breathing for 3 to 5 seconds.

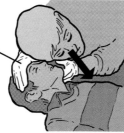

keep the head tilted

place your ear just above the casualty's nose and mouth

look... for chest movement

listen... for sounds of breathing

feel... for breath on your cheek

if If there is no breathing, go to step 6.
- -

6 Breathe into the casualty twice. For a child casualty, blow for 1 to 1½ seconds. Use just enough air to make the chest rise.

If the chest doesn't rise when you blow:

♦ reopen the airway by tilting the head

♦ pinch the nose again

♦ make a better seal around the mouth

♦ try blowing again

If the chest still doesn't rise, give first aid for choking—see page 3-20, step 7.

take a deep breath and seal your mouth around the casualty's mouth

pinch the nostrils

blow slowly and watch for the chest to rise

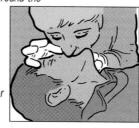

move your mouth away and release the nostrils to allow the air to escape

look for the chest to fall, listen for air sounds and feel for air being exhaled against your cheek

give another breath and go to step 7

7 Check for a pulse at the neck. There is a carotid pulse on either side of the neck—feel for a pulse on the side closest to you—**do not feel or compress both sides at the same time**

First aider's view of the pulse check

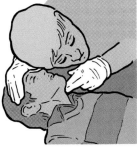

keep the head tilted

slide 2 fingers into the groove of the neck just down from the Adam's apple

press gently to detect the pulse, take 5 to 10 seconds

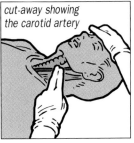

cut-away showing the carotid artery

4

If there is no pulse, start CPR—see page 5-24, step 8.

If there is a pulse, continue AR—see step 8, below.

8 Breathe into the casualty once every three seconds (20 times a minute). After one minute of AR, recheck the pulse for five seconds, and at the same time, look, listen and feel for breathing:

♦ if there is no pulse, start CPR—see page 5-24, step 8

♦ if there is a pulse and breathing, continue the primary survey—see page 2-9, step 2

♦ if there is a pulse and still no breathing, continue AR. Recheck the pulse and breathing every few minutes. Keep giving AR until the casualty starts to breathe on his own, medical help takes over or you are too tired to continue

if

If you are alone, see page 1-19 for information on when to go for medical help.

Don't blow too hard

If you blow into a casualty too hard or too fast, the air may go into the stomach instead of the lungs. This can cause a few problems—see page 4-28 for more on this. Only blow hard enough to make the chest rise.

4

Don't blow too hard – gastric distention and vomiting

Gastric distention

If you blow into a casualty too quickly or too hard, air will go into the stomach causing the stomach to swell. This is called **gastric distention**, and it can make it harder to give AR and increase the chances that the casualty will vomit.

If the stomach becomes a little distended, try to prevent further distention by:

♦ repositioning the head and opening the airway again

♦ blowing more slowly, with less air

♦ making sure the airway is held fully open

It is unusual, but the stomach can become so distended that the lungs cannot expand. In this case, the air you blow won't go into the lungs, so you have to relieve the gastric distention by forcing the air in the stomach out. **Only relieve gastric distention when the lungs cannot expand and AR is ineffective.**

Turn the casualty onto her side with face downwards. Press on her stomach—this should force the air out. The casualty will probably vomit when you do this. If she vomits, quickly wipe out her mouth to keep

the airway clear. Reposition the casualty, reassess breathing and pulse, and continue AR if necessary.

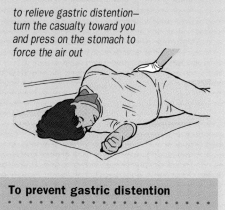

to relieve gastric distention—turn the casualty toward you and press on the stomach to force the air out

To prevent gastric distention

♦ give slow breaths

♦ only blow enough air to make the chest rise

♦ make sure the airway is fully open— keep the head tilted well back (but not over-extended)

Vomiting

Vomiting is a common complication both during AR and when the casualty starts to breathe on her own again. If the casualty vomits during AR, turn her to the side and wipe out her mouth. Once the airway is clear, reposition the casualty and continue AR.

If you suspect the casualty has a head or spinal injury, turn her to the side as a unit, so the head and spine stay in the same relative position.

if the casualty vomits, turn her towards you and quickly wipe out her mouth

reposition the casualty, reassess breathing and pulse, and continue AR

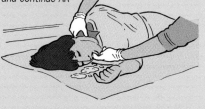

How to give AR to someone who breathes through the neck

Some people breathe through an opening at the base of the neck. This opening, called a **stoma**, is the result of a previous medical operation called a laryngectomy (lar-en-jec-toe-me).

4

How to recognize that a person breathes through the neck

You may not know a person breathes through the neck when you try to give AR. If the air seems to go down the airway when you blow, but the chest doesn't rise, check the neck for a stoma. You may also hear air coming out of the stoma as you blow.

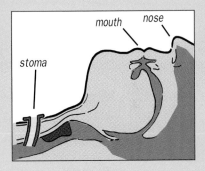

stoma

mouth   nose

Giving AR to a neck breather

The first aid rescue sequence does not change. Once you recognize a person breathes through a stoma, do the following:

◆ expose the entire neck and remove all coverings over the stoma. If there is a tube coming out of the stoma, don't remove it

◆ put a pad under the shoulders to keep them slightly elevated (if you have one close by)

◆ keep the head in line with the body and keep the chin raised

◆ seal the mouth and nose with the hand closest to the head

◆ seal your mouth around the stoma and blow directly into it, or seal your pocket mask over the stoma and blow into the pocket mask

◆ watch the chest rise (look, listen and feel for air movement)

◆ let the air escape from the stoma between breaths

◆ maintain a clean air passage, using a cloth to clean the opening; never use paper tissues

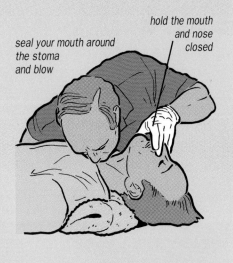

hold the mouth and nose closed

seal your mouth around the stoma and blow

How to give mouth-to-nose AR

Mouth-to-nose AR

Use this method when:

◆ the mouth cannot be opened

◆ there are injuries in or around the mouth, including burns or poisoning

◆ your mouth doesn't fully cover the casualty's mouth, and you can't get a good seal

Mouth-to-nose AR is exactly the same as mouth-to-mouth AR except you hold the mouth closed and you blow into the nose, as shown in the illustration.

Open the casualty's mouth between breaths to help let the air out of the lungs.

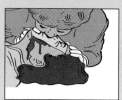

hold the mouth closed

blow into the nose— here, a face shield is being used to reduce the risk of infection

Mouth-to-mouth and nose artificial respiration – infant casualty

You arrive at a scene and there is an unconscious infant (a baby under one year old)...

If there could be a head or spinal injury, continue as shown on page 4-22 and 4-23.

1 Begin ESM—start the scene survey (see page 2-3). Ask a parent or guardian for consent to help, if present.

2 Assess responsiveness.

Baby, baby! Can you hear me?

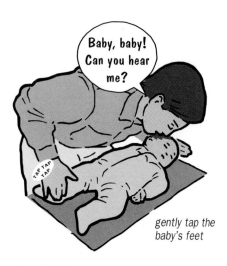

gently tap the baby's feet

3 Send a bystander for medical help. If you are alone, keep giving first aid for one minute before going for medical help.

Get medical help. Call an ambulance and tell them an infant is unconscious.

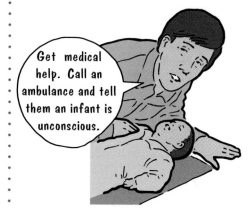

4 Place the baby face up, protecting the head and neck during any movement. Open the airway by tilting the head.

to open the airway push backward on the forehead and lift the jaw

If you suspect a head or spinal injury, don't move the baby. See page 4-22 for how to open the airway and check for breathing.

4

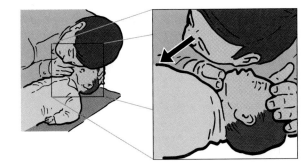

airway closed   *airway open*

when the head is tilted back, the tongue is lifted off the back of the throat, opening the airway

5 Keep the head tilted and place your ear near the baby's mouth and nose. Check for breathing for 3 to 5 seconds.

look... for chest movement

listen... for sounds of breathing

feel... for breath on your cheek

The back of an infant's head is quite large compared to the rest of his body. When lying on his back, a baby's head will come forward and close off his airway.

When giving AR or CPR, it may be helpful to put a thin pad under the shoulders to help keep the airway open—but don't waste time looking for a pad.

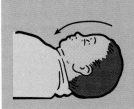

an infant's head flexes forward when he's lying on his back

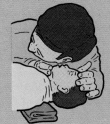

place a thin pad under the shoulders to help keep the airway open

6   Breathe into the casualty twice. For an infant casualty, blow for 1 to 1½ seconds, using just enough air to make the chest rise.

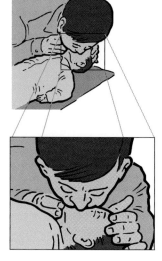

4

if

If the chest doesn't rise when you blow, try again

◆ reopen the airway by tilting the head

◆ make a better seal around the mouth and nose

◆ try blowing again

If the chest still doesn't rise, give first aid for choking—see page 3-27, step 7.

take a deep breath and seal your mouth around the baby's mouth and nose

blow slowly and watch for the chest to rise

move your mouth away and release the nostrils to allow the air to escape

look for the chest to fall, listen for air sounds and feel for air being exhaled against your cheek

give another breath and go to step 7

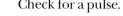

7   Check for a pulse.

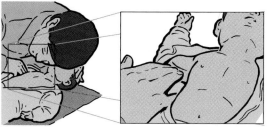

keep the head tilted

press gently with two fingertips on the inside of the arm between the large muscles and the bone

take 5 to 10 seconds

If there is no pulse, start CPR—see page 5-28, step 8.

If there is a pulse, continue AR—see step 8 on the next page.

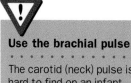

Use the brachial pulse

The carotid (neck) pulse is hard to find on an infant, so the brachial (upper arm) pulse is used instead.

8   Breathe into the casualty once every three seconds (20 times a minute). After one minute of AR, recheck the pulse for five seconds, and at the same time, look, listen and feel for breathing:

◆ if there is no pulse, start CPR—see page 5-28, step 8

◆ if there is a pulse and breathing, continue the primary survey—see page 2-3

◆ if there is a pulse and still no breathing, continue AR. Recheck the pulse and breathing every few minutes. Keep giving AR until the casualty starts to breathe on his own, medical help takes over or you are too tired to continue

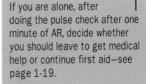

If you are alone, after doing the pulse check after one minute of AR, decide whether you should leave to get medical help or continue first aid—see page 1-19.

4

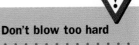

Don't blow too hard

If you blow into a casualty too hard or too fast, the air may go into the stomach instead of the lungs. This can cause a few problems—see page 4-28 for more on this. Only blow hard enough to make the chest rise.

How to give assisted breathing

Assisted breathing helps a casualty with severe breathing difficulties to breathe more effectively. It is most useful when the casualty shows very little or no breathing effort. If breathing effort is good, the casualty will likely breathe better on his own. Start assisted breathing when you recognize the signs of severe breathing difficulties (see page 4-5).

The technique for assisted breathing is the same as for artificial respiration except for the timing of the ventilations. You seal your mouth around the casualty's mouth and/or nose and blow air into the lungs (use a face mask or shield if you have one). If the casualty is breathing too slowly, give a breath each time the casualty inhales, plus

an extra breath in between the casualty's own breaths. Give one breath every five seconds for a total of 12 to 15 breaths per minute.

If the casualty is breathing too fast, give one breath on every second inhalation by the casualty. This will hopefully slow down the casualty's own breathing. Give a total of 12 to 15 breaths per minute.

If the casualty is conscious, explain what you are going to do and why. Reassure the casualty often and encourage him to try tobreathe at a good rate with good depth. If the casualty doesn't want you to assist his breathing, explain why it is important. If the casualty still doesn't want you to assist his breathing, don't.

How to help
with medication for anaphylaxis

Anaphylaxis medication is injected into the body with a needle. The two most popular products are explained here. Both of these are designed for simple use and give the right amount of medication with each injection. If the casualty cannot give the injection to himself, you may have to do it.

EpiPen® Auto-Injector

The EpiPen® Auto-Injector is a disposable drug-delivery system with a spring-activated, concealed needle. An EpiPen® Auto-Injector delivers a single dose of medication. A casualty may have more than one auto-injector for multiple doses.

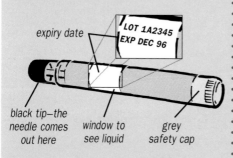

expiry date

LOT 1A2345
EXP DEC 96

black tip—the
needle comes
out here

window to
see liquid

grey
safety cap

To use the EpiPen® Auto-Injector

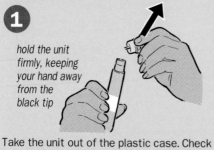

1

hold the unit
firmly, keeping
your hand away
from the
black tip

Take the unit out of the plastic case. Check the expiry date and pull off the grey safety cap—once this is off, any pressure on the black tip will activate the unit.

♦ If the liquid in the syringe is brown, do not use it. It should be clear and have no colour.

♦ If the device has expired (check the expiry date) do not use it.

♦ If you or anyone else is injected by mistake, get medical help.

2

only use the auto-injector on the fleshy part of the outer thigh

EpiPen® Auto-Injector can be given through lightweight clothing

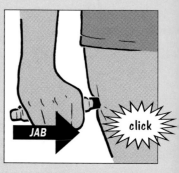

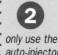
JAB

click

Firmly jab the black tip into the outer thigh until the unit activates—you'll feel and hear a "click." Hold the EpiPen® Auto-Injector in place for ten seconds, then pull it straight out.

3 After the injection, keep the casualty warm and avoid any exertion. If the casualty's condition doesn't get better in 10 minutes, give another dose if the casualty has one. The medication will begin to wear off within 10 to 20 minutes—get medical help right away.

Throw away the EpiPen® Auto-Injector

Bend the needle now coming out of the black tip of the unit against something—never touch it. Put the broken needle and the used unit back in the plastic case and throw this in the garbage.

Ana-Kit® Anaphylaxis Emergency Treatment kit

The Ana-Kit® is more complex than the Epipen® Auto-Injector, and for this reason, you should be trained in its use by a qualified health professional. The steps below show how to give the Ana-Kit® injection. Refer to the kit instructions for information on how to use all the contents of the kit.

Contents of the Ana-Kit®

complete instructions for the Ana-Kit®

alcohol wipes for cleaning the injection site

4 antihistamine tablets

tourniquet to prevent insect venom from spreading

syringe with 2 single, adult doses of medication

4

To use the Ana-Kit®

1

check the expiry date

LOT: XY123 G EXP.: 96 SE

2

remove red rubber needle cover

hold syringe upright and press plunger to push out any air

3

rotate the plunger a ¼ turn to the right so the plunger shaft is aligned with the slot

4 choose an injection site in the fleshy part of the thigh

clean the injection site with an alcohol wipe

push the needle at least half way into the thigh

push the plunger until it stops, and then pull out the needle

Doses for casualties under 13 years old

The Ana-Kit syringe is marked in 0.1 ml sections so smaller doses can be given. If the casualty is a child or an infant, give the dose according the table below.

Age range	Dose*
infants to 2 years	0.05 – 0.1 mL
2 to 6 years	0.15 mL
6 to 12 years	0.20 mL

* verify these doses with the instructions in the kit

5 After the injection, keep the casualty warm and avoid any exertion. Get the needle ready to give a second injection by turning the plunger another quarter turn to the right. If the casualty's condition doesn't improve in 10 minutes, give a second dose. The medication will begin to wear off within 10 to 20 minutes—get medical help right away. Put the used syringe back in the case. Dispose of the used kit as directed by the casualty's doctor.

4

How to help a casualty take medication for a severe asthmatic attack

• •

> Often, a person with asthma carries medication in the form of a metered-dose **inhaler** (puffer). Usually the person can give himself this medication without help. But a person could need help during a severe asthmatic attack. A first aider can help a casualty to take his medication.

An inhaler delivers a premeasured amount of medication. For all medication to reach the lungs, it must be used properly. Always read and follow the manufacturer's instructions.

To help a casualty with asthma medication

1 Shake the container, then remove the cap.

2 Tell the casualty to breathe out completely in a relaxed manner. Then tell her to breathe in slowly and deeply—as she does, press the canister to release the medication.

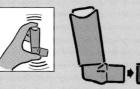

3 Tell the casualty to hold her breath for 10 seconds so the medication can spread out in the lungs. Then tell her to breathe normally so the medication won't be expelled. If more doses are needed, wait 30 seconds before repeating these steps.

Using a spacer

When the medication comes out of the inhaler, it is cold. This may cause the casualty to stop inhaling as the medication hits the back of the throat. To reduce this problem, use a spacer. It traps the particles of the spray, allowing the casualty to inhale more effectively.

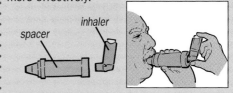

spacer   *inhaler*

Small children and other casualties who have difficulty coordinating their inhaling with your releasing the medication, will find a spacer helpful. It allows them to inhale two or three times before the medication is completely dispelled. A mask can be attached to the device to make taking the medication easier.

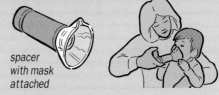

spacer with mask attached

If the casualty complains of throat irritation after using the inhaler, have her gargle or rinse her mouth with water.

If the casualty is unable to breathe in deeply before using the inhaler, using the spacer and having the casualty take three or four normal breaths from the spacer will help.

Pneumothorax–
a serious complication of a chest injury

The **pleural space** is the space between the lungs and the chest wall that is usually not a space at all—it is filled with the lungs. The lungs are sucked into this space because there is no air in it. But if air gets into the space, the lung on that side won't be sucked into it, and it will collapse. A **pneumothorax** (pronounced "new-mow-thor-ax") occurs when air gets into the pleural space. It is life threatening because the lungs can collapse and cause the person severe breathing difficulties.

Open pneumothorax

An open pneumothorax occurs when there is a penetrating wound to the chest and air is going through the wound into the pleural space. It is called "open" because the pneumothorax is "open" to the outside through the wound. A sucking chest wound is an open pneumothorax.

Closed pneumothorax

There doesn't have to be an external chest wound for a pneumothorax. Air can enter the pleural space from inside the body through a damaged lung or airway. This can happen by itself without any obvious cause (called a "spontaneous" pneumothorax), or from an injury, like a broken rib piercing the lung.

Tension pneumothorax

If air keeps going into the pleural space and can't get out, it builds up—this is a **tension pneumothorax**. As the air builds up, it collapses the lung and puts pressure on the heart which then can't pump blood as well as it should. If the air keeps building up, the casualty's condition will worsen. A tension pneumothorax is a serious medical emergency.

Sealing a sucking chest wound with an airtight dressing can cause a tension pneumothorax. If there is also a wound inside the chest, air can get into the chest cavity through the lung or airway, but it can't get out because you've sealed the wound, so it builds up. This is where the flutter-valve of the sucking chest wound dressing is important. It allows the air building up inside the chest to escape as the casualty exhales, but it doesn't let air into the chest as the casualty inhales.

If air is getting into the chest cavity through a damaged lung, and there is no chest wound, the first aider cannot stop any build-up of air in the pleural space. Get medical help as quickly as possible and make the casualty as comfortable as you can.

4

pneumothorax

normal lung

collapsed lung

air has entered the space between the lungs and chest wall and caused the lung to collapse–this is a pneumothorax

tension pneumothorax

air is building up in the chest cavity on the injured side

the air puts pressure on the heart and other lung–this is a tension pneumothorax

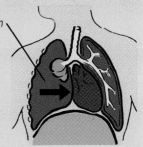

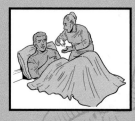

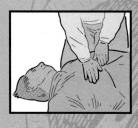

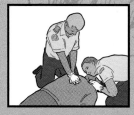

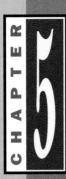

CHAPTER 5

CARDIOVASCULAR DISEASE AND CPR

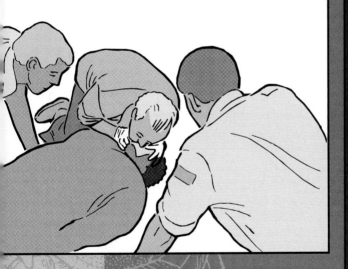

◆ *Introduction*

◆ *You and the "Chain of Survival"*

◆ *First aid for angina/heart attack*

◆ *First aid for heart failure*

◆ *First aid for stroke/ TIA*

◆ *Cardiac arrest*

◆ *Cardiopulmonary resuscitation (CPR)*

◆ *How to take over CPR from another rescuer*

◆ *One-rescuer CPR*

◆ *Two-rescuer CPR*

Introduction

Cardiovascular disease kills more Canadians than any other cause of death. Some of these deaths could be prevented if appropriate first aid were given. Even more of these deaths could be prevented if individuals adopted a heart-healthy lifestyle that reduces the risk of cardiovascular disease. This chapter describes:

◆ cardiovascular disease

◆ how to reduce your risk of cardiovascular disease

◆ first aid for cardiovascular emergencies, including

❖ first aid for stroke

❖ first aid for angina/heart attack

❖ first aid for cardiac arrest, which is CPR

Cardiovascular disease

Cardiovascular disease refers to disorders of the heart and blood vessels. High blood pressure and atherosclerosis are cardiovascular disorders. Over time, they can lead to cardiovascular emergencies such as angina, heart attack, congestive heart failure, transient ischemic attack, stroke and cardiac arrest. Each of these is described below. Appropriate first aid starts on page 5-6 under *First aid for angina/heart attack.*

High blood pressure

Blood pressure is the pressure of the blood against the inside walls of the blood vessels. Blood pressure goes up and down naturally. When a person is excited or emotionally stressed, blood pressure goes up, but it usually comes down once the excitement has passed. In some people, their blood pressure stays high all the time. This condition of constant high blood pressure is called **hypertension**. Over time, hypertension damages the tissues of the cardiovascular system. The walls of the blood vessels become thick and lose their elasticity and the heart becomes enlarged.

The changes caused by high blood pressure increase the risk of stroke, heart attack, kidney or eye problems. Unfortunately, hypertension does not always give warning signals—you may feel perfectly well but still have high blood pressure. This is why it is called the **silent killer**.

Narrowing of the arteries

Arteries are the blood vessels that carry blood away from the heart. They become diseased when fatty deposits build up inside them, making the passage for blood narrower. This process of fat deposition and narrowing of the arteries is called **atherosclerosis**. In the coronary arteries, which carry oxygenated blood to the heart, it is called **coronary artery disease**.

normal artery

As an artery gets narrower, less and less blood gets through. When the artery gets too narrow , the tissues on the other side of the narrowing don't get enough oxygenated blood to function normally. Although the signs and symptoms of hardening of the arteries usually don't appear until middle age or later, atherosclerosis often begins in childhood.

blocked artery

Angina

If one of the coronary arteries becomes hardened, the blood supply feeding that part of the heart muscle becomes limited. When the heart works harder and needs more blood (e.g. when you run for a bus or shovel snow), it can't get the oxygenated blood it needs through the narrowed coronary artery. This causes pain or discomfort in the chest which may spread to the neck, jaw, shoulders and arms. This pain is called **angina pectoris** (or "angina"). Angina pain doesn't usually last long, and goes away if the person rests or takes prescribed medication. Many people with angina live normally by taking medication that increases blood flow to the heart.

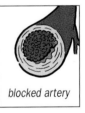

5

You and the "Chain of Survival"

The "Chain of Survival"

CPR is often what comes to mind when people think of first aid for a heart attack or cardiac arrest. But CPR is only part of the picture. Five steps should be followed to give a casualty of a cardiovascular emergency the best chance for survival:

1. **early recognition** of a cardiovascular emergency
2. **early access** into the community emergency medical services (EMS) system. This means calling for help . . .quickly
3. **early CPR** if required
4. **early defibrillation** if required (defibrillation is an electrical shock given to a quivering heart to make it beat properly again)
5. **early advanced care** given by medical personnel

This sequence is known as the **chain of survival**. Each step or "link" is as important as the others. None of them alone will give the casualty the best chance for survival. Time is a vital ingredient. To give a casualty with no pulse a reasonable chance of survival, CPR must be given within four minutes of the heart stopping. Defibrillation is needed within eight to ten minutes. For both procedures, the sooner they happen, the better.

You, the first trained person on the scene, are responsible for the first three steps. You must recognize the cardiovascular emergency, call for medical help and start CPR if needed. You are the crucial first three links in the chain of survival.

Don't worry, it's just indigestion.

I'm perfectly fit, I jog a mile a day. . . it's not my heart!

You watch, we'll wait a few minutes and the pain will go away.

A cup of tea and I'll be fine.

Early recognition and denial

The first link in the chain of survival is recognizing a cardiovascular emergency. This may be the toughest job you have to do. It's not easy to accept that someone is having a heart attack and could die very soon. This is especially true if the person is a family member or a close friend (family members and friends are often present during a heart attack). The person could still be talking to you and not *look* as if he is about to die. And perhaps the person is denying anything serious is happening, which often occurs.

On average, heart attack casualties take 4½ hours to get to a hospital from the time they first start feeling poorly. One reason for this is that it takes a long time to accept that something serious could be wrong. It is this wasted time that prevents many lives from being saved. When someone complains of chest pain, you should consider it a serious problem—that's early recognition. The first thing you sould do is call for medical help—that's early access.

By getting the casualty to the hospital quickly, you will have given her the best chance for survival. If there is no serious problem, you will still have done the right thing and the casualty will have had a complete check-up. On the other hand, if there is a serious problem, you may have saved a life.

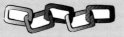

Heart attack

A heart attack happens when heart muscle tissue dies because its supply of oxygenated blood has been cut off. Usually, a blood clot gets stuck in a coronary artery that has been narrowed through atherosclerosis. The supply of blood is cut off and the heart tissue beyond the clot is starved of oxygen. A heart attack can feel just like angina, except the pain doesn't go away with rest and medication. If the heart attack damages the heart's electrical system, or if a lot of the heart muscle is affected, the heart may stop beating. This is cardiac arrest.

5

Doctors now have drugs to dissolve a blood clot, but they work best if given right away. This is why you have to get a casualty with a suspected heart attack to the hospital right away—the longer medical help is delayed, the more likely the heart will be damaged or stop beating. The medical term for a heart attack is **myocardial infarction** (my-o-car-dee-al in-fark-shun).

coronary arteries

blocked coronary artery

damaged heart tissue

Signs and symptoms of angina and a heart attack

the pain may feel like:

- heaviness
- tightness
- squeezing
- pressure
- crushing
- indigestion
- aching jaw
- sore arms

a heart attack can feel like indigestion

other signs and symptoms include:

- denying anything is wrong
- fear
- pale skin
- nausea
- vomiting
- sweating
- shortness of breath
- fatigue
- shock
- unconsciousness
- cardiac arrest

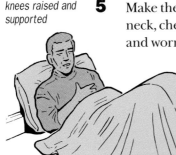

First aid for angina/heart attack

A first aider may *understand* the difference between angina and a heart attack, but a first aider cannot *decide* whether a casualty is having angina pain or a heart attack—only a medical doctor can do this. For this reason, the first aid for angina and heart attack is the same.

1   Begin ESM—do the scene survey (see page 2-3) Ask the casualty questions to determine the scene history:

"Can you show me where it hurts?"

"Have you had this pain before?"

"Do you have medication for this pain?"

2   Do a primary survey (see page 2-5).

3   As soon as you recognize the signs and symptoms of angina/heart attack, call, or have a bystander call, for medical help. If you have to leave to call, place the casualty at rest (step 4) before you go.

4   Place the casualty at rest to reduce the work the heart has to do. The most comfortable position for the casualty is best. Usually this is semisitting, as shown below.

In some cases, the semisitting position will increase the pain. Let the casualty try what has helped before, but don't delay calling medical help while trying different positions to ease the pain.

head and shoulders raised and supported

knees raised and supported

5   Make the casualty comfortable—loosen tight clothing at the neck, chest and waist. Reassure the casualty to lessen fear and worry—these cause the heart to work harder.

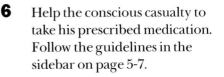

6   Help the conscious casualty to take his prescribed medication. Follow the guidelines in the sidebar on page 5-7.

7   If breathing stops, start AR. If there is no pulse, start CPR.

Congestive heart failure

Heart failure means the heart can't pump blood effectively any more. Chronic heart disease or a previous heart attack may have led to this condition. Since the blood isn't pumped forward properly, it begins to back up in the lungs, causing breathing problems. The blood also backs up in the rest of the body and causes swelling, as in the ankles.

Signs and symptoms of heart failure

◆ inappropriate shortness of breath, especially when exercising

◆ difficulty breathing when lying flat

◆ blueness around the lips, fingernail beds, ears and other parts of the body

◆ swelling of the ankles

◆ coughing up frothy, pink fluid

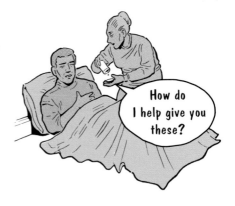

How do I help give you these?

First aid for heart failure

1 Begin ESM—do the scene survey (see page 2-3). Ask the casualty questions to determine the scene history.

"Have you had this pain before?"

"Do you have medication for this pain?"

Do a primary survey (see page 2-5).

2 Call for medical help.

3 Place the casualty at rest in a semisitting position (see illustration opposite page) and loosen tight clothing.

4 Reassure the casualty and monitor breathing closely.

Helping a casualty take his medication

Only assist a casualty with medication if he is conscious and specifically asks for your help. Nitroglycerine tablets are a common medication for relief of angina pain. Ensure the medication is prescribed for this person. Place these tablets under the tongue—they aren't to be swallowed. When helping with medication, always read and follow the instructions on the container.

blocked artery

ruptured artery

5

Stroke

If a blood clot blocks a narrowed artery in the brain and the part of the brain beyond the clot doesn't get the oxygen it needs, the brain tissue dies. This is called a **stroke** or **cerebrovascular accident** (CVA). A severe stroke can cause death. A less severe stroke may cause brain damage, which impairs certain body functions, depending on the part of the brain affected. In both heart attack and stroke, hardening of the arteries is the main cause. Over time, the arteries become narrowed and finally a clot blocks a narrowed artery. The difference between the heart attack and the stroke is the final resting place of the clot. A stroke can also be caused by a ruptured artery.

A condition similar to a stroke is a **transient ischemic attack** (TIA). A TIA is caused by a lack of oxygen to part of the brain. It has the same signs and symptoms as a stroke. A TIA lasts from a few minutes to 24 hours and leaves no permanent brain damage. Although a TIA by itself is not life threatening, it is a warning sign that a stroke may follow. Advise anyone who has a TIA to get medical help.

Signs and symptoms of a stroke/TIA

The signs and symptoms of a stroke/TIA depend on what part of the brain is affected. Often, only one side of the body shows signs because only one side of the brain is affected. The signs may include:

more common

paralysis of face muscles

difficulty speaking, swallowing e.g. slurred speech, drooling

dizziness or a sudden fall

loss of coordination

numbness or weakness of the arms or legs, especially on one side

decrease in level of consciousness

mental confusion

double vision or loss of vision

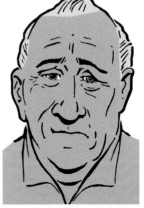

less common

loss of bladder and bowel control

unequal size of pupils

severe headache

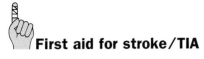

First aid for stroke/TIA

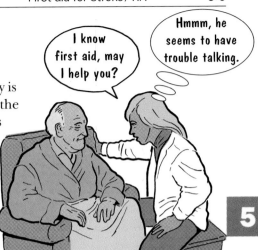

A first aider can't tell whether the casualty is having a stroke or a TIA, so the first aid is the same for both. If the signs and symptoms pass after a short while, suggesting the problem was a TIA, tell the casualty to see a doctor. A stroke could soon follow.

1 Begin ESM—do the scene survey (see page 2-3). Ask the casualty questions to determine the scene history. Do a primary survey.

2 Call for medical help.

3 Place the casualty at rest in the most comfortable position—usually semisitting.

4 Give nothing by mouth. If the casualty is thirsty, moisten the lips with a wet cloth.

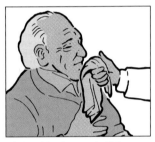

give nothing by mouth; if the casualty complains of thirst, moisten lips with a wet cloth

5 Protect the casualty from injury when he is lifted, moved or during convulsions.

6 Reassure the casualty and keep him warm.

7 If the casualty becomes semiconscious or unconscious, place him in the recovery position. If there is paralysis, place the paralyzed side down. This will make breathing easier.

8 If breathing stops, start AR. If there is no pulse, start CPR.

Which side is paralyzed?

If the casualty becomes unconscious, it may be hard to tell if there is any paralysis. The mouth and cheek on the paralyzed side may droop more than the non-paralyzed side—the face may look "crooked."

If you can, place the casualty in the recovery position with the non-paralyzed side up. The casualty will be able to breathe better with the good muscles on the upper side.

non-paralyzed side up

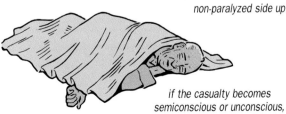

if the casualty becomes semiconscious or unconscious, place him in the recovery position

5

Cardiac arrest

When the heart stops pumping, it is in **cardiac arrest**. A cardiac arrest can happen suddenly or may follow a period of stopped or ineffective breathing, when much of the oxygen in the body is used up. A heart attack causes cardiac arrest when so much heart tissue is damaged that it can't pump blood anymore. Other reasons for cardiac arrest include severe injuries, electrical shock, drug overdose, drowning, suffocation and stroke. When a person's heart has stopped, he is considered **clinically dead** even though he may still be resuscitated. The first aid for cardiac arrest is cardiopulmonary resuscitation (CPR) as described in the sequence below.

. . . .

Cardiopulmonary resuscitation (CPR)

CPR is two basic life support skills put together—artificial respiration and artificial circulation. Artificial respiration provides oxygen to the lungs. Artificial circulation causes blood to flow through the body, but flows only enough to give a person a chance for survival. The purpose of CPR is to circulate oxygenated blood to the brain and other organs until either the pulse returns, or medical help takes over.

Ages in CPR

. . . .

In CPR, AR and first aid for choking, the following age guidelines are used:

◆ adult = 8 years and older

◆ child = between 1 and 8 years old

◆ infant = under 1 year old

These ages are guidelines only; the casualty's size must also be considered. For example, you would give adult CPR to a tall, husky seven-year-old.

The CPR sequence follows from the scene survey and primary survey outlined in Chapter 2, *Emergency Scene Management*. When you find an unresponsive casualty, send for help immediately (scene survey). Then, start the primary survey by opening the airway and checking for breathing. If there is no breathing, give two breaths (AR rescue sequence). Next, check for a pulse. If there is no pulse, begin CPR. Variations in the CPR sequence are described for situations involving an adult casualty, a child casualty, an infant casualty or where two rescuers are available to assist. To show complete scenarios, the CPR sequences repeat many of the steps of the scene survey, primary survey and AR sequence.

CPR – adult casualty

You arrive at a scene… an unconscious adult (someone eight years or older) is lying on the floor…

1   Begin ESM—start the scene survey (see page 2-3).

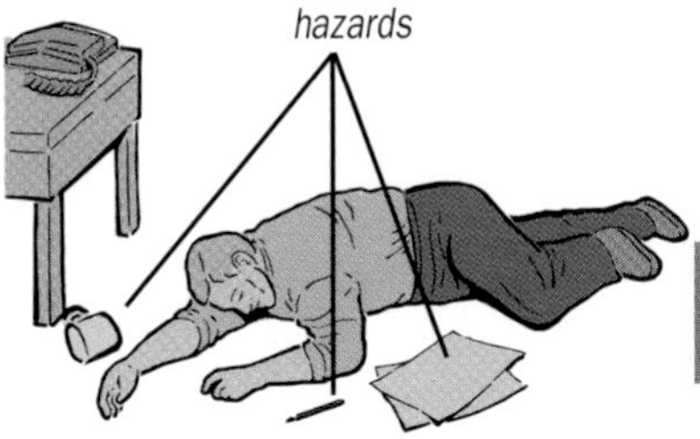

hazards

5

. . . .

2   Assess responsiveness.

ask the casualty if he is O.K. Assess any response

gently tap the shoulders

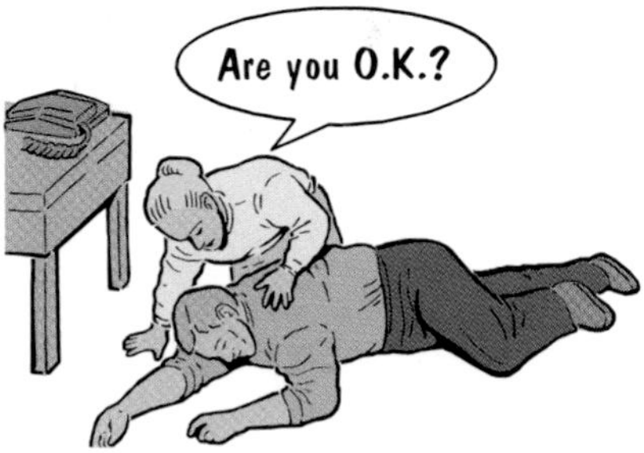

Are you O.K.?

If there is no response, go to step 3.

. . . .

3   Send or go for medical help. If you are alone, see page 1-19 for information on when to go for medical help.

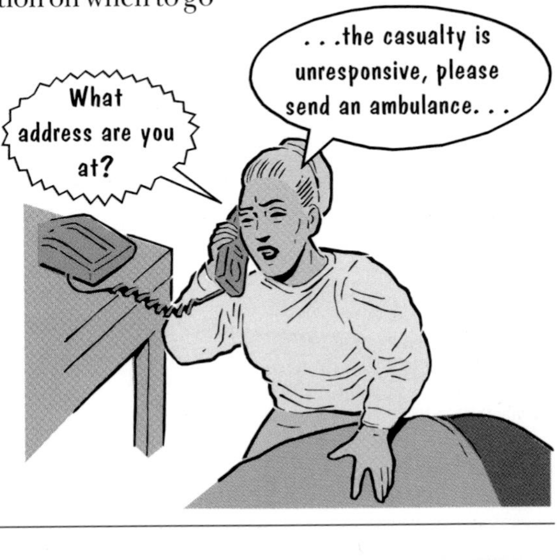

What address are you at?

. . .the casualty is unresponsive, please send an ambulance. . .

4   Place the casualty face up, protecting the head and neck during any movement. Open the airway by tilting the head.

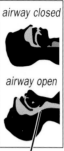

airway closed

airway open

to open the airway push backward on the forehead and lift the jaw

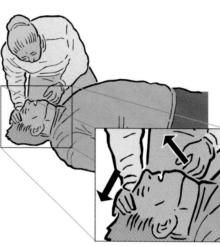

when the head is tilted back, the tongue is lifted off the back of the throat, opening the airway

5

if

If you suspect a head or spinal injury, don't move the casualty. See page 4-22 for how to open the airway and check for breathing.

5   Check breathing for 3 to 5 seconds.

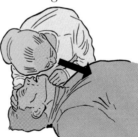

keep the head tilted

place your ear just above the casualty's nose and mouth

look. . . for chest movement

listen. . . for sounds of breathing

feel. . . for breath on your cheek

if

If there is no breathing, go to step 6.

6   Breathe into the casualty twice. For an adult casualty, blow for 1½ to 2 seconds. Use enough air to make the chest rise.

If the chest doesn't rise when you blow:

♦ reopen the airway by tilting the head

♦ pinch the nose again

♦ make a better seal around the mouth

♦ try blowing again

If the chest still doesn't rise, give first aid for choking—see page 3-9.

take a deep breath and seal your mouth around the casualty's mouth

pinch the nostrils

blow slowly and watch for the chest to rise

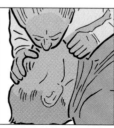

move your mouth away and release the nostrils to allow the air to escape

look for the chest to fall, listen for air sounds and feel for air being exhaled against your cheek

give another breath and go to step 7

7 Check for a pulse at the neck. There is a carotid pulse on either side of the neck—feel for a pulse on the side closest to you—**do not feel or compress both sides at the same time**

First aider's view of the pulse check

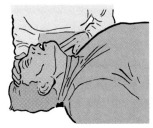

keep the head tilted

slide 2 fingers into the groove of the neck just down from the Adam's apple

press gently to detect the pulse, take 5 to 10 seconds

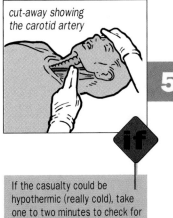

cut-away showing the carotid artery

5

if

If there is a pulse, start AR—see page 4-24, step 8.

If there is no pulse, continue CPR—see step 8.

If the casualty could be hypothermic (really cold), take one to two minutes to check for a pulse.

· ·

8 Make sure the casualty is on a firm, flat surface and landmark to position your hands on the chest for chest compressions.

1. kneel so your hands can be placed mid-chest

locate the bottom edge of the rib cage with the fingers of the hand closest to the feet—this is the landmarking hand

2. slide fingers to the notch where the ribs meet

place the heel of the other hand midline on the breastbone above the fingers

3. place the landmarking hand on top and raise the fingers off the chest

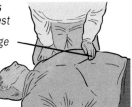

use the hand position you find easiest

- fingers interlocked
- fingers straight
- holding wrist

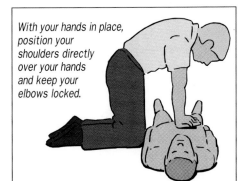

With your hands in place, position your shoulders directly over your hands and keep your elbows locked.

9 Give CPR for one minute, which is about four cycles of CPR. Give 15 compressions...

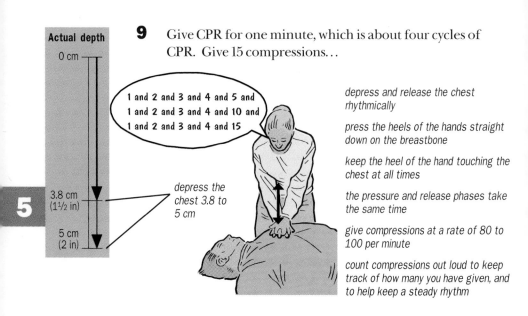

Actual depth

0 cm

1 and 2 and 3 and 4 and 5 and
1 and 2 and 3 and 4 and 10 and
1 and 2 and 3 and 4 and 15

depress the chest 3.8 to 5 cm

3.8 cm (1½ in)

5 cm (2 in)

depress and release the chest rhythmically

press the heels of the hands straight down on the breastbone

keep the heel of the hand touching the chest at all times

the pressure and release phases take the same time

give compressions at a rate of 80 to 100 per minute

count compressions out loud to keep track of how many you have given, and to help keep a steady rhythm

... and two ventilations—this is one **cycle** of 15:2 (15 compressions to 2 ventilations).

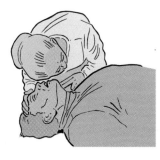

blow slowly for 1½ to 2 seconds

watch for the chest to fall, feel air being exhaled

blow slowly for 1½ to 2 seconds

Give three more cycles of 15:2. This will be about one minute of CPR.

· ·

10 Reassess the pulse and breathing to see if the casualty's heart has started to beat, and if breathing has also started.

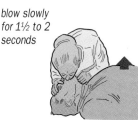

If there is a pulse but no breathing, continue first aid by giving AR, see page 4-24, step 8.

If there is both a pulse and breathing, continue the primary and secondary surveys.

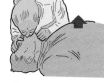

check for a pulse and look, listen and feel for breathing at the same time

take five seconds for this

If there is still no pulse and no breathing, continue CPR, see step 11.

11 Continue compressions and ventilations in the ratio of
15 : 2, starting with compressions. Landmark for
correct hand position at the beginning of each new
cycle of compressions. Check the pulse and breathing every few minutes. Continue CPR until either the
casualty's pulse returns, another first aider takes
over, medical help takes over or you are exhausted and cannot continue.

5

How to take over
CPR from another rescuer

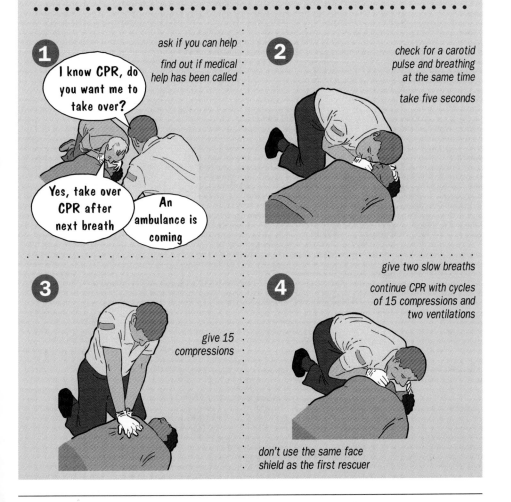

1   ask if you can help
find out if medical
help has been called

*I know CPR, do
you want me to
take over?*

*Yes, take over
CPR after
next breath*   *An
ambulance is
coming*

2   check for a carotid
pulse and breathing
at the same time

take five seconds

3   give 15
compressions

4   give two slow breaths

continue CPR with cycles
of 15 compressions and
two ventilations

don't use the same face
shield as the first rescuer

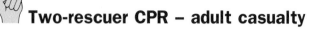

Two-rescuer CPR – adult casualty

Two people trained in two-rescuer CPR can work together as a team to give CPR. Two-rescuer CPR can be more effective in circulating oxygenated blood and it is not as tiring as one-rescuer CPR. The following instructions focus on the different tasks of each rescuer and the communication between them. The specific first aid skills are detailed in *CPR – adult casualty* on page 5-11.

One-rescuer CPR in progress

When a two-rescuer team gets to a scene where a rescuer is doing one-rescuer CPR, they should try to take over without interrupting CPR. The following sequence shows how to do this.

1 As you and your partner arrive on the scene, begin ESM— do the scene survey (see page 2-3).

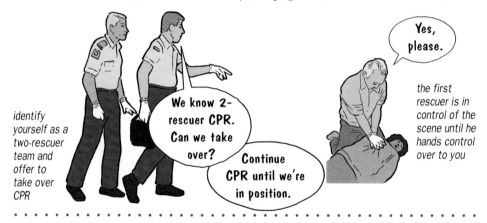

identify yourself as a two-rescuer team and offer to take over CPR

We know 2-rescuer CPR. Can we take over?

Continue CPR until we're in position.

Yes, please.

the first rescuer is in control of the scene until he hands control over to you

2 If you have to, tell the rescuer that you'll take over after two breaths. Get into position, ready to take over.

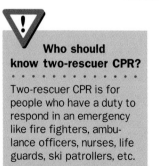

Who should know two-rescuer CPR?

Two-rescuer CPR is for people who have a duty to respond in an emergency like fire fighters, ambulance officers, nurses, life guards, ski patrollers, etc.

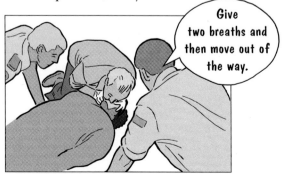

Give two breaths and then move out of the way.

3 The original rescuer moves out of the way
and should go to call medical help if this has
not been done. The ventilator assesses the
casualty. The compressor gets
into position.

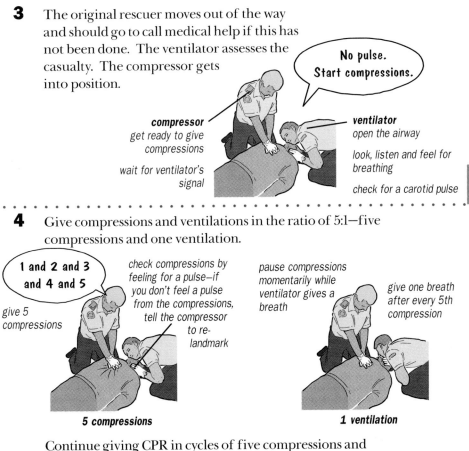

> No pulse.
> Start compressions.

compressor
*get ready to give
compressions*

*wait for ventilator's
signal*

ventilator
open the airway

*look, listen and feel for
breathing*

check for a carotid pulse

4 Give compressions and ventilations in the ratio of 5:1—five
compressions and one ventilation.

> 1 and 2 and 3
> and 4 and 5

*give 5
compressions*

*check compressions by
feeling for a pulse—if
you don't feel a pulse
from the compressions,
tell the compressor
to re-
landmark*

*pause compressions
momentarily while
ventilator gives a
breath*

*give one breath
after every 5th
compression*

5 compressions   **1 ventilation**

Continue giving CPR in cycles of five compressions and
one ventilation. Reassess the carotid pulse and breathing
every few minutes.

One-rescuer CPR not in progress

When two rescuers arrive at an emergency scene, they do the
scene survey and the lead rescuer starts the primary survey. The
other rescuer asks any bystanders what happened and whether
medical help has been called. Once the lead rescuer determines
the casualty is unresponsive, he either starts one-rescuer CPR or
two-rescuer CPR. Start one-rescuer CPR if:

◆ medical help has not been called and there is no bystander to
send. One-rescuer CPR is started and the other rescuer goes
to call for medical help. When the other rescuer returns, two-
rescuer CPR is started

◆ medical help has been called, or there is a bystander to send, but the second rescuer is busy getting equipment, controlling the scene, etc. One-rescuer CPR is started by the lead rescuer and two-rescuer CPR starts when the second rescuer is available

They start two-rescuer CPR if:

◆ medical help has been called

◆ medical help has not been called but there is a bystander to send to call

5

One-rescuer CPR becomes two-rescuer CPR

1   As the rescuers arrive on the scene, they begin ESM, doing the scene survey (see page 2-3).

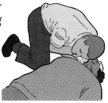
assess hazards and make the area safe

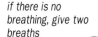
assess responsiveness

Are you O.K.?

get medical help

Go call an ambulance.

2   The lead rescuer starts the primary survey (see page 2-5).

open the airway and check for breathing

if there is no breathing, give two breaths

check the carotid pulse

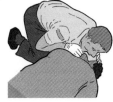
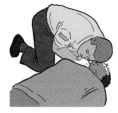
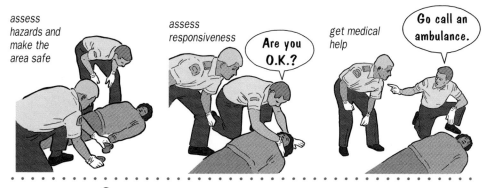

3 If there is no pulse, start one-rescuer CPR.

landmark for proper hand position for compressions

give 15 chest compressions

give 2 slow breaths

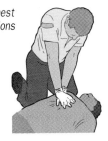
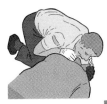

Continue CPR in cycles of 15 compressions to two ventilations.

4 When the second rescuer returns, he gets ready to become the ventilator.

lead rescuer

second rescuer

After this breath I'll reassess the casualty

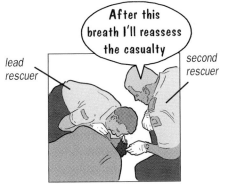

5 The second rescuer checks for a pulse and breathing while the first rescuer gets ready to continue compressions.

No pulse. Start compressions.

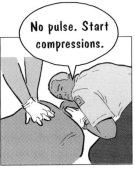

6 Continue CPR with the two-rescuer method. Give cycles of five compressions and one ventilation.

ventilator checks the compressions by feeling for a pulse.

1 and 2 and 3 and 4 and 5

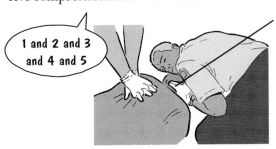

Continue giving CPR in cycles of five compressions and one ventilation. Reassess the carotid pulse and breathing every few minutes.

⚠ Use a second mask or face shield

If possible, the second rescuer should use a different face mask or face shield than the first rescuer.

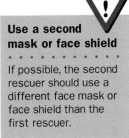

5

Two-rescuer CPR

Start two-rescuer CPR when both rescuers are available to give care to the casualty.

1   As the rescuers arrive on the scene, they begin ESM, doing the scene survey (see page 2-3).

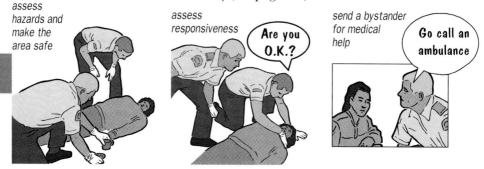

assess hazards and make the area safe

assess responsiveness — **Are you O.K.?**

send a bystander for medical help — **Go call an ambulance**

2   Start the primary survey (see page 2-5).

open the airway and check for breathing

if there is no breathing give two breaths

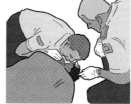

the second rescuer takes his position as the compressor

check the carotid pulse

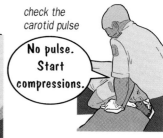

No pulse. Start compressions.

compressor is in position, waiting for ventilator's signal

3   Compressor gives five compressions and then pauses while the ventilator gives a breath. Continue two-rescuer CPR in cycles of five compressions and one ventilation. Reassess the carotid pulse and breathing every few minutes.

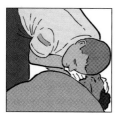

give 5 compressions

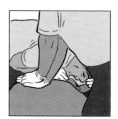

give 1 breath

How to switch positions while giving two-rescuer CPR

You might want to switch positions when giving two-rescuer CPR. Usually the compressor wants to switch first, since giving compressions is more tiring. The following switch-over method helps ensure that CPR is given continuously.

5

①

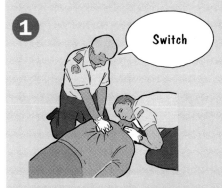

Switch

The compressor says "Switch" after giving five compressions. While the ventilator gives a breath, the compressor moves into position beside the casualty's head to become the new ventilator.

②

the new compressor landmarks for hand position and waits for the ventilator's command

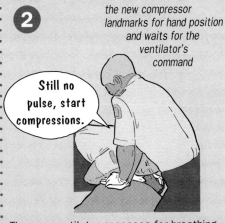

Still no pulse, start compressions.

The new ventilator assesses for breathing and a pulse for five seconds.

③

ventilator checks effectiveness of compressions by feeling for a pulse

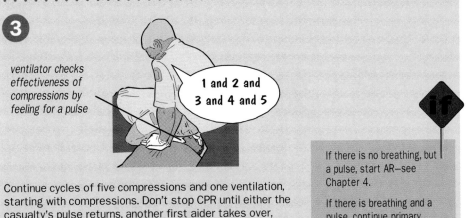

1 and 2 and 3 and 4 and 5

Continue cycles of five compressions and one ventilation, starting with compressions. Don't stop CPR until either the casualty's pulse returns, another first aider takes over, medical help takes over or both rescuers are exhausted and cannot continue two-rescuer or one-rescuer CPR.

if

If there is no breathing, but a pulse, start AR—see Chapter 4.

If there is breathing and a pulse, continue primary survey—see Chapter 2.

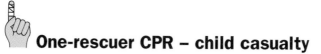

One-rescuer CPR – child casualty

You arrive at a scene…an unconscious child (someone between one and eight years old) is lying on the floor…

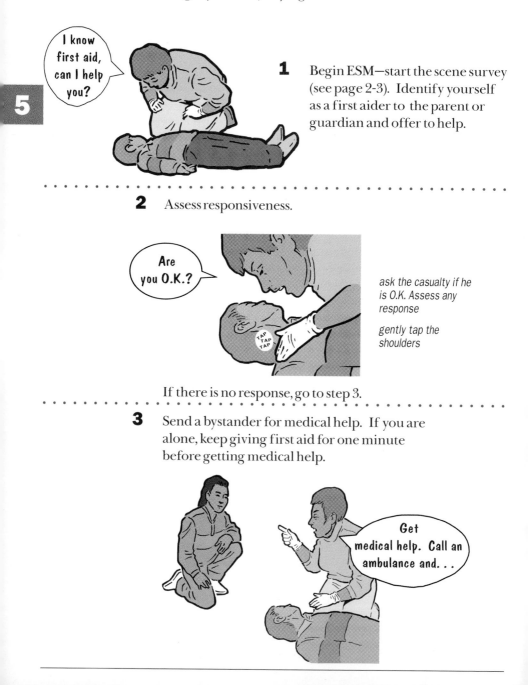

1   Begin ESM—start the scene survey (see page 2-3). Identify yourself as a first aider to the parent or guardian and offer to help.

I know first aid, can I help you?

2   Assess responsiveness.

Are you O.K.?

ask the casualty if he is O.K. Assess any response

gently tap the shoulders

If there is no response, go to step 3.

3   Send a bystander for medical help. If you are alone, keep giving first aid for one minute before getting medical help.

Get medical help. Call an ambulance and…

4   Place the casualty face up, protecting the head and neck during any movement. Open the airway by tilting the head.

to open the airway, push backward on the forehead and lift the jaw

If you suspect a head or spinal injury, don't move the casualty. See page 4-22 for how to open the airway and check for breathing.

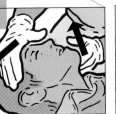

airway closed   *airway open*

when the head is tilted back, the tongue is lifted off the back of the throat, opening the airway

5   Check for breathing for 3 to 5 seconds.

keep the head tilted

place your ear just above the casualty's nose and mouth

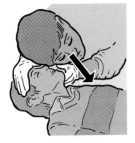

look... for chest movement

listen... for sounds of breathing

feel... for breath on your cheek

If there is no breathing, go to step 6.

6   Breathe into the casualty twice. For a child casualty, blow for 1 to 1½ seconds. Use just enough air to make the chest rise.

take a deep breath and seal your mouth around the casualty's mouth

pinch the nostrils

blow slowly and watch for the chest to rise

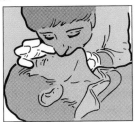

move your mouth away and release the nostrils to allow the air to escape

look for the chest to fall, listen for air sounds and feel for air being exhaled against your cheek

give another breath and go to step 7

If the chest doesn't rise when you blow:

♦ reopen the airway by tilting the head

♦ pinch the nose again

♦ make a better seal around the mouth

♦ try blowing again

If the chest still doesn't rise, give first aid for choking— see page 3-19.

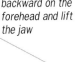

7   Check for a pulse at the neck. There is a carotid pulse on either side of the neck—feel for a pulse on the side closest to you—**do not feel or compress both sides at the same time.**

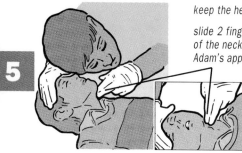

keep the head tilted

slide 2 fingers into the groove of the neck just down from the Adam's apple

press gently to detect the pulse, take 5 to 10 seconds

First aider's view of the pulse check

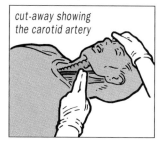

cut-away showing the carotid artery

If there is a pulse, start AR—see page 4-27, step 8.

If there is no pulse, continue CPR—see step 8.

8   Make sure the casualty is on a firm, flat surface and landmark to position your hand on the chest for chest compressions.

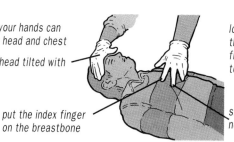

kneel so your hands can reach the head and chest

keep the head tilted with one hand

put the index finger on the breastbone

locate the bottom edge of the rib cage with the fingers of the hand closest to the feet

slide middle finger to the notch where the ribs meet

place the heel of the landmarking hand midline on the breastbone just above the spot where the index finger was positioned

lift the fingers off the chest

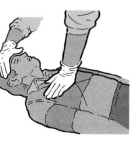

With your hand in place, position your shoulders directly over your hand and keep your elbow locked.

breastbone (sternum)

heart

spine

9   Give CPR for one minute, which is about fifteen cycles of
CPR. Give five compressions...

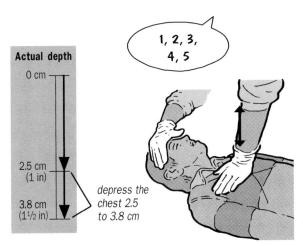

1, 2, 3, 4, 5

Actual depth

0 cm

2.5 cm (1 in)

3.8 cm (1½ in)

depress the chest 2.5 to 3.8 cm

depress and release the chest rhythmically

press the heel of the hand straight down on the breastbone

keep the heel of the hand touching the chest at all times

the pressure and release phases take the same time

give compressions at a rate of 100 per minute

count compressions out loud to keep track of how many you have given, and to help keep a steady rhythm

...and one ventilation—this is one **cycle** of 5:1
(5 compressions to 1 ventilation).

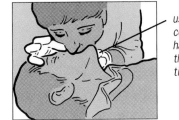

blow slowly with just enough air to make the chest rise

use the compressing hand to hold the chin tilted

Give fourteen more cycles of 5:1. This will be about one
minute of CPR.

10   Reassess the pulse and breathing to see if the
casualty's heart has started to beat, and if
breathing has also started.

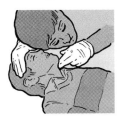

check for a pulse and look, listen and feel for breathing at the same time

take five seconds for this

If there is a pulse but no breathing, continue first aid by giving AR, see page 4-27, step 8.

If there is both a pulse and breathing, continue the primary and secondary surveys.

If you are alone and medical help hasn't been called, decide whether to call medical help— see page 1-19.

If there is still no pulse and no breathing,
continue CPR, see step 11.

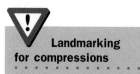

Landmarking for compressions

After each pulse check, landmark for hand position as shown in step 8. At the start of each 5:1 cycle, just landmark by looking for the right hand position.

11 Continue compressions and ventilations in the ratio of 5:1, starting with compressions. Check the pulse and breathing every few minutes. Continue CPR until either the casualty's pulse returns, another first aider takes over, medical help takes over or you are exhausted and cannot continue.

One-rescuer CPR – infant casualty

You arrive at a scene and there is an unconscious infant (a baby under one year old)...

1 Begin ESM—start the scene survey (see page 2-3). Identify yourself as a first aider to the parent or guardian and offer to help.

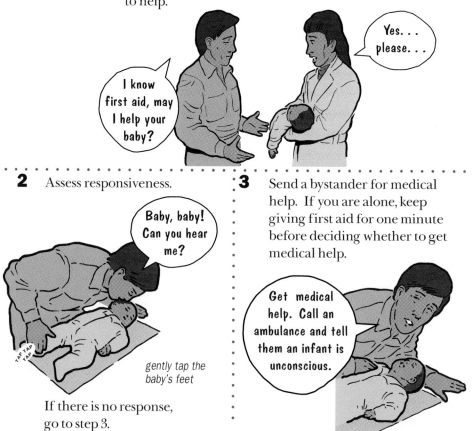

2 Assess responsiveness.

gently tap the baby's feet

If there is no response, go to step 3.

3 Send a bystander for medical help. If you are alone, keep giving first aid for one minute before deciding whether to get medical help.

4   Place the baby face up, protecting the head and neck during any movement. Open the airway by tilting the head.

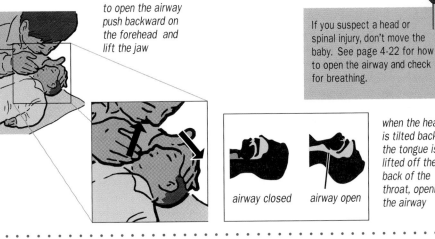

to open the airway push backward on the forehead and lift the jaw

If you suspect a head or spinal injury, don't move the baby. See page 4-22 for how to open the airway and check for breathing.

airway closed   airway open

when the head is tilted back, the tongue is lifted off the back of the throat, opening the airway

5   Keep the head tilted and place your ear near the baby's mouth and nose. Check for breathing for 3 to 5 seconds.

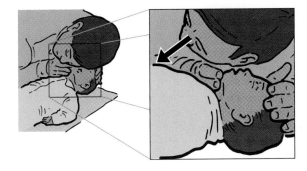

look... for chest movement

listen... for sounds of breathing

feel... for breath on your cheek

The back of an infant's head is quite large compared to the rest of her body. This causes the baby's head to come forward and close off her airway.

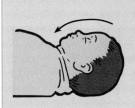

an infant's head flexes forward when she's lying on her back

When giving AR or CPR, it may be helpful to put a thin pad under the shoulders to help keep the airway open—but don't waste time looking for a pad.

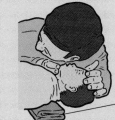

a thin pad under the shoulders helps keep the airway open

6 Breathe into the casualty twice. For an infant casualty, blow for 1 to 1½ seconds using just enough air to make the chest rise.

If the chest doesn't rise when you blow, try again

♦ reopen the airway by tilting the head

♦ make a better seal around the mouth and nose

♦ try blowing again

If the chest still doesn't rise, give first aid for choking— see page 3-26.

seal your mouth around the baby's mouth and nose and blow slowly

move your mouth away and release the nostrils to allow the air to escape

look for the chest to fall, listen for air sounds and feel for air being exhaled against your cheek

give another breath and go to step 7

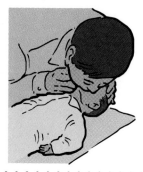

7 Check for a pulse.

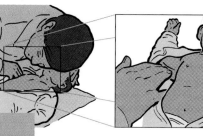

keep the head tilted

press gently with two fingertips on the inside of the arm between the large muscles and the bone

take 5 to 10 seconds

Use the brachial pulse

The carotid (neck) pulse is hard to find on an infant, so the brachial (upper arm) pulse is used instead.

If there is a pulse, start AR— see page 4-33, step 8.

If there is no pulse, continue CPR—see step 8.

8 Make sure the casualty is on a firm, flat surface and landmark to position your fingers on the chest for chest compressions.

keep the head tilted with one hand

place three fingers on the breastbone just below the nipple line

lift the index finger off the chest

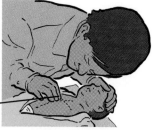

9   Give CPR for one minute. Give five compressions...

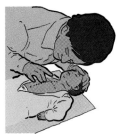

using two fingers, push down on the breastbone

depress the chest 1.3 to 2.5 cm

release the pressure completely but keep your fingers in light contact with the chest

repeat the pressure and release phases rhythmically so that each phase takes the same amount of time

give compressions at a rate of at least 100 per minute

Actual size

0 cm

1.3 cm
(½ in)

2.5 cm
(1 in)

5

...and one ventilation—this is one **cycle** of 5:1 (five compressions to one ventilation).

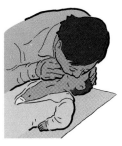

cover the mouth and nose with your mouth

blow slowly with just enough air to make the chest rise

you can keep the fingers used for compressing in light contact with the chest while ventilating the infant

10   Reassess the pulse and breathing to see if the casualty's heart has started to beat, and if breathing has also started.

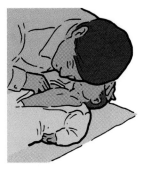

check for a pulse and look, listen and feel for breathing at the same time

take five seconds for this

If there is a pulse but no breathing, continue first aid by giving AR, see page 4-33, step 8.

If there is both a pulse and breathing, continue the primary and secondary surveys.

If you are alone and medical help hasn't been called, decide whether to call medical help— see page 1-19.

If there is still no pulse and no breathing, continue CPR, see step 11.

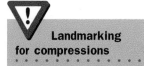

**Landmarking
for compressions**
. . . .

Always keep your fingers
in contact with the chest.
Only landmark for finger
position again if you think
you are not compressing
in exactly the right place.

5

11 Continue compressions and ventilations in the
ratio of 5:1, starting with compressions. Check
the pulse and breathing every few minutes.
Continue CPR until either the casualty's pulse
returns, another first aider takes over, medical
help takes over or you are exhausted and
cannot continue.

How chest compressions work

Chest compressions increase the pressure
inside the chest and may put pressure on
the heart causing blood to flow to the lungs,
heart and brain. The oxygen picked up by the
blood as it passes through the lungs is
carried to the heart and brain. This slows
down the rate of tissue damage. Blood
circulation from CPR is not as effective as a
normal heartbeat—blood circulates only
enough to keep tissues alive a short while.

For chest compressions to be effective, the
casualty has to be on a firm, flat and level
surface. If the head is elevated at all, blood
flow from CPR will be reduced because of
gravity. Compressions have to be given in
the right place, with the right amount of
pressure for the age of the casualty; the
direction of the pressure has to be straight
down.

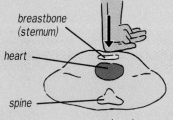

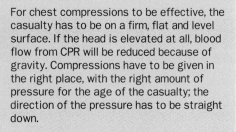

breastbone
(sternum)

heart

spine

compression phase

release phase

Differences in CPR for adults, children and infants

Activity	Adult CPR	Child CPR	Infant CPR
landmarking	2 hands - midline on the lower part of the breastbone	1 hand - 1 finger-width from the bottom of the breastbone	2 fingers - just below the nipple line
depth of compressions	3.8 to 5.0 cm 1.5 to 2 inches	2.5 to 3.8 cm 1 to 1.5 inches	1.3 to 2.5 cm .5 to 1 inch
compression/ ventilation ratio	15 compressions to 2 ventilations	5 compressions to 1 ventilation	5 compressions to 1 ventilation

How to reduce your risk of cardiovascular disease

You can reduce your chances of developing cardiovascular disease by eliminating "risk factors" from your lifestyle. A risk factor is a behavior or trait that increases the likelihood that you will develop cardiovascular disease. Major risk factors are direct contributors to cardiovascular disease. Other factors may contribute indirectly.

Reducing risk factors in young people will have the greatest effect. However, it is very important to assess your present lifestyle and make positive changes wherever possible. Preventative measures may actually reverse arterial disease and will most certainly improve the likelihood of a longer, healthier life.

Major risk factors that cannot be changed include heredity (the presence of a family history of cardiovascular disease), gender, race and age.

The following major risk factors are modifiable. Assess your current status and make an educated decision about what you might do to improve your present condition.

5

Cigarette smoking

Smoking is the single, most important cause of preventable death—but smokers who break the habit can actually return to the risk factor of a non-smoker. Exposure to second-hand smoke (passive smoking) is also directly related to increased rates of heart disease.

Obesity

Obesity is associated with many of the other major risk factors for cardiovascular disease, including hypertension, increased cholesterol levels and diabetes. However, obesity has also been shown to act as an independent risk factor and has a direct effect on the potential for cardiovascular problems.

Consult a physician before undertaking a program of diet and/or exercise to reduce obesity.

Hypertension (high blood pressure)

Increased blood pressure causes damage to blood vessels and enlarges the heart. These changes and related effects of the body may increase the chance of having a heart attack or a stroke.

Have your blood pressure checked regularly by a medical professional. If high blood pressure is detected, follow medical advice on diet and lifestyle changes that will improve the condition. In certain situations, medication may be prescribed to help control blood pressure.

Lack of exercise

One important way to reduce the risk of cardiovascular disease is to include regular physical activity in your lifestyle. The benefits of physical activity over a sedentary lifestyle continue to be supported in research.

Cholesterol

Your overall risk of cardiovascular disease goes up when the level of cholesterol in your blood increases. Where low-density lipoprotein cholesterol has a positive relationship, high-density lipoprotein cholesterol has a negative one. Consult a physician to accurately assess cholesterol levels and obtain advice on recommended changes in diet and/or medications.

Stress

Chronic stress, often characterized by the "fight or flight" response, is often associated with Type A personalities. Recent studies have shown that this association with cardiovascular disease may not be valid; however, stress reduction techniques do help reduce high blood pressure, and improve your general well-being.

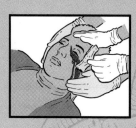

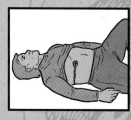

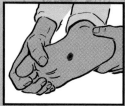

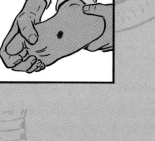

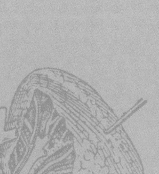

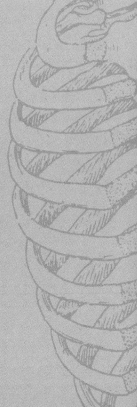

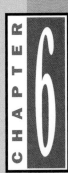

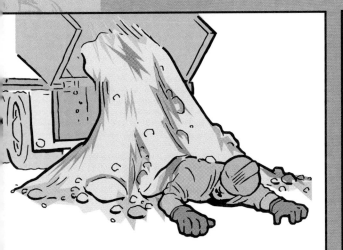

◆ *Dressings and
bandages*

◆ *Slings*

◆ *Types of wounds*

◆ *First aid for severe
external bleeding*

◆ *First aid for
amputations*

◆ *First aid for a
knocked-out tooth*

◆ *First aid for crush
injuries*

◆ *First aid for
puncture wounds*

◆ *First aid for
gunshot wounds*

◆ *First aid for a
contusion (bruise)*

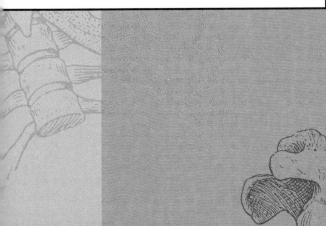

Dressings and bandages

Dressings and bandages are the basic tools of first aid. They are essential for wound care and for the care of injuries to bones, joints and muscles. You should know how to use commercially prepared dressings and bandages, and also be ready to improvise with materials on hand at the emergency scene. Knowing what makes a good dressing and bandage helps you do this.

Dressings

6

A dressing is a protective covering put on a wound to help control bleeding, absorb blood from the wound, and prevent further contamination. A dressing should be:

◆ sterile, or as clean as possible

◆ large enough to completely cover the wound

◆ highly absorbent to keep the wound dry

◆ compressible, thick and soft—especially for severe bleeding so that pressure is applied evenly over the wound

◆ non-stick and lint-free to reduce the possibility of sticking to the wound—gauze, cotton and linen make good dressings; wool or other fluffy materials make poor dressings

Dressings are available in a variety of sizes and designs. The dressings used most often in first aid are:

◆ *adhesive dressings*—prepared sterile gauze dressings with their own adhesive strips. They are sealed in a paper or plastic covering and are available in various sizes and shapes, according to their intended use. They are often used for minor wounds with little bleeding

commercial dressings

◆ *gauze dressings*—in varying sizes, folded and packaged individually or in large numbers—packaged gauze is usually sterile

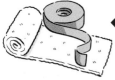

◆ *pressure dressings*—sterile dressings of gauze and other absorbent material, usually with an attached roller bandage. They are used to apply pressure to a wound with severe bleeding

◆ *improvised dressings*—prepared from lint-free sterile or clean material, preferably white. They may be made from a towel, a sheet, a pillow slip or any other clean absorbent material such as a sanitary pad. Plastic wrap or the wrapping from a sterile dressing can be used as an airtight dressing for penetrating wounds of the chest

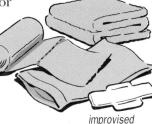

improvised dressings

Follow the guidelines below for putting on dressings:

◆ prevent further contamination as much as you can—use the cleanest material available as dressings, and wear gloves or wash your hands before handling them—see page 6-16 for more on preventing further contamination

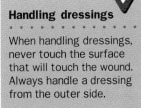

Handling dressings

When handling dressings, never touch the surface that will touch the wound. Always handle a dressing from the outer side.

6

◆ extend the dressing beyond the edges of the wound to completely cover it

◆ if blood soaks through a dressing, leave it in place and cover with more dressings

◆ secure a dressing with tape or bandages

Bandages

A bandage is any material that is used to hold a dressing in place, maintain pressure over a wound, support a limb or joint, immobilize parts of the body or secure a splint. Bandages may be commercially prepared or improvised.

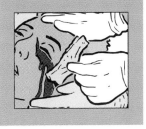

commercial bandages

When using bandages, remember to:

◆ apply them firmly to make sure bleeding is controlled or immobilization is achieved

◆ check the circulation beyond the bandage frequently to ensure the bandage is not too tight

◆ use your bandages only as bandages, not as padding or dressings, when other materials are available—you may need all your bandages for other injuries

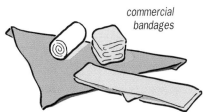

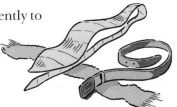

improvised bandages

The triangular bandage

One of the most versatile prepared or improvised bandages is the triangular bandage. It is made by cutting a one-metre square of linen or cotton on the diagonal, producing two triangles. Triangular bandages can be improvised from sheets, garbage bags, canvas, etc. The parts of the triangular bandage, identified for ease of instruction, are:

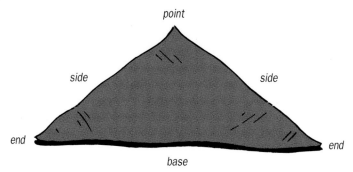

A triangular bandage may be used:

◆ as a **whole cloth**—opened to its fullest extent, as a sling or to hold a large dressing in place

◆ as a **broad bandage**—to hold splints in place or to apply pressure evenly over a large area

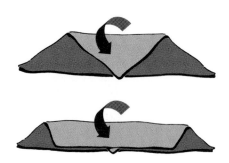

fold the point to the centre of the base with the point slightly beyond the base

fold in half again from the top to the base

◆ as a **narrow bandage**—to secure dressings or splints or to immobilize ankles and feet in a figure-8

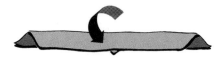

fold a broad bandage in half again from the top to the base

◆ as a **ring pad**—to control bleeding when pressure cannot be applied directly to the wound, as in the case of a short embedded object. Prepare a ring pad for your first aid kit, ready for use

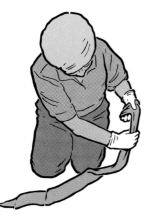

make a narrow bandage

form a loop around one hand by wrapping one end of the bandage twice around four fingers

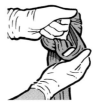

pass the loose end through the loop and wrap it around and around until the entire bandage is used up and a firm ring is made—this is a ring pad

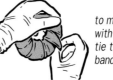

to make a ring pad with a larger loop, tie two narrow bandages together

6

Reef knot—the knot of choice

The reef knot is the best knot for tying bandages and slings because:

◆ it lies flat, making it more comfortable than other knots

◆ it doesn't slip

◆ it is easy to untie

To tie a reef knot:

◆ take one end of a bandage in each hand

◆ lay the end from the right hand over the one from the left hand and pass it under to form a half-knot. This will transfer the ends from one hand to the other

◆ the end now in the left hand should be laid over the one from the right and passed under to form another half-knot. The finished knot looks like two intertwined loops

◆ tighten by pulling one loop against the other or by pulling only on the ends

Place knots so they do not cause discomfort by pressing on skin or bone, particularly at the site of a fracture or at the neck, when tying a sling.

If the knot is uncomfortable, place soft material underneath as padding.

right over left, and under

left over right and under

pull the ends to tighten

Using a triangular bandage to hold a dressing in place

The following bandages are useful for holding dressings or padding in place. The instructions that follow use a full triangular bandage, but this may be too large in some cases. For a smaller casualty, fold a triangular bandage in half, end-to-end, to make a smaller triangular bandage.

Head bandage

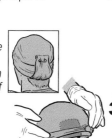

the casualty may be able to hold the dressing in place while the bandage is put on

wrap the ends of the bandage very low on the back of the head

tuck in the remaining ends of the bandage

1   Stand behind the casualty. Use a triangular bandage as a whole cloth with a narrow hem folded along the base. Place the centre of the base in the middle of the forehead, close to the eyebrows.

2   Bring the point over the top of the head to cover the dressing, and down the back of the head. Bring the ends around the back of the head, cross over the point, and around the head to the front. Tie the ends together, using a reef knot, low on the forehead.

3   Steady the head with one hand, and gently pull the point down to put the desired amount of pressure on the dressing. Fold the point up toward the top of the head and secure it carefully with a safety pin or tuck it under the back crisscross.

Knee or elbow bandage

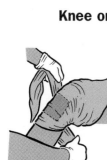

1   Use a triangular bandage as a whole cloth with a narrow hem folded along the base. Place the centre of the base on the leg below the kneecap with the point toward the top of the leg (or to bandage an elbow, on the forearm with the point toward the shoulder).

2   Bring the ends around the joint, crossing over the point in front of the elbow or at the back of the knee.

3 Bring the ends up and tie off over the point. Pull the point up to put the right amount of pressure on the dressing and then fold it down and secure it with a safety pin or tuck it under the knot.

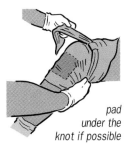

pad
under the
knot if possible

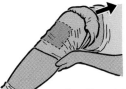

pull on the point
to put pressure on
the dressing

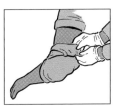

for an elbow, tie the
bandage the same
way as for a knee

6

Foot or hand bandage

1 Use a triangular bandage as a whole cloth. Place it on a flat surface with the point away from the casualty.

fold over
once to
make a
narrow
hem

2 Place the foot or hand on the triangular bandage with the toes or fingers toward the point, leaving enough bandage at the ankle or wrist to fully cover the part. Bring the point up and over the foot or hand to rest on the lower leg or wrist.

3 Bring the ends alongside the foot or hand and crisscross the folded ends up and around the ankle or wrist. Cross over the point and wrap any extra bandage before tying it off.

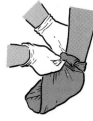

4 Tie off over the point. If the point extends beyond the knot, pull it up to apply the desired pressure. Fold it downward and tuck under the knot.

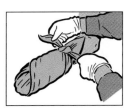

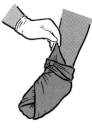

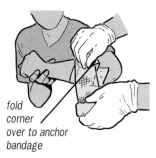

fold
corner
over to anchor
bandage

Roller bandage

Roller bandages, usually made of gauze-like material, are packaged as a roll. Use them to hold dressings in place to secure splints. These are not elasticized roller bandages—see page 7-7 for information on elasticized roller bandages.

Put on a roller bandage in a simple spiral. Starting at the narrow part of the limb, anchor the bandage as follows:

- ◆ place the end of the bandage on a diagonal at the starting point

- ◆ wrap the bandage around the injured part so the corner of the bandage end is left out

- ◆ fold this corner of the bandage over and wrap the bandage around again to cover the corner

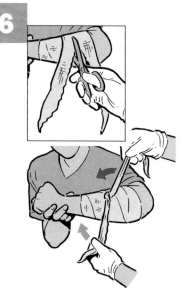

Continue wrapping the bandage, overlapping each turn by one quarter to one third of the bandage's width. Make full-width overlaps with the final two or three turns and secure with a safety pin, adhesive tape or by cutting and tying the bandage as shown. Check circulation below the bandage.

Tubular gauze and elasticized net bandages

When bleeding has been controlled and direct pressure is not required, quick and efficient bandaging can be accomplished with tubular gauze or elasticized net bandages. Both types of bandage come in various sizes to fit different parts of the body. Cut the required length from the roll and either apply it with a specially-designed applicator or stretch it by hand to fit over the dressing.

Tubular gauze and elasticized net are especially useful for holding dressings to the head, shoulder, thigh or finger where roller bandaging is difficult and time-consuming. Instructions on how to put them on are usually included with the bandage.

⚠ Not too tight!

Apply roller bandages firmly, but not too tightly. Check circulation below the injury after putting on the bandage. Check it again every few minutes—as the injured part swells, circulation could be cut off.

Figure-8

A figure-8 bandage is used to tie the ankles and feet, to secure a splint to the ankles/feet, or to support an injured ankle.

To tie a figure-8:

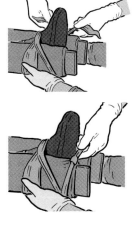

◆ position the centre of a narrow or broad triangular bandage under the ankle (or both ankles if tying the feet together). The bandage may be positioned over a dressing or splint

◆ bring the ends around the ankles, cross over on top of the legs and bring the ends around the feet

◆ tie the figure-8 off where the knot will not put pressure on the foot—either between the feet or on the sole of the shoe

Slings

A sling provides support and protection for an arm. Commercial slings are available but a sling can be easily improvised with a scarf, belt, necktie or other item that can go around the casualty's neck—any material will do as long as it is sturdy enough to support the arm. You can also support the arm by placing the hand inside a buttoned jacket or by pinning the sleeve of a shirt or jacket to the clothing in the proper position.

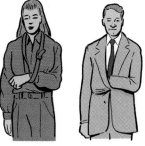

improvised slings

Arm sling

The arm sling is used to support an injured elbow, forearm, wrist or hand. To put on an arm sling:

1 Support the forearm of the injured limb across the body, with the wrist and hand slightly higher than the elbow. Place an open triangular bandage between the forearm and the chest so the point extends beyond the elbow and the base is straight up and down.

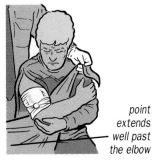

point extends well past the elbow

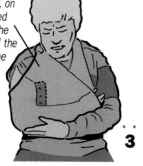

tie the ends together, on the injured side, in the hollow of the collarbone

2 Bring the upper end over the casualty's shoulder on the uninjured side, around the back of the neck to the front of the injured side. While still supporting the forearm, bring the lower end of the bandage over the hand and forearm and tie off on the injured side in the hollow of the collarbone. Place padding under the knot for comfort.

3 Bring the point around to the front of the elbow and secure with a safety pin, or twist the point into a "pigtail" and tuck it inside the sling.

4 Adjust the sling so you can see the fingernails—this way you can watch them to check on circulation.

St. John tubular sling

Use a St. John tubular sling to support the hand and forearm in a well-elevated position that transfers the weight of the arm and hand to the uninjured side. This sling is used for injuries to the shoulder or collarbone, and for bleeding of the hand. To put on a St. John tubular sling:

1 Support the forearm of the injured side diagonally across the chest, with the fingers pointing toward the opposite shoulder.

2 Place a triangular bandage over the forearm and hand with the point extending beyond the elbow and the upper end over the shoulder on the uninjured side.

the casualty may need help supporting the injured arm

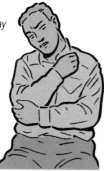

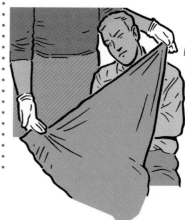

the base is placed vertically in line with the body on the uninjured side

3 Support the forearm and ease the base of the bandage under the hand, forearm and elbow.

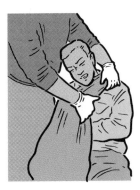

tuck the base of the bandage under the injured arm to make a pocket that runs the full length of the arm

6

4 Gather the bandage at the elbow and bring the lower end across the back and over the shoulder on the uninjured side.

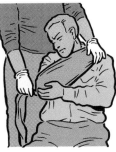

to gather the bandage, twist it around and around towards the body— this closes the pocket at the elbow

5 Gently adjust the height of the arm as you tie off the ends of the bandage so the knot rests in the natural hollow above the collarbone. Place padding under knot, if available.

tie the sling tightly enough to support the weight of the injured arm

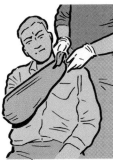

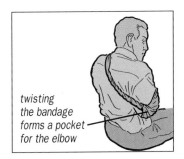

twisting the bandage forms a pocket for the elbow

Wounds and bleeding

A **wound** is any break in the soft tissues of the body. It usually results in bleeding and may allow germs to enter the body. **Bleeding** is the escape of blood from the blood vessels into surrounding tissues, body cavities or out of the body. The soft tissues of the body are the most susceptible to injury, resulting in wounds and bleeding.

A wound can be either open or closed:

- ◆ **open wound**—there is a break in the outer layer of the skin that results in bleeding and may permit germs to enter the body, causing infection

- ◆ **closed wound**—there is no break in the outer layer of skin so there is no external bleeding (but there will be internal bleeding which may be severe) and the risk of infection is low (except in a closed abdominal wound where the risk of infection is high—see page 6-23)

The different types of open and closed wounds to soft tissues are given in the table on the next page. When someone is injured, recognizing the type of wound helps to give appropriate first aid.

The aim in the care of wounds is to stop the bleeding and prevent infection. Although some bleeding may help to wash contamination from the wound, excessive blood flow must be stopped quickly to minimize shock.

Bleeding

Bleeding is the escape of blood from the blood vessels. In **external bleeding**, blood escapes the body through a surface wound—you can see external bleeding. In **internal bleeding**, blood escapes from tissues inside the body—you don't usually see internal bleeding. Also, bleeding is either **arterial**, which is bleeding from the arteries, or **venous**, which is bleeding from the veins.

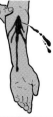

in **arterial** bleeding, the blood is bright red and spurts with each heartbeat— arterial bleeding is serious and often hard to control

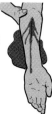

in **venous** bleeding, the blood is dark red and flows more steadily—it is easier to stop than arterial bleeding

Types of wounds

Contusions or bruises	Abrasions or scrapes	Incisions	Lacerations	Puncture wounds	Avulsions & Amputations

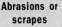

6

Contusions or bruises are closed wounds usually caused by a fall or a blow from something blunt. The tissues under the skin are damaged and bleed into surrounding tissues, causing discolouration. Because there is no break in the skin, there is little chance of infection. A bruise may be a sign of a deeper, more serious injury or illness.

Abrasions or scrapes are open wounds where the outer protective layer of skin and the tiny underlying blood vessels are exposed, but the deeper layer of the skin is still intact. Abrasions are usually due to the skin being scraped across a hard surface (rug burns, road rash). Abrasions do not bleed very much but can be very painful. The risk of infection from dirt and other particles that may be in the wound is high.

Incisions are clean cuts in soft tissue caused by something sharp such as a knife. These wounds may not be as dirty as abrasions, but they may contain fragments of glass or other material.

Lacerations are tears in the skin and underlying tissue. The edges of the wound are jagged and irregular, and dirt is likely to be present, increasing the risk of infection. Lacerations are often caused by machinery, barbed wire or the claws of an animal.

Puncture wounds are open wounds caused by blunt or pointed instruments, such as knives, nails or an animal's teeth. The wound may have a small opening, but often penetrates deep into the tissue. There may be contamination deep in the wound and internal organs may be damaged.

Avulsions are injuries that leave a piece of skin or other tissue either partially or completely torn away from the body. Amputations involve partial or complete loss of a body part and are usually caused by machinery or cutting tools.

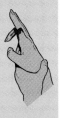

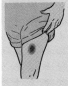

> ⚠️ Gunshot wounds are a special type of wound. The entry wound is often small, and may have burns around it. Sometimes there is an exit wound as well, which is usually larger than the entry wound. Because the bullet may bounce around inside the body, the exit wound may not be directly across from the entry wound.

Signs and symptoms of bleeding

The most obvious sign of external bleeding is blood. You do not always see blood with internal bleeding. General signs and symptoms of bleeding vary depending on how much blood is lost. Severe blood loss will result in the following signs and symptoms of shock:

6

If internal bleeding is severe, signs of shock will be present.

- ◆ pale, cold and clammy skin

- ◆ rapid pulse, gradually becoming weaker

- ◆ faintness, dizziness, thirst and nausea

- ◆ restlessness and apprehension

- ◆ shallow breathing, yawning, sighing and gasping for air

Recognizing internal bleeding

Internal bleeding may not be easy to recognize—a casualty can bleed to death without any blood being seen. Suspect internal bleeding if:

- ◆ the casualty received a severe blow or a penetrating injury to the chest, neck, abdomen or groin

- ◆ there are major limb fractures such as a fractured upper leg or pelvis

Specific signs of internal bleeding

You may recognize internal bleeding by one or more of the following characteristic signs. Blood is:

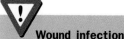

Wound infection

Any wound that becomes infected should be seen by a doctor. Recognize infection in a wound when the wound:

- ◆ becomes more painful
- ◆ becomes red and perhaps swollen
- ◆ feels warmer than the surrounding area
- ◆ shows the presence of pus (whitish fluid)

- ◆ coming from the ear canal or the nose, or it may appear as a bloodshot eye or black eye (bleeding inside the head)

- ◆ coughed up and looks bright red and frothy (bleeding into the lungs)

- ◆ seen in vomitus either as bright red, or brown like coffee grounds

- ◆ seen in the stools, and looks either black and tarry (bleeding into the upper bowel), or its normal red colour (bleeding into the lower bowel)

◆ seen in the urine as a red or smoky brown colour (bleeding into the urinary tract)

If internal bleeding is severe, the casualty will show progressive signs of shock.

First aid for severe external bleeding

The principles of first aid for bleeding and preventing further contamination are on page 6-16. The following sequence shows the principles being used.

1   Begin ESM—do a scene survey (see page 2-3). Assess the mechanism of injury. If you suspect a head or spinal injury, steady and support the head and neck before continuing.

6

2   Do a primary survey (see page 2-5) and give first aid for life-threatening injuries.

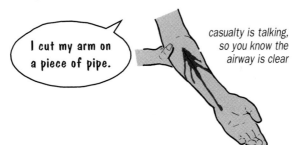

I cut my arm on a piece of pipe.

casualty is talking, so you know the airway is clear

3   To control severe bleeding, apply direct pressure to the wound as quickly as possible. If the wound is large and wide open, you may have to bring the edges of the wound together first.

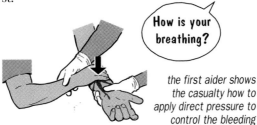

How is your breathing?

the first aider shows the casualty how to apply direct pressure to control the bleeding

continued on page 6-17

Principles of controlling bleeding

The body has natural defences against bleeding. Damaged blood vessels constrict to reduce blood flow and blood pressure drops as bleeding continues. These factors result in reduced force of blood flow. Blood will clot as it is exposed to air, forming a seal at the wound. Even so, the first aider should try to stop all bleeding as soon as possible, following the ABC priorities.

Steps to control bleeding

The following steps will control all but the most severe bleeding—you can often do these all at the same time.

Direct pressure—apply pressure directly to the wound to stop blood flow and allow clots to form. When bleeding is controlled, keep the pressure on the wound with dressings and bandages.

Elevation—raise the injured limb above the level of the heart to use gravity to reduce blood flow to the wound area. Elevate the limb as high as is comfortable.

Rest—place the casualty at rest to reduce the pulse rate. Unless the bleeding is from a head wound, the preferred position is lying down with feet and legs elevated.

Minor cuts and scrapes that cause slight bleeding are easily controlled with pressure, elevation and rest. Severe bleeding must be brought under control quickly to prevent further blood loss and to slow the progress of shock.

Preventing further contamination

All open wounds are contaminated to some degree. From the moment of injury, there is risk of infection that continues until the wound is completely healed. Stopping bleeding is your priority, but do it using the cleanest materials available.

Minor wound care

Follow the principles listed below for cleaning a wound. Tell the casualty to seek medical help if signs of infection appear later (see page 6-14).

◆ wash your hands with soap and water and put on gloves if available

◆ do not cough or breathe directly over the wound

◆ fully expose the wound but don't touch it

◆ gently wash loose material from the surface of the wound. Wash and dry the surrounding skin with clean dressings, wiping away from the wound

◆ cover the wound promptly with a sterile dressing. Tape the dressing in place

◆ remove and dispose of gloves in an appropriate manner (see page 1-10) and wash your hands and any other skin area that may have been in contact with the casualty's blood

Tetanus Infection

Any wound may be contaminated by spores that cause tetanus, a potentially fatal disease characterized by muscle spasms. Tetanus is commonly referred to as "lockjaw."

Deep wounds, especially those caused by animal bites or those that may have been contaminated by soil, dust or animal feces, are at high risk of tetanus infection. Advise a casualty with this type of wound to get medical help.

continued from page 6-15

4   While keeping pressure on the wound, elevate the injury—this will reduce blood flow at the wound.

if injuries permit, elevate the injury above the level of the heart

5   Place the casualty at rest—this will further reduce blood flow.

6   Quickly replace the casualty's hand with dressings (preferably sterile) and continue direct pressure over the dressings.

7   Once bleeding is under control, continue the primary survey, looking for other life-threatening injuries. Give life-saving first aid as needed.

6

8   Before bandaging the wound, check circulation below the injury.

check the temperature and colour of the fingers and use the nailbed test—see page 6-18

9   Bandage the dressing in place.

10   Check the circulation below the injury and compare it with the other side. If it is worse than it was before the injury was bandaged, loosen the bandage just enough to improve circulation.

11   Give ongoing casualty care, including first aid to minimize shock—see page 1-26.

If the dressings become blood-soaked. . .

. . . don't remove them—add more dressings and continue pressure. Removing the blood-soaked dressings may disturb blood clots and expose the wound to further contamination.

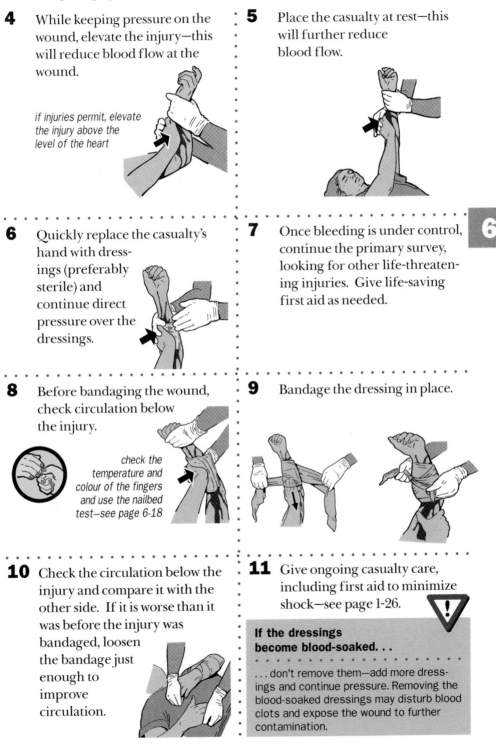

Checking circulation below an injury

Causes of impaired circulation

Certain injuries and first aid procedures may impair (reduce or cut off) circulation to the tissue below the injury (called *distal* circulation). A joint injury or fracture could pinch an artery and restrict the flow of blood to the limb. Bandages tied too tightly will impair distal circulation. Sometimes, a bandage is not too tight when it is put on but as the injury swells, the bandage becomes too tight, impairing circulation.

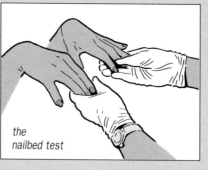

the nailbed test

Effects of impaired circulation

If oxygenated blood does not reach the tissues below the injury, there may be tissue damage that could lead to loss of the limb. Check circulation below an injury before tying any bandages. Check again after tying bandages. If circulation is impaired, take steps to improve it.

How to monitor circulation

For each of the methods below, check both the injured side and the uninjured side of the casualty. If circulation is not impaired, both sides will be the same. Monitor circulation below the injury by:

◆ checking skin colour—if the skin does not have full colour, circulation may be impaired

◆ checking skin temperature—if the skin temperature feels cold, especially if it is colder than the uninjured side, circulation may be impaired

◆ checking for a pulse—in an arm injury, check for a pulse at the wrist— see page 2-16

◆ doing the nailbed test— press on a fingernail or toenail until the nailbed turns white, and then release it. Note how long it takes for normal colour to return. If it returns quickly, blood flow is unrestricted. If it stays white, or if the colour returns slowly, circulation may be impaired

When the injury is on the arm, expose the hands and fingers to check circulation. When the injury in on the leg and there is no reason to remove the shoe, check circulation by placing fingers inside the sock along the side of the foot.

Improving impaired circulation

To improve impaired circulation, loosen tight bandages. If circulation doesn't improve and medical help will be delayed, try moving the limb to restore circulation. By moving the limb, you will hopefully relieve any pressure on blood vessels. If possible, move the limb towards its natural position. Only **move the limb as much as the casualty will let you, or as far as you can without resistance.** Resecure the limb and recheck circulation.

Keep monitoring circulation until medical help takes over. If circulation remains impaired, medical help is urgently needed.

First aid for severe, internal bleeding

As a first aider, you can do very little to control internal bleeding. Give first aid to minimize shock and get medical help as quickly as you can.

1 Begin ESM—do a scene survey (see page 2-3).

2 Do a primary survey (see page 2-5) and give first aid for life-threatening injuries. In this case, you suspect severe internal bleeding.

if the mechanism of injury suggests a severe blow to the body, look further for signs of internal bleeding

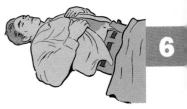

If the casualty is conscious, place him at rest on his back with the feet and legs raised to about 30 cm (12 in).

If the casualty is unconscious, place him in the recovery position (see page 1-32 and 1-33).

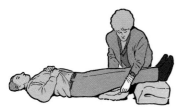 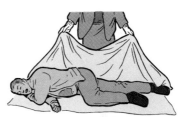

conscious casualty in shock position

unconscious casualty in recovery position

3 Send or go for medical help.

4 Give ongoing casualty care. Do not give the casualty anything by mouth. If he complains of thirst, moisten his lips with a wet cloth. Make the casualty comfortable—loosen all tight clothing at the neck, chest and waist. Keep the casualty warm and protected from extreme temperatures.

Monitor the casualty often. When medical help takes over, make sure you tell them you suspect internal bleeding.

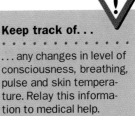

Keep track of. . .

. . . any changes in level of consciousness, breathing, pulse and skin temperature. Relay this information to medical help.

Amputations

An amputation is when a part of the body, such as a toe, foot or leg, has been partly or completely cut off. When this happens, you must control the bleeding from the wound, care for the amputated tissue and get medical help. The first aid for both a completely amputated hand and a partly amputated finger is shown below.

First aid for amputations

1 Begin ESM—do a scene survey (see page 2-3). Do a primary survey (see page 2-5) and give first aid for life-threatening injuries. In this case, there is severe bleeding from an amputation.

2 Control the bleeding—apply direct pressure to the wound. If the bleeding won't stop with direct pressure, use a tourniquet (see next page).

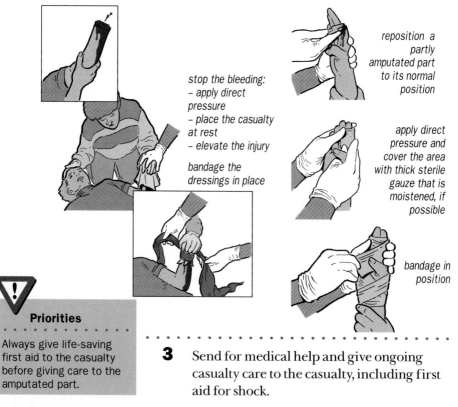

completely amputated hand

stop the bleeding:
– apply direct pressure
– place the casualty at rest
– elevate the injury

bandage the dressings in place

partly amputated finger

reposition a partly amputated part to its normal position

apply direct pressure and cover the area with thick sterile gauze that is moistened, if possible

bandage in position

! Priorities

Always give life-saving first aid to the casualty before giving care to the amputated part.

3 Send for medical help and give ongoing casualty care to the casualty, including first aid for shock.

4 Care for the amputated tissue—completely or partly amputated parts must be preserved, regardless of their condition, and taken to medical help with the casualty. It may be possible to reattach the part—and with the proper care of the part, the chances are even better. Care for the amputated part as follows:

wrap the amputated part in a clean, moist dressing—if you can't moisten the dressing, a dry dressing will do

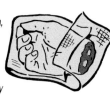

put the amputated part in a clean, watertight plastic bag and seal it

put this bag in a second plastic bag or container partly filled with crushed ice

attach a record of the date and time this was done and send this package with the casualty to medical help

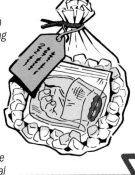

6

5 Keep the amputated part in a shaded, cool place and get the casualty and the amputated part to medical help as soon as possible.

Do not. . .

... try to clean an amputated part. Do not use any antiseptic solutions.

Using a tourniquet to stop bleeding

Direct pressure, elevation and rest should control bleeding, but if bleeding from a limb does not stop, or if you must go to other casualties with life-threatening conditions, use a tourniquet to stop blood flow.

To put on a tourniquet:

◆ use a narrow triangular bandage or an improvised bandage—do not use rope or wire that could cut into the skin

◆ while trying to control bleeding with direct pressure, wrap the bandage tightly twice around the limb above the wound and as close to it as possible. Tie a half-knot

◆ place a stick, or something similar, on the half-knot, and then tie a full knot

◆ twist the stick to tighten the tourniquet just enough to stop the bleeding

◆ secure the stick in place with the remaining ends of the bandage or tape

◆ tag or mark the casualty in a clearly visible place with the letters "TK." If you don't have a tag, mark it on the casualty's forehead. Make a note of the time the tourniquet was applied

Make sure that the tourniquet is always visible. If medical help will be available within one hour, do not loosen it.

If medical help is delayed more than one hour, loosen the tourniquet each hour to assess the bleeding. If bleeding has stopped, leave the loosened tourniquet in place so that it can be tightened quickly if bleeding starts again.

twist this stick to tighten the tourniquet

tie the stick in place

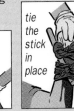

First aid for a knocked-out tooth

A knocked-out tooth can be reimplanted if the casualty receives medical/dental help quickly.

1   Begin ESM—do a scene survey (see page 2-3)—carefully assess the mechanism of injury—was there enough force to cause a head or spinal injury?

2   Do a primary survey (see page 2-5). Assess the airway—is there blood or swelling that could block the airway? Assess breathing and circulation and give first aid for other life-threatening conditions.

3   Apply direct pressure to stop the bleeding from the socket of the tooth.

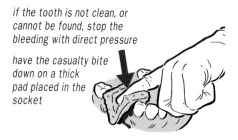

if the tooth is not clean, or cannot be found, stop the bleeding with direct pressure

have the casualty bite down on a thick pad placed in the socket

Seat the casualty with the head forward so blood can drain out of the mouth.

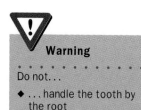

Warning

Do not...

◆ ... handle the tooth by the root

◆ ... try to clean an amputated part, including a knocked-out tooth. Do not use any antiseptic solutions

◆ ... wash out the mouth when the bleeding has stopped—this may disturb the blood clots making the injury bleed again

4   Care for the knocked-out tooth. Place the tooth in a cup of milk. If milk is not available, the tooth may be preserved in a saline solution or wrapped in plastic wrap kept moist with the casualty's saliva. Handle the tooth by the top—don't touch the root.

5   Give ongoing casualty care and get medical help. If the knocked-out tooth is the only injury, get the casualty to a dentist as quickly as possible for the best chance of reimplanting the tooth.

Abdominal injuries

Abdominal wounds may be closed or open. Closed wounds occur when internal abdominal tissues are damaged but the skin is intact. Open abdominal wounds are those in which the skin has been broken. Abdominal organs may protrude out from the wound.

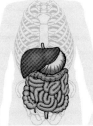

the abdominal organs

Complications from abdominal wounds may include severe bleeding (either internal or external) and contamination from the contents of ruptured abdominal organs. These complications may result in shock and infection.

Assessing an abdominal injury

6

Expose the injured area. Consider the history of the incident, especially the mechanism of injury. Observe the casualty's position and examine the casualty gently. Feel for swelling, rigidity, and pain.

First aid for closed abdominal wounds

If you suspect an abdominal injury, you should also suspect internal bleeding that may be severe. Give first aid for severe internal bleeding—see page 6-19.

First aid for open abdominal wounds

1   Begin ESM—do a scene survey (see page 2-3). Do a primary survey (see page 2-5). In this case you find an open abdominal wound.

2   This wound may be open wide and must be prevented from opening wider. Position the casualty with head and shoulders slightly raised and supported, and with the knees raised.

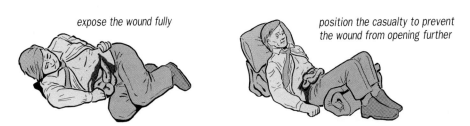

expose the wound fully

position the casualty to prevent the wound from opening further

3   Dress the wound. The method of dressing a wound of the abdominal wall depends on whether or not internal organs are protruding:

♦ if organs are not protruding, apply a dry dressing to the wound and bandage firmly.

♦ if organs are protruding, don't try to put them back into the abdomen. Put on a moist dressing as shown below. The moist dressing helps stop the organs from drying out.

cover the wound and the protruding organs with a large, moist, sterile gauze dressing, or a soft, clean, moist towel

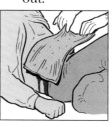

secure the dressing in place without putting any pressure on the protruding organs

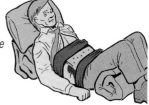

4   Do not give anything by mouth. If the casualty coughs or vomits, support the abdomen with two broad bandages.

5   Give ongoing casualty care and get the casualty to medical help promptly.

Crush injuries

"Crush injury" occurs when a portion of the body is crushed under heavy weight. The crushing force causes extensive bruising of the area, and there may be complications including fractures or ruptured organs. When the crushed area is limited, such as a hand or foot, the injury is considered serious, but is not usually life-threatening. However, a major crush injury may cause severe shock or **crush syndrome**, both of which are life threatening.

Severe shock can develop after a casualty is released from the weight that caused the crush injury. When the crushing force is removed, fluids from the crushed tissues leak into surrounding tissues—this causes shock.

When muscle is crushed, it releases the contents of muscle cells into the blood. If the injury is large, it can cause kidney failure. This is **crush syndrome**, also called post-traumatic acute renal (kidney) failure.

First aid for crush injuries

Give first aid for wounds and fractures to stop bleeding and relieve pain. Stabilize other conditions while waiting for transportation to medical help.

1 Begin ESM—do a scene survey (see page 2-3) and a primary survey (see page 2-5). Move the casualty as little as possible and do what you can to minimize pain.

2 Give first aid for shock right away—even if there are no signs, shock will probably develop.

3 Give ongoing casualty care and transport to medical help as soon as possible.

Puncture wounds

All puncture wounds must be considered serious because of the possibility of serious tissue damage and contamination deep inside the wound.

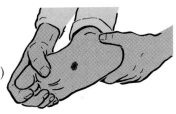

 First aid for puncture wounds

1 Begin ESM—do a scene survey (see page 2-3) and a primary survey (see page 2-5). Wash your hands or put gloves on (if available).

2 Start the secondary survey—expose the wound. Although there may not be much external bleeding, you should suspect internal bleeding, especially if the wound is in the chest or abdomen.

3 Control bleeding with direct pressure, rest and elevation (see page 6-16), dress the wound, and transport the casualty to medical help.

4 Give ongoing casualty care until handover.

Gunshot wounds

A gunshot wound is a special type of wound—see page 6-13 for more on gunshot wounds. First aid for gunshot wounds is below.

First aid for gunshot wounds

The aim of first aid for gunshot wounds is to give life-saving first aid and get the casualty to medical help as quickly as possible.

1   Begin ESM—do a scene survey (see page 2-3). If there is any possibility of danger to yourself, don't go any further. Call the police.

2   Do a primary survey (see page 2-5) and give first aid for life-threatening conditions. When looking for bleeding, examine all parts of the body very carefully. The exit wound may not be where you expect it to be—look for it carefully.

3   Place the casualty at rest and give first aid for shock. Do not give anything by mouth.

4   Give ongoing casualty care and transport the casualty to medical help as soon as possible.

If you suspect a crime...

...has been committed, do not disturb anything at the scene—you may be disturbing evidence.

Wounds with embedded objects

Never remove an object embedded in a wound. Removing the object will probably result in heavier bleeding and could cause further tissue damage. The aim of first aid for a wound with an embedded object is to stop the bleeding, prevent the embedded object from moving and to get medical help. The first aid is slightly different depending on whether the embedded object is short or long.

don't remove the embedded object—this could cause more tissue damage and make bleeding worse

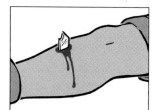

check the circulation below the injury

Bandaging a wound with a short embedded object

1 Wash hands or put gloves on (if available). Expose the injured area and assess the wound.

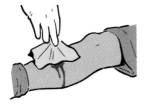

gently place a clean, preferably sterile, dressing over the object

2 To stop the bleeding, you must put pressure around the embedded object. For a short embedded object, a ring pad (see page 6-5) works well. "Tent" the dressing to avoid pressure on the object.

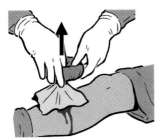

hold the ring pad over the dressing

pull the dressing through the ring pad

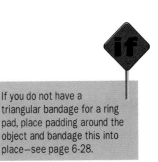

If you do not have a triangular bandage for a ring pad, place padding around the object and bandage this into place—see page 6-28.

3 Secure the ring pad with a narrow bandage.

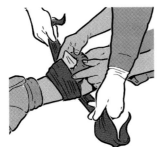

tie the bandage tightly enough to:

– control the bleeding
– keep the ring pad and dressing in place
– cover as much of the ring pad as possible

do not tie the bandage tightly enough to cut off circulation below the injury

4 Elevate the bandaged leg about 30 cm (12 in) if injuries permit. Check the circulation below the injury and give ongoing casualty care. Get medical help.

if circulation below the injury is impaired, and it wasn't before bandaging, loosen the bandage

Bandaging a wound with a long embedded object

check the circulation below the injury

1 Wash hands and put gloves on (if available). Expose the injured area and assess the wound.

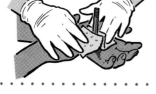

2 Gently place clean dressings around the object.

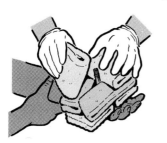

3 Place bulky dressings around the object to keep it from moving. This will apply pressure to the wound but not to the object.

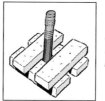

use the log cabin method

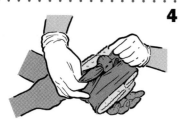

4 Secure the bulky material (dressings) in place with a narrow bandage, taking care that pressure is not exerted on the embedded object.

5 Elevate the injured part if injuries permit. Check the circulation below the injury—if circulation below the injury is impaired, and it wasn't before bandaging, loosen the bandage to restore circulation. Give ongoing casualty care and get medical help.

First aid for a sliver/splinter

Slivers are embedded objects and may be wood, thorns, glass or metal. This type of injury is common in the hands and feet. Although slivers may cause discomfort and pain, in most cases they can be removed easily without complications.

In serious cases, slivers can be disabling and cause serious infections. Organic objects including thorns and wood slivers are particularly likely to result in infection.

Slivers should be removed if there is no threat to the surrounding tissues (the sliver is neither too large, nor embedded too deeply into the flesh).

6

Removing a sliver

1   Clean the area with soap and warm water.

2   With sterile tweezers, grip the sliver as close to the skin as possible.

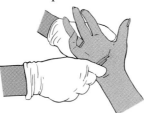

3   Pull the sliver in a straight line in the opposite direction to the angle of entry.

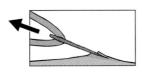

do not pull too quickly or with too much force as this may result in breaking the sliver and leaving part of it in the wound

4   When the sliver is removed, give first aid for a puncture wound (see page 6-25). Get medical help if some of the sliver was not removed, there is more tissue damage than a simple, small puncture wound or if an infection develops (see page 6-14).

Warning

Do not remove any sliver that:

◆ lies over a joint

◆ is deeply embedded into the flesh

◆ is in or close to the eye (see page 6-39)

◆ possesses a barb (e.g. metal slivers and fishhooks). This may result in tissue damage.

◆ cannot be removed easily

In these cases, give first aid for an embedded object (see page 6-26). Reassure the casualty and get medical help.

First aid for a contusion (bruise)

With a contusion or bruise, blood escapes into the surrounding tissue. Relieve the pain and reduce the swelling by following RICE—see page 7-7.

A "bump on the head"

A "bump on the head" is a very common injury, especially in children. Typically, a child falls and bangs his head on a piece of furniture—he cries, is comforted by a parent and finally settles down. Within minutes, there is a big red or purple welt on his fore-head—but in a few hours it disappears and the whole episode is forgotten.

Usually a "bump on the head" is harmless. But as with any injury to the head, it should be taken seriously—there is always the threat of an underlying skull fracture or brain injury. When a child bumps his head, do the following:

Don't pick him up!

When a child falls, an adult's instinct is to pick him up and comfort him. But if there is serious injury, picking the child up could make things worse.

Don't pick up a fallen child, and don't allow a fallen child to move, until you know for sure there is no serious injury.

♦ begin ESM—start a scene survey (see page 2-3). Immediately assess the mechanism of injury—was there enough force to seriously harm the child? If you think there might have been, don't move the child, and don't let him move, until you check further. If you suspect a serious injury, give first aid for a head/spinal injury—see page 7-9

♦ if it appears that there is no serious injury, pick the child up and comfort him. As soon as possible, put a cold compress or ice bag (15 minutes on; 15 minutes off—see page 6-42) on the injury site to relieve pain and control swelling

♦ watch the child for any signs or symptoms of:

   ❖ a skull fracture—see page 7-8

   ❖ a concussion—see page 7-11

   ❖ compression—see page 7-12

If you see any of these signs developing, even after many days, get medical help immediately.

Warning

Any casualty who has lost consciousness for a few minutes should be taken to medical help—follow medical advice on what signs and symptoms to watch for as possible indicators of a head injury.

First aid for bleeding from inside the ear

1   Begin ESM—do a scene survey (see page 2-3) and assess the mechanism of injury. If you suspect a head or spinal injury, tell the casualty not to move.

2   Do a primary survey (see page 2-5) and give first aid for life-threatening conditions.

3   Do a secondary survey if needed—assess the bleeding from the ear. If the blood from the ear is mixed with straw-coloured fluid, suspect a skull fracture—steady and support the head and neck. Place a dressing lightly over the ear and give first aid for a skull fracture—see page 7-9.

6

4   If a head or spinal injury is not suspected, lightly tape a dressing over the ear.

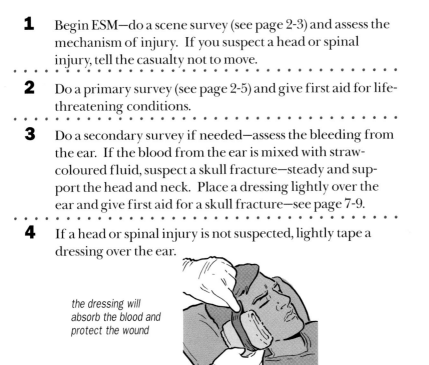

the dressing will absorb the blood and protect the wound

Position the casualty to allow the blood to drain from the ear if injuries permit.

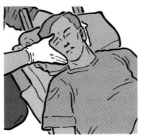

a semisitting position with the head tilted towards the injured side is a good, comfortable position to allow drainage from the ear

If the casualty is unconscious and injuries permit, put dressings over the ear and place him in the recovery position with the injured side down.

5   Give ongoing casualty care until medical help takes over.

Warning

When there is bleeding from the ear canal, don't try to stop the bleeding by putting pressure on the ear or by packing the ear canal with dressings.

To reduce the risk of infection inside the ear, it is best to let the blood drain away.

First aid for a nosebleed

A nosebleed may start for no obvious reason, or may be caused by blowing the nose, an injury to the nose, or in more serious cases, by an indirect injury, such as a fractured skull.

1   Begin ESM—do a scene survey (see page 2-3) and assess the mechanism of injury. If there could be a head or spinal injury, tell the casualty not to move.

2   Do a primary survey (see page 2-5) and give first aid for life-threatening conditions.

3   Do a secondary survey as needed—assess the bleeding from the nose. If the blood from the nose is mixed with straw-coloured fluid, suspect a skull fracture. Allow the nose to bleed and give first aid for a skull fracture—see page 7-9.

4   If a head or spinal injury is not suspected, place the casualty in a sitting position with the head slightly forward.

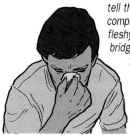

tell the casualty to compress the entire fleshy part below the bridge of the nose firmly with the thumb and index finger for about 10 minutes or until bleeding stops

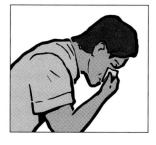

leaning forward allows blood to drain from the nose and mouth instead of back into the throat

5   Loosen clothing around the casualty's neck and chest. Keep the casualty quiet to avoid increased bleeding. Tell the casualty to breathe through his mouth and not blow his nose for a few hours, so that blood clots will not be disturbed. If bleeding does not stop with this first aid, or if it starts again, get medical help.

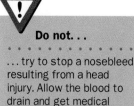

Do not. . .

. . . try to stop a nosebleed resulting from a head injury. Allow the blood to drain and get medical help.

Bleeding from the scalp

Bleeding from the scalp is often severe and may be complicated by a fracture of the skull or an embedded object. When giving first aid for these wounds, avoid direct pressure, probing and contaminating the wound. Care must be taken to:

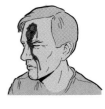

◆ clean away loose dirt

◆ apply a thick, sterile dressing that is large enough to extend well beyond the edges of the wound and bandage it firmly in place with a head bandage—see page 6-6

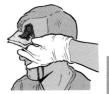

◆ if there is suspected underlying skull fracture, give first aid for a fracture of the skull—see page 7-9

◆ if there is an embedded object, apply a large ring pad over the dressing to maintain pressure around but away from the wound—see page 6-27

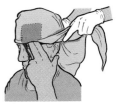

◆ give ongoing casualty care and transport the casualty to medical aid

Bleeding from the cheek, gums or tongue

When there is bleeding from the gums or mouth, first assess the mechanism of injury to determine if there is a chance of a serious head and/or spinal injury. If so, give first aid for a head/spinal injury. Make sure the bleeding in the mouth doesn't block the airway.

bleeding from the gums-this should be treated as a sign of a fractured jaw until proven otherwise—see page 7-9

Control the bleeding in the mouth using direct pressure over a clean, preferably sterile, dressing.

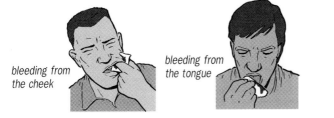

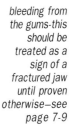

bleeding from the cheek

bleeding from the tongue

Do not wash out the mouth after bleeding has stopped. This may dislodge clots and cause bleeding to start again.

First aid for bleeding from the palm of the hand

1 Start ESM—do a scene survey (see page 2-3). Do a primary survey (see page 2-5) and give first aid for life-threatening injuries. In this case, there is severe bleeding from a wound to the hand. Expose the wound.

2 Control the bleeding—elevate the hand above the level of the heart and apply direct pressure. The casualty can use his other hand to apply direct pressure while you locate a first aid kit. Bandage dressings in place.

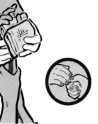

1. put a dressing over the wound and fill the palm with more dressings or a bulky pad

check the circulation in the fingers and compare it with the other hand

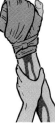

2. bend the fingers over the pad to make a fist and bandage the hand so the fist is held firmly closed

place the middle of a narrow triangular bandage on the inside of the wrist and bring the ends around the back of the hand

3. wrap the bandage over the fingers and around the wrist tightly, but not so tight as to cut off circulation

4. leave the thumb exposed, if possible, to check circulation

tie the bandage off at the wrist and tuck in the ends

3 Support the injured hand and keep it elevated. Use a St. John tubular sling—see page 6-10. Recheck the circulation below the injury.

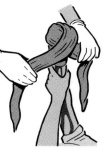

4 Give ongoing casualty care and get medical help.

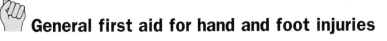

General first aid for hand and foot injuries

Hand and foot injuries are common. The following are first aid guidelines for these injuries.

1   Begin ESM—do a scene survey (see page 2-3). Expose and assess the injury.

2   Give first aid for any severe bleeding—direct pressure, elevation and rest (see page 6-16).

3   Remove any jewellery before swelling occurs.

4   For wounds without severe bleeding, brush away loose debris and cover with dressings. If there are wounds on the fingers or toes, put dressings, preferably non-stick dressings, between the fingers and toes to prevent them from sticking together.

5   If there are signs of fractures, or if there is any significant loss of function, immobilize the hand or foot as shown on pages 7-29 and 7-37.

6   Elevate the limb above the level of the heart and get medical help.

If the injury seems minor, such as a minor sprain or minor wound, and the casualty chooses not to get medical help, tell him that within 48 hours it should be obvious that the injury is well on the way to healing. If this is not the case, and there is still pain, loss of function, or perhaps an infection, tell the casualty he should get medical help to ensure there are no complications and that everything is being done to ensure a full recovery.

Pinched fingernail

When a finger, thumb or toe has been pinched, the pressure from the blood under the nail can cause great pain. You can relieve this pain as follows:

♦ place the injured part under cool running water to reduce pain and swelling

◆ if the pain is severe, and you can see pooled blood under the nail, release the pressure under the nail as follows:

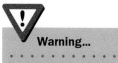

❖ straighten a paper clip and heat one end to red hot, using a stove element or the flame from a lighter— be careful not to burn yourself

❖ place the heated end of the paper clip on top of the nail and let it burn a hole to release the pooled blood

❖ once the pressure has been released, wash the area with soap and water and put on an adhesive dressing

Wounds to the eye

Sight depends on one of the most delicate and sensitive organs of the body, the eye. The eye can be injured very easily, and for this reason, extra care must be taken to protect the eyes from hazards. When an eye is injured, proper first aid given right away may prevent partial or complete loss of eyesight.

Particles in the eye

A particle of sand, grit or a loose eyelash on the eyeball or under the eyelid causes discomfort and inflammation of the tissue around the eye. When this happens, the eye becomes a character- istic pink or reddish colour. Tears may not be enough to loosen and wash away such particles.

 ### First aid to remove a particle from the upper eyelid

pull the upper lid over the lower lid, then let go

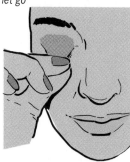

Begin by using the lashes of the lower eyelid to sweep away the particle from the upper eyelid. Tell the casualty to gently hold the eyelashes of the upper eyelid and pull the lid straight out and then down and over the lower eyelid. Let go of the eyelashes. The lashes of the lower lid may sweep away the particle as the upper lid slides over the lower lid.

Try this a couple of times. If it doesn't work, expose the inner surface of the eyelid to locate and remove the loose particle.

1   Begin ESM—do a scene survey (see page 2-3). Wash your hands or put gloves on (if available).

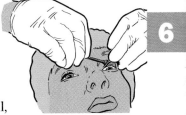

2   Seat the casualty facing a good light. Steady the head and ask the casualty to look down.

> If the casualty is wearing contact lenses, have her remove the lens before trying to remove a particle from the eye.

3   Expose the upper eyelid—place the stick of a cotton-tipped applicator at the base of the upper lid. Press the lid gently backwards.

4   Gently hold the upper eyelashes between the thumb and index finger.

5   Pull the lid away from the eye and up and over the stick. Roll the stick back to turn the eyelid outward and expose the underside.

6   If you can see the particle, and it is not on the coloured part of the eye or sticking to the eyeball, remove it with the moist corner of a facial tissue, clean cloth or a cotton-tipped applicator.

7   Let the upper eyelid return to its proper position. If the pain and discomfort don't go away, put a dressing on the eye (see page 6-38) and get medical help.

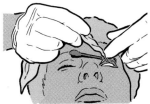

First aid for removing a particle from the lower eyelid

1   Begin ESM—do a scene survey (see page 2-3). Wash hands or put gloves on (if available). Seat the casualty facing a light.

2   Gently draw the lower eyelid down and away from the eyeball while the casualty rolls the eye upward.

3   Wipe the particle away with the moist corner of a facial tissue, clean cloth or a cotton-tipped applicator.

> **Warning...**
>
> Don't try to remove a particle from the eye if it:
> - is embedded in the eyeball or surrounding tissue
> - is sticking to the eyeball
> - cannot be seen—even though the eye is inflamed and painful
>
> See page 6-38 for what to do.

6

First aid for removing a particle from the eyeball

1   Begin ESM—do a scene survey (see page 2-3). Wash hands or put gloves on (if available).

2   Shine a light across the eye, not directly into it—the light will often cast a shadow of the particle, showing its location.

3   If the particle is loose, and not on the cornea, remove it with the moist corner of a facial tissue or clean cloth. If the light fails to locate a particle in the eye, do not continue—further attempts to find and remove the particle may aggravate the eye.

4   Bandage the injured eye as described below.

First aid when you cannot safely remove a particle from the eye

1   Begin ESM—do a scene survey (see page 2-3). Wash hands or put on gloves (if available).

2   Warn the casualty not to rub the eye because this may cause pain and tissue damage.

3   Close the casualty's eye and cover the affected eye with an eye or gauze pad. Extend the covering to the forehead and cheek to avoid pressure on the eye.

4   Secure lightly in position with a bandage or adhesive strips.

5   Give ongoing casualty care and get medical help.

⚠ Do not cover both eyes

Cover only one eye (the most seriously injured eye) to avoid the psychological stress that the casualty may suffer when both eyes are covered. If both eyes must be covered due to serious injury, (e.g. intense light burn from arc welding), reassure the casualty often by explaining what is being done and why.

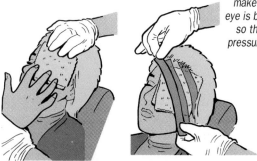

make sure the eye is bandaged so there is no pressure on the eyeball

Wounds in the soft tissue around the eye

Wounds to the eyelid and soft tissue around the eye are serious because there may be injury to the eyeball. If the eyeball is not damaged, vision should not be impaired once the wounds have healed.

Blows from blunt objects may cause bruises and damage the bones that surround and protect the eyes. Blows like this may also rupture the blood vessels of the eye and damage internal eye structures, causing loss of vision. Wounds from sharp objects penetrating the eyeball are serious because of the internal damage they can cause and the infection that can result.

First aid for lacerations and bruises around the eye

Lacerated eyelids usually bleed profusely because of their rich blood supply. A dressing on the area will usually control bleeding. Never apply pressure to the eyeball—this may force fluid out of the eyeball and cause permanent damage to the eye.

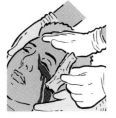 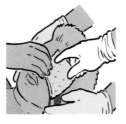 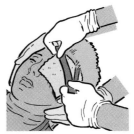

First aid for an embedded object in or near the eyeball

Give first aid for an embedded object in or near the eyeball as for any embedded object—leave the object where it is, stop the bleeding and get medical help. Prevent the embedded object from moving since movement could cause further damage to the eyeball.

1   Begin ESM—do a scene survey (see page 2-3). Lay the casualty down and, if available, have a bystander support the head to reduce movement. Wash your hands or put gloves on (if available).

2   Place a dressing, preferably sterile, around the embedded
object. Place padding or dressings around the object in a
"log cabin" fashion, to stabilize the object.

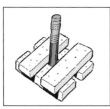

"log cabin" method

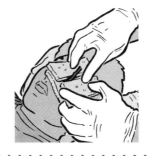

use dressings or
padding to stabilize
the embedded
object

6

3   There are different ways to hold the dressings in place and
to prevent movement of the embedded object. If available,
a drinking cup may work well to hold dressings in place
and protect the object. Two ways to secure the cup are
shown below:

if you have tape
available, tape the
cup into place

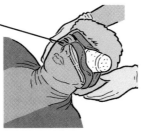

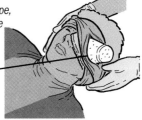

if you don't have tape,
hold the cup in place
with a triangular
bandage

slit a narrow
bandage down the
centre and place
this over the cup

If you don't have a drinking cup, a ring pad can be used to
hold dressings in place, as shown below:

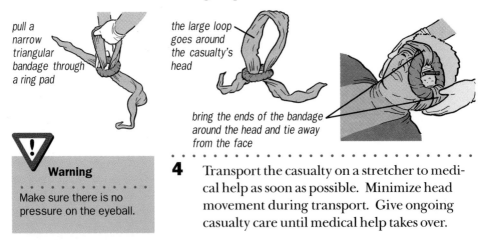

pull a
narrow
triangular
bandage through
a ring pad

the large loop
goes around
the casualty's
head

bring the ends of the bandage
around the head and tie away
from the face

Warning

Make sure there is no
pressure on the eyeball.

4   Transport the casualty on a stretcher to medical help as soon as possible. Minimize head
movement during transport. Give ongoing
casualty care until medical help takes over.

First aid for an extruded eyeball

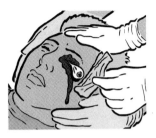

When the eyeball has been thrust out of its socket, it is called "extruded." Do not try to put the eye back into position.

1   Begin ESM—do a scene survey (see page 2-3). Lay the casualty down, and if available, have a bystander support the head to reduce movement. Wash your hands or put gloves on (if available).

2   Gently cover the eyeball and socket with a moist dressing. Hold this in place with tape and more dressings, or use the cup and ring pad bandage shown in step 3 on the opposite page.

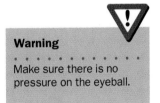

3   Place the casualty face up on a stretcher with the head immobilized for transportation to medical help.

4   Serious injury may result if the casualty is not kept quiet and is not moved carefully by stretcher. Give ongoing casualty care until handover.

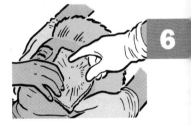

Warning

Make sure there is no pressure on the eyeball.

When and how to use cold on injuries

Applying cold to an injury is generally good first aid and you should do it as soon as possible following the guidelines below.

Use cold:

◆ as soon as possible after an injury has taken place

◆ when pain, swelling and bruising are the dominant factors, as in strains, sprains, bruises, dislocations, or when muscle spasm is present e.g. a "charley horse"

◆ for up to 48 hours after injury

Do not use cold:

◆ on an open injury

◆ if circulation below the injury is impaired or the casualty has known circulatory disorders

◆ if the skin at the injury site is "tented" by pressure from broken bones under the skin

◆ if the casualty is unconscious or semi-conscious, since she cannot tell you if discomfort or frostbite occurs

◆ if the casualty is sensitive to cold (ask the casualty about this) or if the cold causes hives to appear.

Different ways to apply cold

Use a **cold compress**. Soak a towel in cold water, wring out the excess water and wrap the towel around the injured part.

add water to the compress from time to time, or replace it with a fresh one

Use an **ice bag**. Make one by filling a rubber or plastic bag two-thirds full of crushed ice, forcing out any excess air from the bag, and sealing the opening to make it watertight. Wrap the bag in a towel and apply it carefully to the injured part. Replace the ice as necessary.

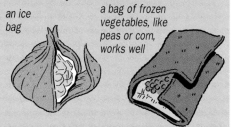

an ice bag

a bag of frozen vegetables, like peas or corn, works well

Use a **commercial cold pack**. Follow the manufacturer's directions to activate the chemicals that make it cold. Wrap the cold pack in a towel before applying it to the injured area. Caution must be used, as these sometimes leak.

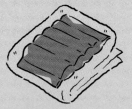

How to use cold

Put the cold compress, ice bag or cold pack on the injured area (with a cloth between the skin and the ice bag or cold pack). Leave the cold in place for 15 minutes. Then take the cold off for 15 minutes. This will help to avoid the casualty suffering frostbite. Repeat this 15-minutes-on 15-minutes-off cycle for the first 48 hours following the injury.

Cold works best when used with rest, compression and elevation—see RICE, page 7-7. Always be alert for signs for frostbite.

FOCUS ON SAFETY

Preventing wounds and bleeding

Wounds are often the result of poor safety practices while using machinery, tools and equipment. The majority of injuries occur in the home and during recreation. Prevent soft tissue injury by eliminating the hazards from the environment. A *what if* approach[*] will help prevent many such injuries. Be safety conscious—think of the consequences:

◆ *what if* knives are stored in a drawer, sharp side up?

◆ *what if* someone uses his fingers to reach into food processors and grinders?

◆ *what if* chain saws, lawnmowers, hedge trimmers, etc. are used without safety guards or personal safety equipment?

◆ *what if* children are allowed to use chain saws and snowblowers?

◆ *what if* helmets, masks, gloves etc. are not worn when playing a hazardous sports?

◆ *what if* guns and ammunition are stored together in an unlocked area?

◆ *What if* guns are left loaded?

Farm tools and machines can be extremely hazardous since they are frequently operated in poor weather conditions, on rough terrain, in poor light and by overtired, untrained or inexperienced people. Adjusting and clearing power takeoffs (PTOs) on tractors while the engine is running has caused many serious injuries. The operator must ensure that the guard remains in place until the power is off and the equipment stops.

Awareness of potential dangers in the home, in industry and on the farm, and a personal commitment to safe practices, can eliminate many causes of injury.

[*] Industrial Accident Prevention Association. *Hazards Recognition and Control Seminar HRC 004*, November 1986.

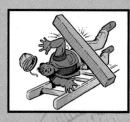

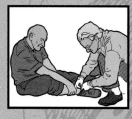

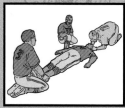

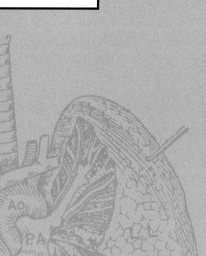

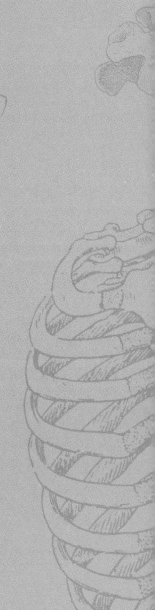

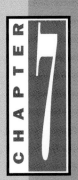

Injuries to Bones, Joints and Muscles

....

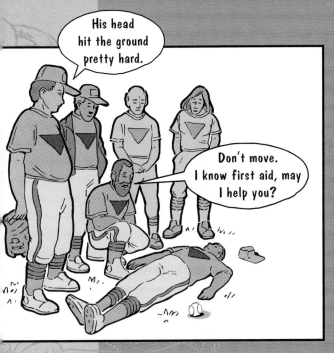

His head hit the ground pretty hard.

Don't move. I know first aid, may I help you?

◆ Introduction

◆ General first aid for injuries to bones and joints

◆ RICE

◆ Head injuries

◆ Spinal injuries

◆ Using hard cervical collars

◆ Immobilizing a fractured pelvis

◆ Splinting materials

◆ Strains

◆ Repetitive strain injury (RSI)

◆ Preventing bone, joint and muscle injuries

Introduction

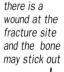

the body has 206 bones

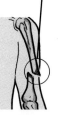

Injuries to bones, joints and muscles can range from minor to very severe. These injuries are common and, as a first aider, you will likely encounter them. Although injuries to bones, joints and muscles are usually not life threatening, they can be painful, debilitating, and can cause life-long aggravation, disability and deformity. Appropriate first aid for these injuries can make the injury more bearable for the casualty and reduce the chances of lifelong effects from the injury.

This chapter describes different types of bone, joint and muscle injuries and the appropriate first aid. The functions of bones, joints and muscles are described in chapter 16, *The body and how it works.*

Injuries to bones

there is a wound at the fracture site and the bone may stick out

Bones break, and broken bones are your concern as a first aider. A break or crack in a bone is called a **fracture**. A fracture is either closed or open:

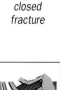

◆ a **closed fracture** is where the skin over the fracture is not broken

◆ an **open fracture** is where the skin over the fracture is broken—this could cause serious infection, even if the wound is very small

open fracture   *closed fracture*

Other terms are used to describe particular types of fractures—some of these are shown below. The first aider often cannot determine the type of fracture that has occurred.

| | | |  | | | 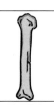 |

depression fracture—skull is fractured inward

complicated fracture—broken bone has caused damage to internal organs

transverse fracture—bone is broken straight across

spiral fracture—bone is broken by twisting

oblique fracture—bone is broken on a steep angle

greenstick fracture—bone is not broken right through

Mechanism of injury

A fracture can be caused by a direct force, such as a blow or kick, a twisting force, or by an indirect force, such as when a bone breaks some distance from the spot where the force is applied. For example, the collarbone can be fractured by falling on an out-stretched arm. Muscular action can also cause fractures. For example, a fracture of the patella (kneecap) can occur from a violent contraction of the muscles attached to it. Certain bone diseases, such as osteoporosis, make bones very brittle and they can break without much force.

Signs and symptoms of a fracture

One or more of the following signs and symptoms will be present when a bone is fractured:

- pain and tenderness—it is worse when the injury is touched or moved

- loss of function—the casualty cannot use the injured part

- a wound—the bone ends may be sticking out

- deformity—any unnatural shape or unnatural position of a bone or joint

- unnatural movement

- shock—this increases with the severity of the injury

- crepitus—a grating sensation or sound that can often be felt or heard when the broken ends of bone rub together (don't test for this)

- swelling and bruising—fluid accumulates in the tissues around the fracture

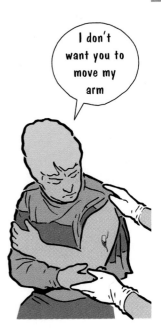

Injuries to joints

A joint is where two or more bones come together. Joints allow the bones to move relative to each other. Joints may be injured when the bones and surrounding tissues are forced to move beyond their normal range. When a joint is forced to move more than it should,

the bones at a joint are held together by tough bands called ligaments

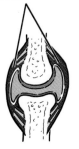

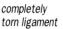

completely torn ligament

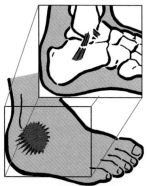

the following can happen:

◆ the bones may break, resulting in a **fracture**

◆ the ligaments may stretch and tear, resulting in a **sprain**

◆ the bone ends may move out of proper position relative to each other, resulting in a **dislocation**

Sprains

A **sprain** is an injury to a ligament. A first-degree sprain is a stretched ligament; a second-degree sprain is a partly torn ligament; and, a third-degree sprain is a completely torn ligament. Without specialized training it is difficult to determine the degree of a sprain—be cautious and give first aid as if the injury is serious. Sprains of the wrist, ankle, knee and shoulder are most common.

The signs and symptoms of sprains may include:

◆ pain that may be severe and increase with movement of the joint

◆ loss of function

◆ swelling and discoloration

Dislocations

When the bone surfaces that come together at a joint are no longer in proper contact, the joint is said to be **dislocated**. A dislocation stretches and tears the fibrous capsule that holds the joint together.

A dislocation can be caused by a severe twist of a joint or by indirect force. The joints most frequently dislocated are the shoulder, elbow, thumb, finger, lower jaw and knee. A shoulder, for example, may be dislocated by a fall on the elbow or on the outstretched arm. Occasionally, a sudden muscular contraction will cause a dislocation. A dislocated bone can put pressure on nearby blood vessels and impair or cut off circulation below the injury—this is a serious complication of dislocation that the first aider should look for.

Signs and symptoms of a dislocation

The signs and symptoms of a dislocation are similar to those of a fracture, and may include:

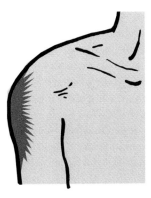

- ◆ deformity or abnormal appearance, a dislocated shoulder may make the arm look longer

- ◆ pain and tenderness aggravated by movement

- ◆ loss of normal function; the joint may be "locked" in one position

- ◆ swelling of the joint

General first aid for injuries to bones and joints

Below is general first aid for injuries to bones and joints. The methods of immobilizing different bones and joints follow this general approach.

The aims of first aid for bone and joint injuries are to prevent further tissue damage and to reduce pain.

1 Begin ESM—do a scene survey (see page 2-3). Assess the mechanism of injury. If you suspect a head or spinal injury, call for medical help, then steady and support the head before continuing.

2 Do a primary survey (see page 2-5) and give first aid for life-threatening injuries.

3 Steady and support any obvious fractures or dislocations found in the primary survey (during the rapid body check). Dress any obvious wounds to prevent further contamination. Protect any protruding bones.

4 Do a secondary survey to the extent needed. When you find a bone or joint injury, carefully and gently expose the injured area. You may have to cut clothing to

Cautions

- ◆ All fractures, dislocations and sprains should be immobilized before the casualty is moved, unless the casualty is in immediate danger.

- ◆ Check circulation below the injury site before and after immobilizing (see page 6-18 for how to do this). If circulation is impaired before immobilizing, the casualty needs medical help urgently. If circulation is impaired after immobilizing, loosen tight bandages.

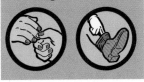

Warnings

◆ Do not give a casualty with a fracture anything to drink, this could complicate medical treatment. If the casualty complains of thirst, moisten his lips with a damp cloth.

◆ Only straighten injured joints as far as you can without causing increased pain or until there is resistance. Splint the limb in the most comfortable position if it won't straighten easily.

7

More information on:

head injuries 7-8

skull injuries 7-9

facial bones and jaw 7-9

spinal injuries 7-13

pelvis fracture 7-20

rib and breastbone
    injuries 7-21

collarbone/shoulder
    blade injuries 7-22

joint dislocation 7-23

upper arm fracture 7-24

elbow injuries 7-25

forearm/wrist 7-27

hand injury 7-29

finger/thumb injuries 7-30

upper leg fracture 7-31

knee injury 7-33

lower leg fracture 7-34

ankle fracture/sprain 7-36

foot/toe injuries 7-37

do this without moving the injured part. Take a good look at the entire injured area to determine the extent of the injury. Look for a wound indicating an open fracture. Most open fractures have only a small wound, but there is still danger of serious infection.

Check the circulation below the injury. If circulation is impaired, medical help is needed urgently.

5 Steady and support the injured part—you can do this, a bystander can do this, or the casualty may be able to do this. Maintain support until medical help takes over, or the injury is immobilized.

6 Now decide what action is best. If medical help is on the way and will arrive soon, steady and support the injury with your hands until they arrive. If medical help will be delayed, or if the casualty needs to be transported, immobilize the injury. Consider the following when making your decision:

◆ are there other risks to the casualty? Are there risks to yourself or others?

◆ if medical help can get to the scene, how long will it take?

◆ do you have the materials needed to properly immobilize the injury?

◆ how long will it take to immobilize the injury compared to how long it will take for medical help to arrive?

7 Apply cold and compression to the injury, as appropriate, and elevate the injured part— see *RICE*, opposite page.

8 Give ongoing casualty care until medical help arrives. Monitor circulation below the injury site.

Use *RICE* for injuries to bones, joints and muscles

Most injuries to bones, joints and muscles benefit from **RICE**, which stands for:

◆ **R**est

◆ **I**ce

◆ **C**ompression

◆ **E**levation

Rest means stopping the activity that caused the injury and staying off it until a doctor tells you it's O.K. For a minor injury, gentle use of the injured part is okay provided you can easily tolerate the pain.

Ice means applying cold to the injury as soon as you can once the injury has been immobilized. The cold narrows the blood vessels, reducing pain, swelling and bruising. Use a commercial cold pack, an improvised ice pack or a cold compress— see page 6-42 for more about using cold.

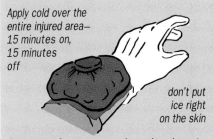

Apply cold over the entire injured area— 15 minutes on, 15 minutes off

don't put ice right on the skin

Compression means using a bandage to apply compression to the injury. This will help limit swelling. An elasticized roller bandage works well, if put on the right way. To put on an elasticized roller bandage:

◆ start about 5 cm below the injury

◆ wrap towards the injury, overlapping by 1/3 of the bandage width with each wrap

◆ start with the bandage quite tight, but not so tight that the circulation is cut off. As you wrap over and above the injury, gradually reduce the tightness of the bandage

◆ wrap the bandage to about 5 cm above the injury

After you secure the bandage, check to see if the circulation has been cut off:

◆ ask the casualty if it feels too tight

◆ use the nailbed test (see page 6-18) and check the skin temperature and colour below the injury . Compare it to the other limb if possible

Recheck circulation every few minutes as swelling may cause the bandage to become too tight. If the bandage is too tight, rewrap the injury using less compression.

Elevation means raising the injured part— preferably to a level above the heart. Elevation helps to reduce swelling and makes it easier for fluids to drain away from the injury. This in turn, helps reduce swelling (don't elevate a "locked" joint).

When to use RICE

Use RICE while waiting for medical help to arrive or while transporting a casualty to medical help. RICE is especially useful for minor sprains and strains when the casualty is not convinced the injury is bad enough to see a doctor. Even the most minor injuries will benefit from RICE.

RICE warnings

◆ Do not put an ice bag directly on the skin; always have a layer of cloth between the ice and the skin.

◆ Do not use cold when there is an open wound or if the skin is "tented" or pushed up from underneath by an injured bone.

◆ Do not use ice if the casualty is sensitive to the cold—ask the casualty if she is sensitive to cold and check for a skin reaction, such as a rash or blisters.

◆ Do not use compression on a fracture, or if the casualty has a disease of the blood vessels or diabetes.

Head injuries

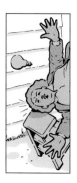

A "head injury" refers to a serious injury of the head where brain function is, or may be, affected. Head injuries include skull fractures, brain concussion and brain compression. Such injuries are frequently complicated by unconsciousness. Fractures at the base of the skull often involve injury to the cervical spine. For this reason, when you suspect a head injury, you should also suspect a neck injury.

Signs and symptoms of head injuries

The following signs and symptoms indicate a possible fracture of the skull or facial bones, concussion or compression

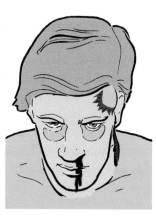

deformed skull

swollen, bruised or bleeding scalp

straw-coloured fluid or blood coming from the nose or ear(s)

bruising below the eyes (black eye) or behind the ears

nausea, vomiting, especially in children

confused, dazed

semi-conscious or unconscious

stopped breathing

very slow pulse rate

pupils are of unequal size

pain at the injury site

weakened or paralysed arms and/or legs

pain when swallowing or moving the jaw

wounds in the mouth

knocked-out teeth

shock

convulsions

Skull fracture

Fractures of the skull may be the result of direct force or an indirect force that is transmitted through the bones. Fractures may occur in the cranium, at the base of the skull, or in the face. Facial fractures include the nose, the bones around the eyes, the upper jaw and the lower jaw. Fractures of the jaw are often complicated by wounds inside the mouth.

different sites of skull fractures

First aid for head injury, including fracture of the skull

Warning
. . . .
An unconscious casualty with a head injury may vomit. Be ready to turn the casualty to the side (as a unit if possible) and clear the airway quickly.

First aid for fractures of the skull depends on the fracture site and the signs. Whenever there is a skull fracture, a spinal injury should be suspected—give first aid as if there was a fractured neck. The head and neck should be immobilized accordingly.

1   Begin ESM—start the scene survey (see page 2-3). When you recognize that there may be a head injury, tell the casualty not to move and get medical help. Steady and support the head with your hands as soon as possible.

2   Assess responsiveness and do a primary survey (see page 2-5). If there is no breathing, open the airway using the jaw-thrust without head-tilt (see page 4-22) and give AR if required.

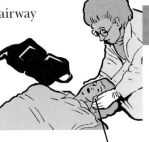

3   If blood or fluid is coming from the ear canal, secure a sterile dressing lightly over the ear, making sure fluids can drain.

4   Protect areas of depression, lumps, bumps, or scalp wounds where an underlying skull fracture is suspected. Use thick, compressible, soft dressings bandaged in place. Avoid pressure on the fracture site.

lightly cover the ear with a sterile dressing when blood or fluid is coming from the ear canal

5   Warn the casualty not to blow her nose if there is blood or fluid coming from it. Do not restrict blood flow. Wipe away any external, trickling blood to prevent it from entering the mouth, causing breathing difficulties.

6   Give ongoing casualty care until medical help takes over (see page 7-12). If you must transport the casualty, immobilize her for a neck injury—see page 7-14.

First aid for fractures of the facial bones and jaw

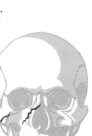

If the bones of the face or jaw are broken, assess the mechanism of injury for a head or spinal injury.

1   Begin ESM—start the scene survey (see page 2-3).

If you suspect a head injury, tell the casualty not to move and get medical help. Steady and support the head with your hands as soon as possible.

2   Do a primary survey (see page 2-5). Check the airway and make sure there is nothing in the mouth. Remove any knocked-out teeth or loose dentures and maintain drainage for blood and saliva.

3   Position the casualty. If there is no suspected head or spinal injury:

◆ place the conscious casualty in a sitting position with head well forward to allow any fluids to drain freely

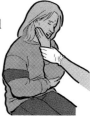

   support the jaw with a soft pad held in place by hand, not with a bandage—don't bandage the mouth closed

◆ if the casualty cannot sit comfortably, place her in the recovery position

◆ place the unconscious casualty in the recovery position. If the casualty vomits, support the jaw with the palm of your hand and turn the head to the uninjured side

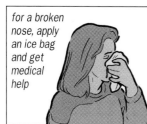

for a broken nose, apply an ice bag and get medical help

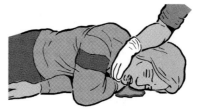

keep the jaw well forward to allow free drainage of fluids

If there is a suspected head or spinal injury, steady and support the casualty in the position found until medical help takes over, or immobilize as for a spinal injury—see page 7-14.

4   Get medical help and give ongoing casualty care. Check the casualty's level of consciousness and airway often.

If transporting the casualty on a stretcher, ensure good drainage from the mouth and nose so that breathing will not be impaired.

Concussion and compression

Concussion is a temporary disturbance of brain function usually caused by a blow to the head or neck. The casualty may become unconscious but usually for only a few moments. The casualty may say he "sees stars." Common causes of concussion include traffic collisions, falls and sports injuries. The casualty usually recovers quickly, but there is a chance of serious brain injury.

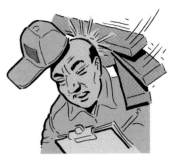

Use both the mechanism of injury and the signs and symptoms below to assess for concussion or compression.

Signs and symptoms of concussion

◆ partial or complete loss of consciousness, usually of short duration

◆ shallow breathing

◆ nausea and vomiting when regaining consciousness

◆ casualty says she is (or was) "seeing stars"

◆ loss of memory of events immediately preceding and following the injury

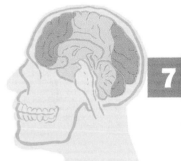

concussion results when there is a temporary disturbance of brain function, but no permanent damage

Compression is a condition of excess pressure on some part of the brain. It may be caused by a buildup of fluids inside the skull, or by a depressed skull fracture where the broken bones are putting pressure on the brain. Compression is a form of elevated intracranial pressure. For example, if a blow to the head causes bleeding in the brain, and the blood cannot drain, it builds up and puts pressure on the brain. This may happen immediately after a blow to the head, or it may take a few hours, days or even weeks for the signs of compression to show. It is very important to monitor a casualty's vital signs and look for other symptoms after a blow to the head.

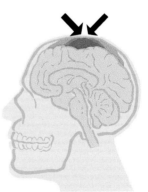

compression results from buildup of fluid inside the skull that puts pressure on the brain—this can be life-threatening

Signs of compression

The signs of compression are progressive—they usually get worse as time goes on, as more and more pressure is put on the brain.

◆ decreasing level of consciousness

◆ unconsciousness from the time of injury, may be deeply unconscious

◆ nausea and vomiting

◆ unequal size of pupils

◆ one or both pupils don't respond to light

Ongoing casualty care for head injury

When a casualty has received a blow to the head or neck that causes unconsciousness or semi-consciousness, immediately suspect a neck injury. Tell the casualty not to move, steady and support the head, and take precautions for a neck injury.

A casualty with a concussion may appear to recover quickly, but there is always the threat of serious injury. Check the casualty for signs of compression. Tell the casualty to get medical help right away for a full evaluation of the injury.

If the casualty is unconscious, place her in the recovery position, carefully supporting the head and neck during any movement. If injuries make it better for the casualty to be face up, monitor breathing continuously. If necessary, hold the airway open using the jaw-thrust without head-tilt (see page 4-22, step 3). Send for medical help and give ongoing casualty care.

Any casualty who shows signs of compression following a blow to the head, even after many days, needs medical help immediately.

Spinal injuries

The spine may be injured anywhere along its length, ,from the base of the skull to the coccyx. Injury to the spine threatens the spinal cord that runs through it and the nerves that branch out from the cord. Damage to the spinal cord or nerves can result in complete and permanent loss of feeling and paralysis below the point of injury. Injury to the spinal cord at the lower spine may affect only the legs. Damage to the spinal cord in the neck could result in paralysis of the muscles that help control chest movement in breathing. In every emergency situation, assess the possibility of a spinal injury. If it exists at all, give first aid for a spinal injury.

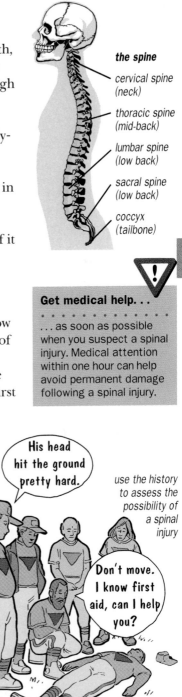

the spine

cervical spine (neck)

thoracic spine (mid-back)

lumbar spine (low back)

sacral spine (low back)

coccyx (tailbone)

7

Recognizing spinal injuries

Spinal injuries, even serious ones, often do not show obvious signs and symptoms. Rely on the history of the scene, especially the mechanism of injury, to decide if there is a chance of a spinal injury. If the history of the scene suggests a spinal injury, give first aid for a spinal injury even if the signs and symptoms below are not present.

Get medical help. . .

. . . as soon as possible when you suspect a spinal injury. Medical attention within one hour can help avoid permanent damage following a spinal injury.

Signs and symptoms of spinal injuries

His head hit the ground pretty hard.

◆ swelling and/or bruising at the site of the injury

◆ numbness, tingling or a loss of feeling in the arms and legs on one or both sides of the body

◆ not able to move arms and/or legs on one or both sides of the body

◆ pain at the injury site

◆ signs of shock—see page 1-26

use the history to assess the possibility of a spinal injury

Don't move. I know first aid, can I help you?

First aid for a head or spinal injury

The aim of first aid for spinal injuries is to prevent further injury, especially to the spinal cord. Further injury is caused by moving the injured area. The first aid is to prevent spinal movement. When moving the casualty is necessary, support her in a way that minimizes movement of the head and spine.

1 Begin ESM—start the scene survey (see page 2-3). As soon as you suspect a head or spinal injury, tell the casualty not to move.

· ·

2 Steady and support the casualty's head and neck as soon as you can—show a bystander how to do this. Show a second bystander how to steady and support the feet. The head and feet should be continuously supported until either the casualty is fully immobilized or medical help takes over.

elbows on the ground to keep arms steady

hands firmly holding the head with fingers along the line of the jaw

support the feet

· ·

3 Assess responsiveness and then do a primary survey (see page 2-5). If the casualty is unresponsive, check for breathing **before** opening the airway. If there is no breathing, open the airway using the jaw-thrust without head-tilt (see page 4-22, step 3) and check for breathing again:

◆ if breathing starts, hold the airway open with the jaw-thrust without head-tilt, or use an oropharyngeal airway—see page 7-16

◆ if there is still no breathing, give AR—see page 4-23, step 5

Check circulation— look for signs of severe bleeding and shock.

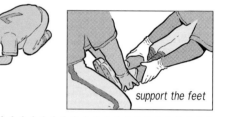

rapid body survey to check for severe bleeding

As much as possible, give first aid in the position found. But, if you cannot properly open the airway, assess breathing, or give AR, you will have to reposition the casualty. Do this quickly, but try to keep the head and neck from moving relative to each other. If there are bystanders, have them help. See page 2-8.

4   Do a secondary survey to the extent needed, but do not move the casualty or poke and probe any possible spinal injury. If you suspect a pelvic injury, don't "test for it" by squeezing the hips together.

5   Decide whether you will need to transport the casualty. If medical help will arrive at the scene, it is probably best to steady and support the casualty in the position found and give ongoing casualty care.

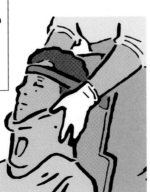

> We're just going to keep you still until the ambulance arrives...

steady and support the casualty in the position found

If medical help will be delayed, or is not available, immobilize the casualty onto a spine board—see step 6.

6   Continue to steady and support for the head and feet until the casualty is completely immobilized on a long spine board. Gather the materials and people you will need to immobilize the casualty before you begin—see sidebar.

7   If you have a hard cervical collar, and are trained to apply it, consider using it to immobilize the head and neck—see page 7-16.

hard cervical collar before it is put on

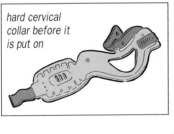

hard cervical collar on a sitting casualty

Materials for spinal immobilization

- ◆ hard cervical collar
- ◆ a full-length spine board or other rigid flat surface like a door or piece of plywood
- ◆ at least 12 triangular bandages or straps, etc.
- ◆ at least 1 blanket plus two small pillows or another blanket
- ◆ 4 people plus yourself

Using hard cervical collars

• •

The best way to immobilize the head and neck is to use a hard cervical collar. When a hard cervical collar is put on a casualty who is not fully conscious, or is at risk of losing consciousness, additional equipment is needed to keep the airway open. A first aider may use this equipment if she is properly trained and has the right equipment, in the correct sizes, available.

Hard cervical collars

The hard cervical collars used by emergency personnel, including first aiders, are especially designed for use at emergency scenes. Although they are quite simple, you need special training before using them. With training, you will learn:

♦ how to choose the right size collar

♦ how to properly move the head to align it with the neck

♦ how to put the collar on

♦ complications that may arise when using a hard cervical collar

There are different manufacturers of hard cervical collars and you should have training for the specific brand of collar you will be using.

Hard cervical collars and the airway

Before using a hard cervical collar, consider the casualty's airway. Remember that if the casualty is not fully conscious, the tongue may fall back and block the airway—and with a hard cervical collar, you won't be able to use the jaw-thrust, or even tilt the head back, to open the airway. To keep the airway open when using a hard cervical collar you need to use an oropharyngeal airway (OPA).

An OPA is a device medical professionals use to keep an unconscious person's airway open. When properly sized and inserted, an OPA prevents the tongue from blocking the airway. However, even with an OPA, saliva and other fluids may pool in the

back of the throat and block the airway. The only way to remove this fluid, while keeping the casualty face up, is with suction equipment designed specifically for use with an OPA. Only use an OPA when you have suctioning equipment available.

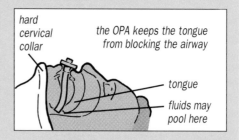

hard cervical collar — the OPA keeps the tongue from blocking the airway — tongue — fluids may pool here

When to use a hard cervical collar and OPA

First, only use this equipment if you are trained. The points below note when to use what equipment:

♦ if the casualty is fully conscious and there is no head injury or other risk of losing consciousness, use a hard cervical collar even if you don't have an OPA

♦ if the casualty is not fully conscious, or has an injury that could cause loss of consciousness, only use a hard cervical collar if you have an OPA and appropriate suctioning equipment

Remember the ABCs

• •

When using a hard cervical collar, always be aware of the risk to the airway and remember that the ABCs are the priority. In a bad situation, you may have to loosen or remove a cervical collar to keep the airway open with the jaw-thrust. You may have to turn the casualty to the side to keep fluids from blocking the airway. You must do whatever is necessary to keep the airway open and to give first aid for the ABCs.

8 Place the casualty on the spine board using the logroll, a method of rolling a casualty onto his side so the whole body moves as a unit. This reduces the chance of further tissue damage. Get the casualty ready by tying his wrists and legs together. This makes it much easier to roll him as a unit.

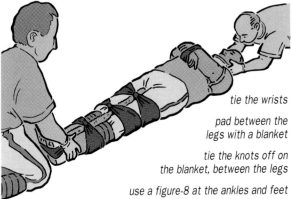

tie the wrists

pad between the legs with a blanket

tie the knots off on the blanket, between the legs

use a figure-8 at the ankles and feet

As you are preparing the casualty for transportation, keep talking to him, explaining what you are doing and why.

More on spine boards

· ·

A long spine board is usually the size shown below. It should be smooth, varnished and highly waxed so you can easily slide a casualty into position.

The long spine board is usually made of sturdy plywood. Holes along the sides and ends of the board serve as hand-holds and places to tie bandages and straps. Runners, tapered at each end and attached to the bottom of the board, make it easier to slide the board along rough surfaces. The runners also lift the board off the ground, making it easier to grasp the hand-holds.

Prepare a spine board for use by passing narrow bandages through the hand-holds as shown.

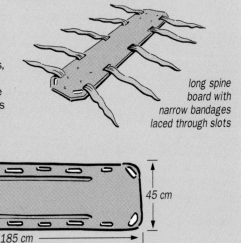

long spine board with narrow bandages laced through slots

long spine board

runners

45 cm

185 cm

9   Position the prepared spine board beside the casualty. Position the assisting rescuers and yourself (first aider) as follows.

- ◆ you, the **first aider,** will pay particular attention to the neck and upper back for the entire procedure

- ◆ rescuers should already be positioned at the head and feet

- ◆ position a rescuer beside you at the casualty's hips and upper legs

- ◆ if you have another rescuer, she can be positioned beside the spine board, ready to move it into position

the first aider controls the rescue team from his position at the casualty's shoulders

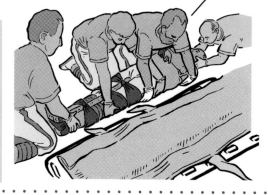

To prepare the spine board

. . . .

Lace bandages through the holes. Centre a blanket on the spine board and fold the sides toward the centre so you can move the spine board, bandages and blanket easily.

10 Give detailed instructions on how the logroll will proceed:

- ◆ tell the rescuers at the head and feet that they will apply gentle pull (traction) at the command, "pull." This traction will be maintained until the casualty is finally secured to the spine board. On the command, "roll," they will lift and turn the head and feet as the rest of the body rolls, so that the whole body turns as a unit

- ◆ tell the rescuer beside you that on the command, "roll," he will roll the casualty toward himself, using a firm grip to control the casualty

- ◆ tell the rescuer at the spine board that on the command, "spine board," she will position the spine board alongside the casualty

◆ tell the group that when the spine board is in position, you will give the command, "roll," and slowly but firmly, you will all roll the casualty back onto the spine board

Emphasize that the casualty must always be turned as a unit. Ask the rescuers if there are any questions.

11 Tell the rescuers to get ready, making sure each has a good, firm grip on the casualty. Logroll the casualty and position the spine board.

12 When the spine board is properly positioned, direct the bearers to roll the casualty back onto the board. Position the casualty in the centre of the spine board by pulling on the blanket.

13 When the casualty is positioned on the spine board, pad around the head and wrap the blanket around him. Secure him to the spine board with narrow bandages and/or ties.

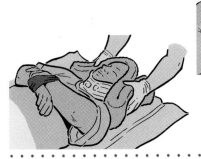

14 Give ongoing casualty care—monitor breathing often. Get medical help quickly and as smoothly as possible. Carry the spine board as explained on page 14-13.

Although a casualty with a spinal injury must be transported to medical help as soon as possible, remember that more harm may result from a fast, rough ride than from a slow, smooth one.

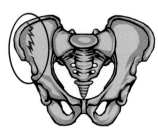

 Immobilizing a fractured pelvis

When you suspect a fractured pelvis, you should also suspect a spinal injury. If there was enough force to fracture the pelvis, the spine may also have been injured. Give first aid as you would for a spinal injury (see page 7-14) but include the following:

◆ the pelvic area may not be stable—if you suspect a pelvic injury, do not squeeze the hips together when examining the casualty

◆ if medical help is coming to the scene, steady and support the casualty in the position found

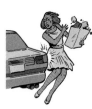

possible
mechanisms
of injury

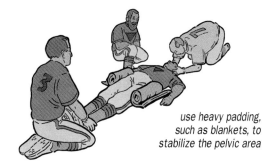

use heavy padding,
such as blankets, to
stabilize the pelvic area

Pelvic injury

Signs & symptoms

◆ signs of shock (casualty could be bleeding internally

◆ casualty cannot stand or walk

◆ urge to urinate

◆ casualty cannot urinate or there is blood in the urine

◆ sharp pain in the groin and small of the back

◆ increased pain when moving

Complications

◆ injury to the lower spine

◆ injury to the bladder that could lead to infection

◆ if the casualty will be transported:

❖ immobilize the casualty on a spine board with added support in the pelvic area

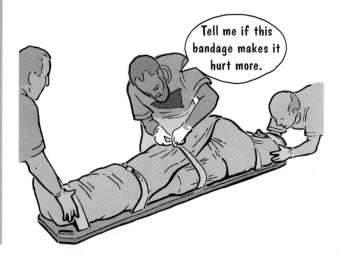

Tell me if this bandage makes it hurt more.

Other bone and joint injuries

First aid for injured ribs or breastbone

First aid for injured ribs or breastbone aims to reduce the chance of further injury, to minimize pain and to make breathing easier.

1 Start ESM—do a scene survey (see page 2-3).
Do a primary survey (see page 2-5).
Give first aid for life-threatening injuries.

2 Expose the injured area and look for a wound. If there is a wound, check for a sucking chest wound (see page 4-7). Put an appropriate dressing on the wound and get medical help quickly.

3 Place the casualty in a semisitting position, leaning slightly toward the injured side—this should help breathing. Hand support over the injured area may make breathing easier.

4 Support the arm on the injured side in a St. John tubular sling to transfer its weight to the uninjured side.

5 Give ongoing casualty care—monitor breathing often. Get medical help.

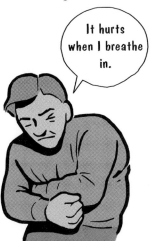

> It hurts when I breathe in.

a conscious casualty will guard the injury and say it hurts to breathe

---

Warning

A fracture of one or two ribs is very painful and causes shallow breathing, but the casualty does not usually have severe breathing difficulties, nor show signs of shock. If these are present, see 4-6 for severe breathing emergencies.

Rib or breastbone injury

Signs & symptoms

◆ pain at injury site when casualty moves, coughs or breathes deeply

◆ shallow breathing

◆ casualty guards injury

◆ deformity and discolouration

◆ may be a wound

◆ may cough up frothy blood (if lung punctured)

◆ may show signs of shock

Complications

◆ pneumothorax or tension pneumothorax

◆ punctured lung

◆ severe breathing difficulties

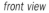

front view

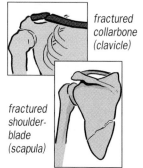

fractured collarbone (clavicle)

fractured shoulder-blade (scapula)

back view

Immobilizing a collarbone or shoulder blade*

The collarbone (clavicle) and shoulder blade (scapula) form and support the shoulder. These bones can be fractured by either direct force, like a blow to the shoulder, or by indirect force like falling on an outstretched hand. Immobilize the injury as shown below.

1   Check circulation below the injury. If circulation is impaired, get medical help quickly.

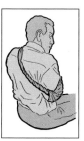

2   Immobilize the arm in the position of most comfort. A St. John tubular sling may work well—see page 6-10.

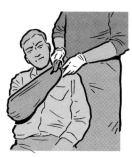

the St. John tubular sling transfers the weight of the arm to the uninjured side

---

Collarbone/shoulder blade fracture

Signs & symptoms

◆ pain at injury site
◆ swelling and deformity
◆ loss of function of the arm on the side of the injury
◆ casualty holds and protects the arm if he can, and may tilt the head to the injured side

head tilted to injured side

Complications

◆ circulation to the arm below the injury may be impaired or cut off

3   Secure the arm to the chest with a broad bandage to prevent movement of the arm.

pad under the elbow, if necessary, to keep the arm in the most comfortable position

tie the bandage on the uninjured side—don't tie it so tightly that the arm is pulled out of position

pad under the knots for comfort

4   Check circulation below the injury. If circulation is impaired, and it wasn't before, loosen the sling and bandage.

---

* This is immobilization only—also see page 7-5 *General first aid for injuries to bones and joints*

Immobilizing a dislocated joint*

Padding, bandages, slings and splints may be used to immobilize a dislocation. Usually the dislocated joint won't move very easily in any direction, and any movement causes pain. Immobilize the limb in the position of most comfort—usually the position found.

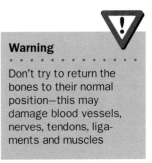

Warning

Don't try to return the bones to their normal position—this may damage blood vessels, nerves, tendons, ligaments and muscles

The illustrations below show two suggestions for immobilizing a dislocated shoulder, or the casualty may want to hold the injured arm herself. If the casualty's arm will bend into position for a St. John tubular sling, as shown on the left, this may be the most comfortable position.

if the arm will bend

use a St. John tubular sling to transfer the weight of the arm to the other side—see page 6-10

use broad bandages to prevent movement

pad under the elbow for support

if the arm will not bend

support the weight of the arm with a bandage around the neck

bandage the arm to the body to prevent movement

pad under the elbow, if necessary, to keep the arm in the most comfortable position

apply cold to the injury if possible

The success of the method you use depends on whether it stops the injured limb from moving—which causes pain and could cause further injury. Often, the "trick" is to use just the right amount of padding between the arm and body so the bandages hold the arm in the most comfortable position. Tie the bandages securely but not so tightly they put pressure on the injured limb.

Once the injury is immobilized, apply cold to help reduce pain and swelling—see page 6-42.

Monitor circulation below the injury often—check the skin colour and temperature, use the nailbed test and check for a pulse. Compare the injured side with the uninjured side. If circulation becomes impaired after immobilizing the injury, loosen the bandages. If circulation remains impaired, get medical help quickly.

check circulation below the injury

---

* This is immobilization only—also see page 7-5 *General first aid for injuries to bones and joints*

Immobilizing the upper arm*

The following shows how to immobilize an open fracture of the upper arm (humerus). Immobilize a closed fracture of the upper arm as shown in step 3.

1   Expose the injury site. Cover the wound with a sterile dressing and check circulation—see page 7-34 for more on dressing an open fracture wound.

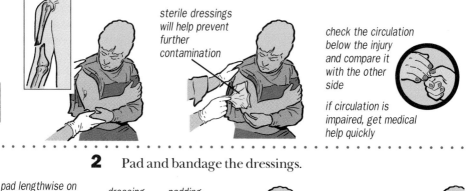

sterile dressings will help prevent further contamination

check the circulation below the injury and compare it with the other side

if circulation is impaired, get medical help quickly

2   Pad and bandage the dressings.

pad lengthwise on both sides of the fracture site

padding should be bulky enough to protect any protruding bone ends

hold padding in place with tape if needed

dressing   padding

bandage dressings tightly enough to hold padding and dressings in place

bandage shouldn't put any pressure on bone ends

3   Immobilize the arm with a sling (see page 6-9) and broad bandages.

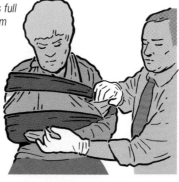

arm sling provides full support for the arm

broad bandages above and below fracture site prevent arm movement

pad under the elbow as needed to hold the arm in the position of comfort

check circulation below the injury and compare it with the other side— if it is impaired, and it wasn't before, adjust the sling and/or bandages

---

* This is immobilization only—also see page 7-5 *General first aid for injuries to bones and joints*

Immobilizing an injured elbow*

The elbow can be severely sprained, fractured or dislocated. Immobilize the injury in the position found, if possible, or in the position of greatest comfort.

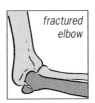

fractured elbow

1 Expose the injury and look for any open wounds. Check circulation below the injury and compare it with the other side. If circulation is impaired, get medical help quickly.

2 If the elbow is bent so the arm is in front of the chest, immobilize the arm in an arm sling—see page 6-9.

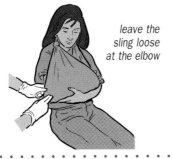

leave the sling loose at the elbow

pad under the elbow, if necessary, to keep the arm in the most comfortable position and use a broad bandage to limit movement

3 If the elbow will not bend, support the arm at the wrist and use broad bandages and padding to immobilize the arm.

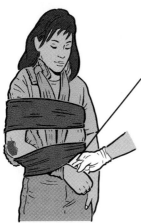

place broad bandages above and below the injury

check circulation below the injury and compare it with the other side—if it is impaired, and it wasn't before, adjust the sling and/or bandages

Injured elbow

Signs & symptoms

- ◆ pain at injury site
- ◆ swelling and deformity
- ◆ loss of function of the arm on the side of the injury
- ◆ casualty holds and protects the injury

Complications

- ◆ circulation and/or nerve function to the arm below the injury could be impaired or cut off

---

* This is immobilization only—also see page 7-5 *General first aid for injuries to bones and joints*

Splinting materials

Definition

A splint is any material used to prevent fractured bones from moving unnecessarily. Fractured arms, hands, fingers, legs, feet and toes can all be splinted.

A good splint is. . .

◆ rigid enough to support the injured limb
◆ well padded for support and comfort
◆ long enough, which means:
  – for a fracture between 2 joints, it extends beyond the joints above and below the fracture
  – for an injured joint, it's long enough for the limb to be secured so the joint can't move

There are many commercial splints available. You may have access to one of these if the incident happened at a workplace, sporting event, etc. Be trained in using these splints and follow the manufacturer's directions.

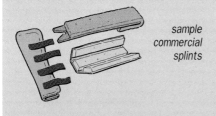

sample commercial splints

A splint can be improvised from any material, as long as it works to immobilize the injury.

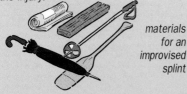

materials for an improvised splint

The casualty's own body can be used as a splint. One leg can be splinted to the other. Fingers and toes can be splinted to the next finger or toe. This is called a "natural" splint.

Other materials needed for splinting

To put the splint on you will need materials for padding and bandages.

Padding does two things:
◆ it fills in the natural hollows between the body and the splint, ensuring the injured limb is properly supported
◆ it makes the splint more comfortable

Always pad between a splint and the injured limb, and between two body parts to be bandaged together.

Bandages are used to secure the splint to the body. If you have triangular bandages, fold and use them as broad bandages (see page 6-4). When using bandages:
◆ make sure they are wide enough to provide firm support without discomfort
◆ pass them under the natural hollows of the body—go under the knee, the small of the back, the hollow behind the ankles
◆ tie them tightly enough to prevent movement, but not so tight they cut off circulation. Check circulation below any bandages you've tied every 15 minutes

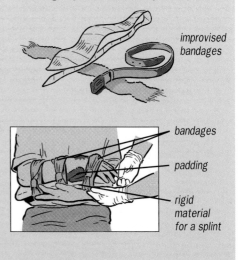

improvised bandages

bandages

padding

rigid material for a splint

Immobilizing the forearm and wrist*

Immobilize the forearm and wrist as shown below when you suspect the forearm or wrist is fractured, or the wrist is badly sprained.

1 Examine the injury and decide the best position for splinting—this is usually in the position found. Have the casualty or a bystander steady and support the injured arm as you gather and prepare the supplies you will need.

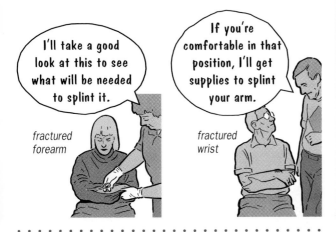

I'll take a good look at this to see what will be needed to split it.

If you're comfortable in that position, I'll get supplies to splint your arm.

fractured forearm

fractured wrist

2 Measure the splint against the uninjured arm to make sure it is the right size. Pad the splint for comfort and to support the fracture. Position the arm on the splint with as little movement as possible.

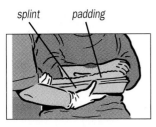

splint *padding*

this splint extends from beyond the elbow to the fingers, and is padded along the full length for firm support of the fractured arm

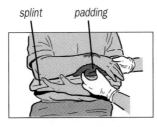

splint *padding*

this splint supports the elbow, forearm and hand, and is padded to keep the fractured wrist in the position found

Splinting helps prevent:

◆ movement of the broken bones
◆ further damage to soft tissues like nerves, the spinal cord and blood vessels
◆ a closed fracture from becoming an open fracture
◆ impaired circulation below the injury
◆ excessive bleeding into the tissues at the fracture site

Splinting also:

◆ helps to reduce pain
◆ makes transporting the casualty easier

When splinting:

◆ expose the injury before splinting so you can fully assess it
◆ check circulation below the injury both before and after splinting
◆ if not sure whether to splint an injury, splint it
◆ dress and bandage any wounds before splinting
◆ realign a severely deformed limb before splinting—see page 7-31 on when to use traction
◆ before putting a splint on, measure it against the uninjured limb
◆ don't cover wounds with splints, if possible
◆ only use commercial splints if you are trained in their use
◆ after splinting, check all the bandages and the circulation below the last bandage

7

---

3   Once the splint is in position, have the casualty or bystander support it while you secure the splint.

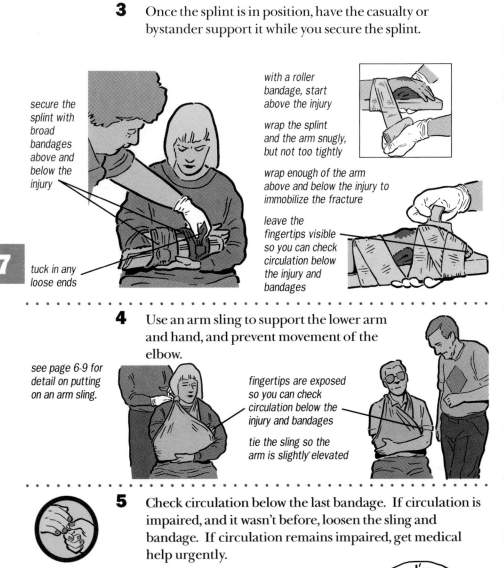

secure the splint with broad bandages above and below the injury

tuck in any loose ends

with a roller bandage, start above the injury

wrap the splint and the arm snugly, but not too tightly

wrap enough of the arm above and below the injury to immobilize the fracture

leave the fingertips visible so you can check circulation below the injury and bandages

4   Use an arm sling to support the lower arm and hand, and prevent movement of the elbow.

see page 6-9 for detail on putting on an arm sling.

fingertips are exposed so you can check circulation below the injury and bandages

tie the sling so the arm is slightly elevated

5   Check circulation below the last bandage. If circulation is impaired, and it wasn't before, loosen the sling and bandage. If circulation remains impaired, get medical help urgently.

I'm checking the circulation below the injury. If the bandages start feeling too tight, or if your hand gets cold, tell me right away.

Immobilizing an injured hand*

Immobilize an injured hand as shown below when you suspect bones in the hand are fractured.

1   Examine the injured hand and decide the best position for splinting—this is usually in the position of function (see sidebar). Have the casualty or a bystander steady and support the injury as you gather and prepare the supplies you will need. If there are open wounds, place non-stick sterile dressings between the fingers to prevent the fingers sticking together.

2   Measure the splint against the uninjured hand and arm to make sure it is the right size. Position the arm on the splint with as little movement as possible. The illustrations below show two types of splints, a pillow and a board.

Position of function

The position of function is the position the uninjured hand naturally takes. This position is safer and more comfortable than trying to flatten the hand against a flat surface.

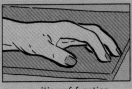

position of function

7

using a pillow

a pillow works well because:
- it lets the hand rest in the position of function
- it is padded but also firm
- it fully supports the wrist and lower arm

secure the pillow with 2 broad bandages, making sure there is no pressure on the hand

using a board

a board works well because it is rigid, but, you must use padding to keep the hand in the position of function

padding

secure the splint with a roller bandage

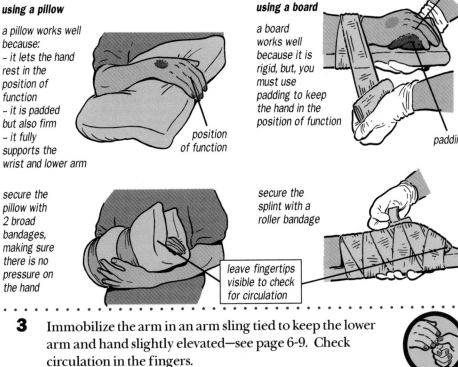

position of function

leave fingertips visible to check for circulation

3   Immobilize the arm in an arm sling tied to keep the lower arm and hand slightly elevated—see page 6-9. Check circulation in the fingers.

Immobilizing an injured finger or thumb

Immobilize a fractured or dislocated finger or thumb in the position found.

1 Expose the injury. Check the circulation below the injury.

2 Immobilize the finger in the position of most comfort, which is usually the position of function. Use a splint, as shown below, or if a splint is not available, secure the injured finger to the uninjured finger beside it.

fractured finger *fractured thumb*

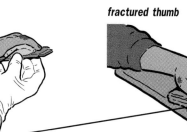

use padding to support the injured finger in the position of function

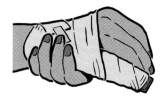

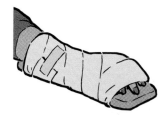

3 Put on a tubular sling to keep the injury elevated. Be careful not to put pressure on the injury. Check circulation below the injury.

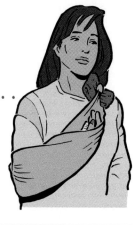

4 Give ongoing casualty care and get medical help.

Immobilizing an injured upper leg (femur)*

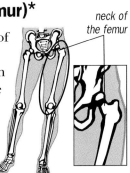

neck of
the femur

A common fracture of the upper leg is a break at the neck of the femur. This is often referred to as a broken hip, and most commonly happens to elderly people during a fall. In a younger, healthy person, great force is needed to fracture the upper leg—always assess for a head or spinal injury.

1   If you suspect a fractured upper leg, realign the leg and show a bystander how to maintain gentle, firm traction.

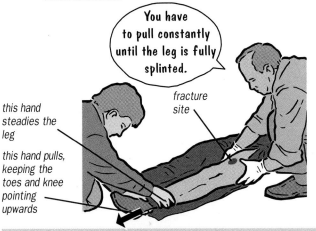

You have to pull constantly until the leg is fully splinted.

this hand steadies the leg

this hand pulls, keeping the toes and knee pointing upwards

fracture site

Fractured upper leg

Signs & symptoms
- pain, perhaps severe
- the foot and leg roll outward
- deformity and shortening of the leg

Complications
- there can be internal bleeding, causing severe shock

Traction in first aid

When a bone breaks, the muscles attached to it contract. This can cause the broken ends to slip past one another and lodge in surrounding tissue, causing further pain and damage to muscles, nerves and blood vessels. This muscular action is a particular problem in leg fractures because the leg muscles are so strong. To minimize this, traction is used in first aid for leg fractures.

Traction means a gentle, firm pull on the leg below the fracture. When traction is needed it is best applied by two people—one supporting the limb above the fracture and the other gently but firmly pulling below the fracture to bring the limb into alignment. Also use traction to realign a fractured limb that is severely deformed. **Never use traction for an injury at or near a joint.**

Take the following precautions when applying traction:

- check circulation below the injury before and after applying traction
- apply only enough traction to align the limb and to relieve the pressure of the broken bone ends on nerves and muscles. More traction may be needed to realign a severely deformed limb, but do not use force. If the limb doesn't move easily, or if pain increases, stop traction and immobilize in the deformed position
- once traction is started it has to be continued until the fracture is fully immobilized with a splint

Tell whoever takes over that traction has been applied.

---

* This is immobilization only—also see page 7-5 *General first aid for injuries to bones and joints*

2 Choose one of the splinting techniques shown below. Gather the splinting materials. Measure the splint(s) against the uninjured leg. Put bandages into position.

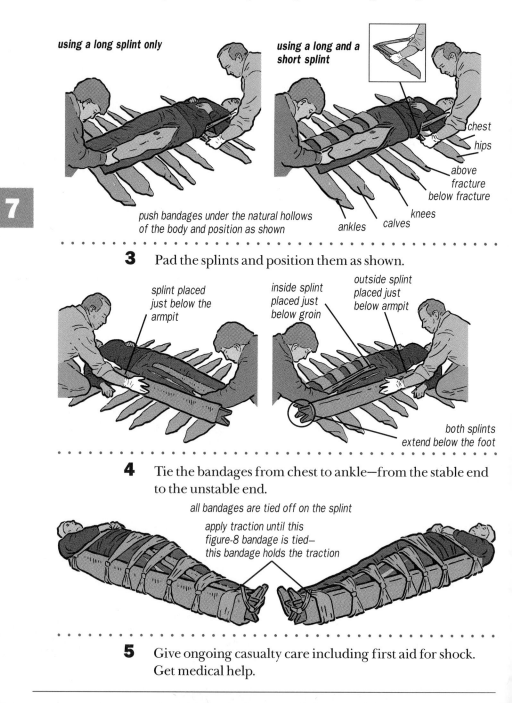

using a long splint only

using a long and a short splint

chest

hips

above fracture

below fracture

push bandages under the natural hollows of the body and position as shown

knees

ankles   calves

3 Pad the splints and position them as shown.

splint placed just below the armpit

inside splint placed just below groin

outside splint placed just below armpit

both splints extend below the foot

4 Tie the bandages from chest to ankle—from the stable end to the unstable end.

all bandages are tied off on the splint

apply traction until this figure-8 bandage is tied— this bandage holds the traction

5 Give ongoing casualty care including first aid for shock. Get medical help.

Immobilizing an injured knee

Have a bystander steady and support the injured leg. Expose and assess the injury. If the leg is straight, splint as shown below. If the leg is bent, try to straighten it. Depending on the injury, the casualty may be able to straighten the leg with your help. With a more severe injury, gently move the leg into a straightened position. If the leg won't straighten (see warning box), splint the leg in the position found.

Warnings

Don't use any traction on a knee injury.

Don't straighten the leg if:
◆ the pain increases
◆ the leg doesn't move easily

If the leg is straight

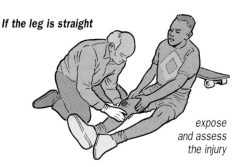

expose
and assess
the injury

If the leg is bent

expose
and assess
the injury

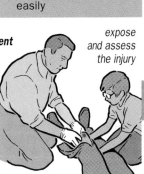

7

carefully lift the injured leg and position a padded splint

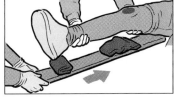

position five broad bandages under the leg—two above the knee and three below

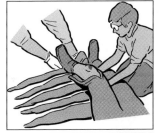

adjust the pads to fit the natural hollows of the leg

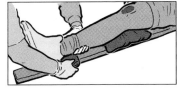

position padded splints on the inside and outside of the leg

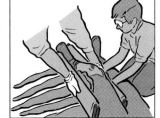

secure the splint with 2 broad bandages and a figure-8 at the ankle

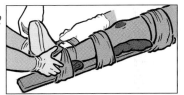

secure the splint with the bandages, keeping the leg in the bent position

* This is immobilization only—also see page 7-5 *General first aid for injuries to bones and joints*

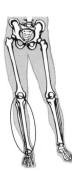

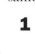 # Immobilizing a fractured lower leg (tibia and/or fibula)

A fractured lower leg is a common sports injury. The example here shows an open fracture. Immobilize a closed fracture the same way but without the dressings and bandages over the wound.

1   Expose the injury. Here the first aider discovers the injury is an open fracture.

clothing is removed by cutting to minimize movement of the injured leg

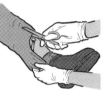

a fracture is "open" when the skin is broken— the bone may stick out

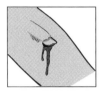

2   Show a bystander how to steady and support the leg, and apply gentle traction. Check the circulation below the injury. Give first aid for the open fracture wound.

cover the wound with a sterile dressing

the dressing should extend well beyond the edges of the wound

leave the shoe on unless there is a wound to be examined

traction is applied from the heel

put bulky padding lengthwise on both sides of the fracture, over the dressing, to protect the bone end

it may help to tape the padding in place

dressing

⚠ Dressing an open fracture wound

When there is an open fracture, give first aid for the wound first and then immobilize the fracture. For the wound, apply a sterile dressing to prevent further contamination. To stop bleeding from the wound, apply pressure around the fracture, but not on it. Apply a dressing with padding on both sides of the fracture site. Secure this with a broad bandage tied tightly enough to put pressure on the padding. Always check circulation before and after dressing a wound of this type.

tie a broad bandage over the padding and dressing tightly enough to put pressure on the padding, but not tight enough to cut off circulation—check circulation below the injury once the bandage is tied

make sure there is no pressure on the bone ends

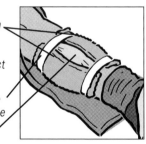

---

* This is immobilization only—also see page 7-5 *General first aid for injuries to bones and joints*

3 Immobilize the lower leg. Position the bandages and splints.

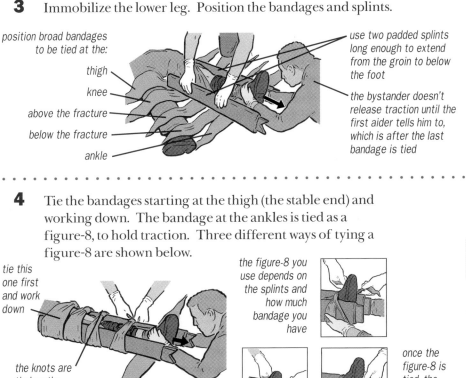

position broad bandages
to be tied at the:

thigh

knee

above the fracture

below the fracture

ankle

use two padded splints
long enough to extend
from the groin to below
the foot

the bystander doesn't
release traction until the
first aider tells him to,
which is after the last
bandage is tied

4 Tie the bandages starting at the thigh (the stable end) and working down. The bandage at the ankles is tied as a figure-8, to hold traction. Three different ways of tying a figure-8 are shown below.

tie this
one first
and work
down

the knots are
tied on the
splint for
comfort

the figure-8 you
use depends on
the splints and
how much
bandage you
have

once the
figure-8 is
tied, the
bystander can
release the
traction

5 Check the circulation below the injury, elevate the injured leg and give ongoing casualty care. Get medical help.

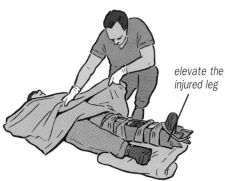

elevate the
injured leg

If you don't have splints. . .

. . .use the uninjured leg as a "natural" splint by tying the legs together.

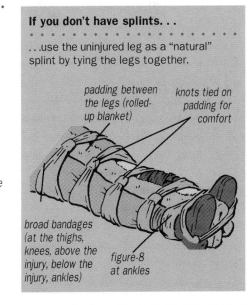

padding between
the legs (rolled-
up blanket)

knots tied on
padding for
comfort

broad bandages
(at the thighs,
knees, above the
injury, below the
injury, ankles)

figure-8
at ankles

Immobilizing an injured ankle

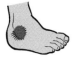

The ankle should be immobilized whenever you suspect a sprain or a fracture. If you suspect a serious injury, including an open fracture, immobilize the lower leg as shown on page 7-34. If the injury doesn't seem serious, or if the journey to medical help will be smooth, use a blanket splint or pillow splint to immobilize the ankle, as shown below.

1   Check circulation below the injury. If circulation is impaired see page 6-18.

2   Loosen footwear and immobilize the ankle.

blanket/pillow splint

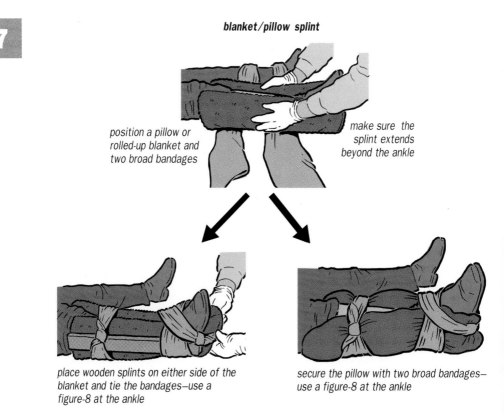

position a pillow or rolled-up blanket and two broad bandages

make sure the splint extends beyond the ankle

place wooden splints on either side of the blanket and tie the bandages—use a figure-8 at the ankle

secure the pillow with two broad bandages— use a figure-8 at the ankle

3   Check circulation below the injury. Elevate the injured limb and apply cold—see RICE, page 7-7. Give ongoing casualty care and get medical help.

---

* This is immobilization only—also see page 7-5 *General first aid for injuries to bones and joints*

Immobilizing an injured foot or toe

1   Check circulation below the injury. If circulation is impaired, get medical help quickly.

2   Immobilize the ankle using a double figure-8.

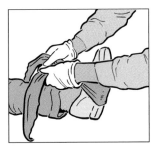

1. untie shoe laces and tie the first figure-8 beginning at the sole of the foot and tying toward the leg

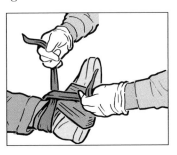

2. tie the second figure-8 by wrapping the ends around the leg, crossing in front of the ankle and tying off on the sole of the foot

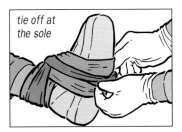

tie off at the sole

3. every few minutes ask the casualty if the bandage feels tight—this may happen as the injured area swells

Immobilizing a toe

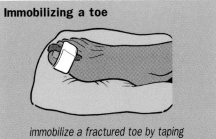

immobilize a fractured toe by taping it to an adjacent, uninjured toe

When is medical help needed?

It is always safest to get medical help for any injury. Injuries that appear minor can be more serious than they seem, and minor injuries can benefit from medical treatment.

First aiders may be in the awkward position of trying to convince a casualty to get medical help. The following points indicate when all activity should be stopped and medical help consulted.

Stop activity and get medical help when:

◆ there is any loss in the range of motion, meaning the injured area doesn't move the way it usually does

◆ the casualty complains of pain during normal activity

This means if the casualty limps, favours the injured side, or shows any sign of injury, medical help should be consulted.

* This is immobilization only—also see page 7-5 *General first aid for injuries to bones and joints*

Strains

When a muscle or tendon is over-stretched or forcefully short-ened, it can result in a stretch or tear injury, called a *strain*. This injury is called a strain. There are different degrees of strains, from mildly uncomfortable to disabling, but it is difficult for a first aider to determine the exact degree of a strain. Muscles strains of the lower back are common.

Signs and symptoms

The signs and symptoms of a strain often show up many hours after the injury.

◆ sudden sharp pain in the strained muscle

◆ swelling of the muscles causing severe cramps (e.g. charley horse)

◆ bruising and muscle stiffness

◆ casualty may not be able to use the affected body part (loss of function)

First aid for strains

1   Begin ESM—do a scene survey (see page 2-3). Have the casualty stop the activity that caused the injury.

2   Place the casualty in a position of comfort and assess the injury. If there is loss of function, immobilize the injury as for a fracture. Use RICE—see page 7-7.

3   Give ongoing casualty care. Get medical help.

Causes/mechanisms of injury for strains

◆ sudden pulling or twisting of a muscle

◆ poor body mechanics during lifting

◆ not warming up muscles before physical activity

◆ repetitive, long-term overuse of a muscle and/or tendon

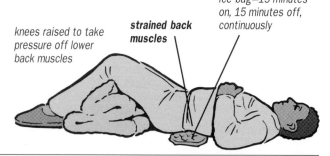

knees raised to take pressure off lower back muscles

strained back muscles

ice bag—15 minutes on, 15 minutes off, continuously

FOCUS ON SAFETY

Preventing bone, joint and muscle injuries

Preventing fractures

Most fractures can be prevented by adopting good safety habits.

Motor vehicle collisions are the cause of many bone injuries. Defensive driving reduces the number of accidents, and the use of seat belts decreases the incidence and severity of injuries.

Adopt a **what if** attitude*to every hazardous condition in the workplace and at home. Potential falls exist on every working and walking surface. Prevent the fall—avoid the injury. Ask yourself:

◆ **what if** work areas are cluttered and untidy? What if tools, hoses, extension cords are left lying about?

◆ **what if** floors are wet, greasy and slippery? What if floor coverings— carpets, rugs at the tops and bottoms of stairs, tiles and floorboards are loose?

◆ **what if** stairs are poorly lit, cluttered with shoes, toys or newspapers, have no handrails, are covered with ice and snow? What if chairs are used to reach high places, stepladders are in poor repair, ladders are not secured?

◆ **what if** life-lines and safety belts are not used when working in high places? What if children are left on balconies unattended?

The appropriate safety action in each of the above situations will take only a moment, but could save someone many days, weeks or months of pain and suffering from a preventable fall.

Preventing strains, sprains and dislocations

Strains, sprains and dislocations are caused by sudden excessive pulling or twisting of a muscle or joint. Strains or sprains are often the result of poor body mechanics or of inadequate conditioning of the body for a particular sport or physical activity. Dislocations are usually caused by violent movements.

◆ use proper body mechanics when lifting—see page 14-3

◆ if you are not sure if you can manage lifting a load or moving a heavy object, don't try, get help

◆ warm up before exercising and don't push your limits while exercising

Repetitive strain injury (RSI)

Muscles and tendons can be injured when they do the same movements over and over again, especially when the movement causes stress on the tissues. These injuries develop over a period of time—days, weeks or months—but can be very disabling.

RSI injuries are also called **overuse injuries**; examples include tennis elbow, bursitis and carpal tunnel syndrome.

First aid for RSI

◆ stop the activity causing the injury

◆ use RICE—see page 7-7

◆ refer the casualty to medical help

---

* Industrial Accident Prevention Association. *Hazards Recognition and Control Seminar HRC 004*, November 1986.

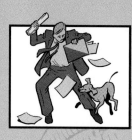

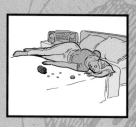

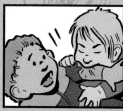

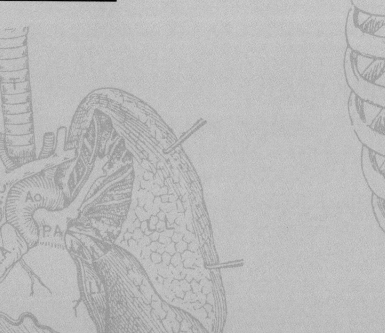

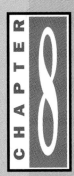

CHAPTER 8

POISONS, BITES AND STINGS

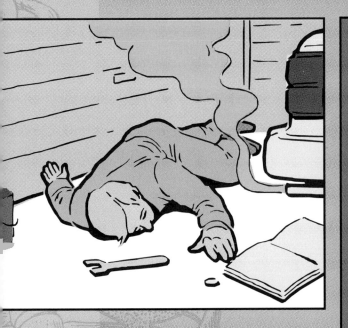

- ◆ *Types of poisons*
- ◆ *Signs and symptoms of poisoning*
- ◆ *General first aid for poisoning*
- ◆ *First aid for animal/human bites*
- ◆ *First aid for snakebite*
- ◆ *First aid for an insect bite or sting*
- ◆ *First aid for bites from ticks*
- ◆ *First aid for lesions from leeches*
- ◆ *How to prevent poisoning*

Poisons

poison symbol

A poison is any substance that can cause illness or death when absorbed by the body. There are poisonous substances all around us. Poisonous consumer products have poison symbols on their labels, but there are many other poisonous substances that don't carry warnings. Examples include alcohol, some common household plants, contaminated food, and medications when not taken as prescribed. Many substances that are not harmful in small amounts are poisonous in large amounts.

Types of poisons

The four types of poisons are classified according to how they enter the body:

◆ **swallowed poisons**—through the mouth

◆ **inhaled poisons**—through the lungs

◆ **absorbed poisons**—through the skin and mucous membranes

◆ **injected poisons**—through a hollow needle or needle-like device (e.g. a snake's fangs)

An important part of the first aid for poisoning is telephoning the Poison Information Centre for advice on what to do. Before calling, the first aider must quickly gather as much information about the incident as possible. Use the history of the scene and the signs and symptoms of the casualty to gather the information you'll need to answer the questions asked by the Poison Information Centre.

History of the scene

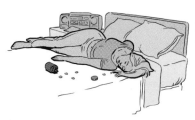

Poisoning may occur despite all reasonable precautions. When it does, act quickly but do not panic. You need to know four basic facts to give appropriate first aid for poisoning:

◆ what poison was taken—container labels should identify the poison; otherwise, save vomit and give it to medical help for analysis

◆ how much poison was taken—estimate the quantity that may have been taken based on what you see or are told—the number of pills originally in the container, the amount of chemical in the bottle, etc.

◆ how the poison entered the body—first aid may differ for poisons taken by mouth, absorbed through the skin, injected into the blood or breathed into the lungs

◆ when the poison was taken—the length of time the poison has been in the body will help determine the first aid and medical care needed

Signs and symptoms of poisoning

If the history does not reveal what poison was taken, or by what means it was taken, signs and symptoms may be helpful in answering these questions. All poisons may affect consciousness, breathing and pulse. Other signs and symptoms may vary depending on how the poison was taken. Poisons that have been:

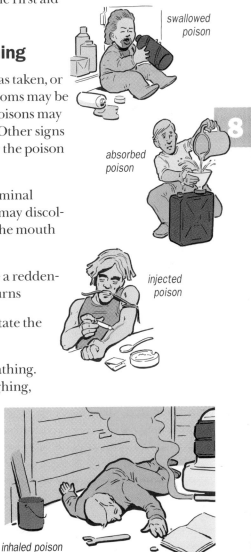

swallowed poison

absorbed poison

injected poison

◆ **swallowed** usually cause nausea, abdominal cramps, diarrhea and vomiting. They may discolour the lips, cause burns in or around the mouth or leave an odour on the breath

◆ **absorbed through the skin** may cause a reddening of the skin, blisters, swelling and burns

◆ **injected through the skin** usually irritate the point of entry

◆ **inhaled** may cause problems with breathing. Signs and symptoms may include coughing, chest pain and difficulty breathing. Prolonged exposure to natural gas used for heating or carbon monoxide (CO) from combustion engines will cause headache, dizziness, unconsciousness, stopped breathing and cardiac arrest.

inhaled poison

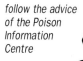

*follow the advice
of the Poison
Information
Centre*

⚠ **Poison
Information Centre**

The phone number for your
local Poison Information
Centre is listed at the
beginning of your
telephone directory.

8

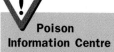

General first aid for poisoning

1 Begin ESM—do a scene survey (see page 2-3).
Gather any information about the suspected
poison. Assess the casualty's responsiveness.

◆ if the casualty is responsive, call the Poison
Information Centre in your region, your
hospital emergency department, or your
doctor. Answer any questions and follow
their advice on first aid

◆ if the casualty is unresponsive, call
medical help (e.g. an ambulance)
immediately and go to step 2

2 Do a primary survey (see page 2-5). If
breathing is stopped and you need to give
artificial respiration, check for poisonous
material around the mouth first.

If there is poisonous material around or in
the mouth, wipe it off and use the mouth-to-
nose method of artificial respiration. Use a
barrier device if you have one.

3 Place the unconscious breathing casualty
into the recovery position.

⚠ **For more
first aid information**

There is more first aid
information for each type
of poisoning on the pages
listed below:
◆ swallowed
   poisons .... page 8-5
◆ inhaled
   poisons .... page 8-6
◆ absorbed
   poisons .... page 8-7
◆ injected
   poisons .... page 8-8

*monitor
breathing
often*

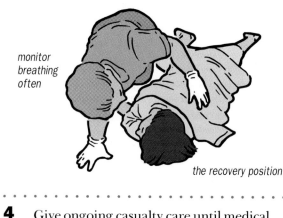

the recovery position

4 Give ongoing casualty care until medical
help takes over.

First aid for swallowed poisons

1 Begin ESM—do a scene survey (see page 2-3) and a primary survey (see page 2-5).

2 Do not dilute a poison that has been swallowed (do not give fluids) unless told to do so by the Poison Information Centre or a doctor.

3 If the casualty is conscious, wipe poisonous or corrosive residue from the casualty's face and rinse or wipe out the mouth.

4 Never induce vomiting except on the advice of the Poison Information Centre or a doctor—many poisons will cause more damage when vomited.

If you do not have syrup of ipecac, a doctor may instruct you to induce vomiting by giving the conscious casualty 30 to 45 mL (2-3 tablespoons) of liquid dish detergent in 250 mL (8 oz.) of water to drink.

Check the expiry date on the bottle of syrup of ipecac on a regular basis and replace if necessary.

If syrup of ipecac freezes, or reaches a temperature above 30°C, do not use it—replace it with a newer bottle.

8

Syrup of ipecac

If you are told to make the casualty vomit, you can do this by giving syrup of ipecac. Syrup of ipecac is an emetic, which means it makes the person who takes it vomit. It comes in sealed, one-dose bottles and is available at most pharmacies without a prescription. Keep at least two bottles in the home, out of reach of children, for emergency use.

Use syrup of ipecac only on the advice of the Poison Information Centre or a doctor. You will be instructed to give a quantity of clear fluids to drink—water or juice—to increase the effectiveness of the syrup of ipecac.

Don't give the casualty any milk after giving syrup of ipecac. The milk will stop the action of the syrup of ipecac.

Do not use syrup of Ipecac if the casualty:

♦ has decreased level of consciousness

♦ has no gag reflex or has suspected head/spinal injuries

♦ has ingested petroleum-based poisons (like paint thinner and gasoline) or strong acid or alkali poisons (like drain cleaners)

♦ is less than six months old or over 70 years old

syrup of ipecac comes in sealed one-dose bottles

First aid for inhaled poisons

1 Begin ESM—do a scene survey (see page 2-3). Assess hazards with particular attention to the possible presence of a poisonous gas or vapour. Make the area safe.

2 Inhaled poisons, such as gases, should be cleared from the lungs as quickly as possible. Move the person to fresh air and away from the source of the poison.

move the casualty to fresh air as quickly as possible

3 If the casualty is unresponsive, call for medical help right away.

4 Do a primary survey (see page 2-5) and give first aid for the ABCs. Monitor breathing closely and give mouth-to-mouth artificial respiration if needed. If the poison could affect you while giving first aid, use a face mask or shield with a one-way valve.

5 If the casualty vomits, keep the airway open by clearing out the mouth and putting the casualty into the recovery position.

6 If the casualty goes into convulsions, prevent him from injuring himself.

7 Get medical help. Give ongoing casualty care, monitoring the casualty closely.

carbon monoxide is a clear odourless gas that kills many people every year—there is carbon monoxide in car exhaust

silo gas (nitrogen dioxide) is a hazard in a farming environment

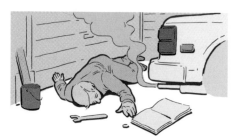

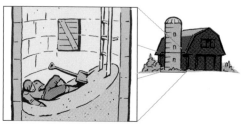

First aid for absorbed poisons

Most poisons absorbed by the skin cause irritation at the place of contact, but don't affect the rest of the body. The irritation, called **contact dermatitis**, includes redness, itching and blisters.

Some chemicals, however, do affect the rest of the body when absorbed by the skin, and these can cause life-threatening emergencies.

1   Begin ESM—do a scene survey (see page 2-3).

2   Do a primary survey (see page 2-5) and give first aid for life-threatening conditions.

3   Flush the affected area with large amounts of cool water.

   ◆ if the poisonous substance is a powder, brush off excessive amounts with a dry cloth before flushing

4   Remove any clothing that has been in contact with the poison. Don't touch the clothing until it has been thoroughly washed. Try not to touch the affected part of the body to any other part of the body.

5   Wash the affected skin thoroughly with soap and water.

   ◆ pay careful attention to hidden areas such as under the fingernails and in the hair

6   Give ongoing casualty care until medical help takes over.

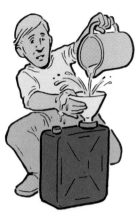

any substance that irritates the skin is a poison

8

poison ivy, a common woodland plant, produces an oil that is very irritating to the skin of many people

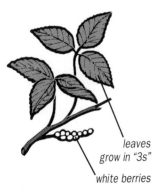

leaves grow in "3s"

white berries

First aid for injected poisons

Follow the general first aid for poisoning—see page 8-4. Injected poisons should be contained near the injection site. Delay the circulation of the poison throughout the body by placing the casualty at rest and keeping the affected limb below heart level.

Bites and stings

Animal and human bites

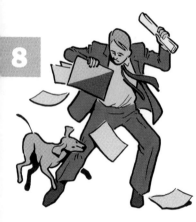

Animal and human bites that cause puncture wounds or lacerations may carry contaminated saliva into the body. Human bites and the bites of domestic animals are dangerous because of the risk of infection. The most common human bites in adults are to the hand and knuckles. Bites from wild animals, such as bats, foxes, skunks and raccoons, may carry the rabies virus which could be fatal if the casualty does not get medical help quickly. To be safe, always give first aid for an animal bite as if the animal had rabies, until it is proved otherwise. Any bite that breaks the skin is serious.

More about rabies

Rabies is an acute viral disease of the nervous system that is always fatal if not treated. Rabies should be suspected in domestic animals if they behave in an unusual way (the gentle dog or cat that attacks for no apparent reason and shows no fear of its owner) and in all attacks by wild animals. The rabies virus can be transmitted to anyone who handles a diseased animal or who touches the area of the wound that carries the virus.

Be especially careful when giving first aid to anyone you suspect may have been exposed to rabies and in handling the live or dead animal involved. Wear gloves and/or scrub your hands thoroughly after contact to reduce the risk of infection.

If the animal can be captured without risk to you or others, it should be kept for examination. If the animal must be killed, try to keep the head intact so that the brain can be examined for the rabies virus.

Even if a person has been exposed to a rabid animal, full-blown rabies can be prevented if immunization against the disease is given quickly.

First aid for animal/human bites

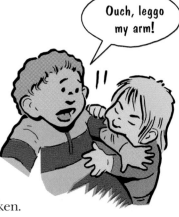

> Ouch, leggo my arm!

1 Start ESM—do a scene survey—see page 2-3. Protect yourself by wearing gloves when giving first aid or handling an animal that may be infected.

2 Do a primary survey and give first aid for any life-threatening conditions— see page 2-5.

3 Examine the wound to see if the skin was broken.

4 If there is bleeding, allow moderate bleeding of the wound—this helps to cleanse the wound.

5 Wash the wound with an antiseptic soap or detergent. Apply a dressing and bandage.

6 If the skin was broken, get medical help as soon as possible.

All animal and human bites that break the skin should be seen by a doctor.

8

Snakebite

Rattlesnakes are the only poisonous snakes found in the wild in Canada. Varieties of this snake are found in parts of British Columbia, Alberta, Saskatchewan and Ontario but they are not numerous, and snakebites are not common. If you are travelling to areas where there are other poisonous snakes, learn the first aid for snakebites in that area.

A rattlesnake's bite leaves one or two puncture holes in the skin. Venom is usually, but not always, injected into the casualty. If it is, the casualty will feel a burning sensation. This is followed by swelling and discoloration, severe pain, weakness, sweating, nausea, vomiting and chills. Breathing may be affected.

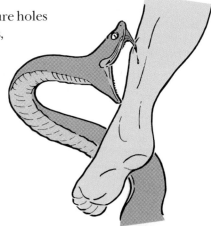

Precautions when dealing with snakes and snakebites

- most snakes will be within 10 metres of the place where the bite took place—be careful
- do not let a snakebite casualty walk if there is any other method of transportation to medical help
- do not give the casualty alcoholic beverages
- do not cut the puncture marks or try to suck poison out with your mouth
- do not apply ice—this could cause more damage
- if the snake is killed, bring it to medical help for identification, but do not touch the snake directly. Avoid the snake's head—a dead snake still may have a bite reflex

First aid for snakebite

1 Begin ESM—do a scene survey (see page 2-3). Make sure there is no danger of a second snakebite to either the casualty or yourself.

2 Do a primary survey (see page 2-5).

3 Place the casualty at rest in a semisitting position and keep the affected limb below heart level. By placing the casualty at rest, the venom won't spread as quickly.

4 Flush the bite with soapy water, if available, but do not apply cold compresses or ice.

5 Immobilize the limb as for a fracture—see chapter 7.

6 Give ongoing casualty care and transport the casualty to medical help as soon as possible.

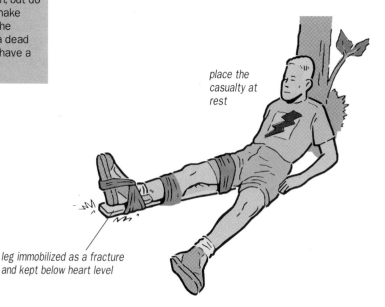

place the casualty at rest

leg immobilized as a fracture and kept below heart level

Insect bites and stings

In most people, an insect bite or sting causes only a painful swelling with redness and itching at the site of the sting. But some people are severely allergic to these stings and being stung may cause a life-threatening allergic reaction.

Ask the casualty if he has ever had an allergic reaction to a sting before. Also look for the signs of an allergic reaction. If you suspect the casualty is having an allergic reaction to a sting, place him at rest and give first aid for a severe allergic reaction—see page 4-16.

First aid for an insect bite or sting

1 Begin ESM—do a scene survey (see page 2-3). Do a primary survey and give first aid for the ABCs (see page 2-5). Examine the sting site closely, looking for the stinger that may still be in the skin. If it is there, remove it by carefully scraping it and the attached poison sac from the skin. Don't use tweezers, fingers or anything that may squeeze more poison into the body.

2 For the irritation at the site of the sting, apply rubbing alcohol, a weak ammonia solution or a paste of baking soda and water. Ice can also be used. Don't use alcohol or ammonia near the eyes.

Signs and symptoms at the site of a bite or sting

◆ sudden pain
◆ swelling
◆ heat
◆ redness
◆ itching

Signs and symptoms of an allergic reaction to a bite or sting

◆ general itching, rash
◆ a bump on the skin that may be white, pink, reddish or blotchy
◆ generalized swelling—especially of the airway
◆ weakness, headache
◆ fever
◆ breathing difficulties that may be severe
◆ anxiety, abdominal cramps, vomiting

8

stinger and poison sac

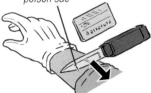

scrape the stinger from the skin with a sharp edge like a knife blade or a credit card

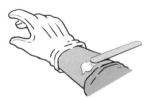

use a paste of baking soda and water to relieve the irritation

If the sting is in the mouth, give the person a mouthwash of one teaspoonful of baking soda in a glass of water, or a piece of ice to suck on. If there is swelling in the mouth, or if there is difficulty breathing, monitor the person closely and get medical help.

Ticks

ticks

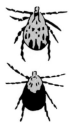

Ticks are found in abundance throughout the forests in some parts of Canada. They drop from the foliage onto animals and humans, biting through the skin and anchoring themselves to the tissue with barbed mouth parts. A tick will suck the host's (the person or animal) blood for many hours and may become quite large. At the end of the meal, the tick detaches itself and drops off.

Poison from the tick may be harmful. They sometimes carry disease that can be transmitted to humans. A tick on the body should be removed. If one tick is found, check your body and clothing thoroughly for others.

actual size before a blood meal

First aid for bites from ticks

1   Begin ESM—do a scene survey (see page 2-3).
Remove the embedded tick. Grasp it as close to the casualty's skin as possible and pull away from the skin with even, steady pressure. Avoid squashing an engorged tick during removal. Infected blood may spurt into your eyes, mouth, or a cut on the surface of your skin.

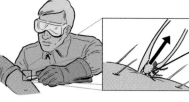

wear gloves

if the tick is full of blood, wear eye protection too

grasp the tick as close to the skin as possible and pull straight out with firm, steady pressure

If you don't have tweezers, use your fingers covered with gloves, a plastic bag or tissue paper.

2   Keep the dislodged tick and bring it to medical help for identification.

3   Clean the area with soap and water and apply an antiseptic to prevent infection. Wash your hands.

4   Tell the casualty to get medical help to find out if there is a risk of disease transmission by the ticks in your area. If the site of the bite shows any sign of infection, or there are other worrisome signs or symptoms within the next week, the casualty should get medical help.

Leeches

Leeches live in swamps, ponds, lakes and stagnant water. Some feed on the warm blood of animals or humans. A leech makes a tiny cut in the skin, which may not be felt at the time, and attaches itself to feed on blood. Once a leech is attached, trying to pull it off often doesn't work—the leech may tear into smaller parts, making it even harder to remove those parts still attached. This may increase the risk of infection.

First aid for lesions from leeches

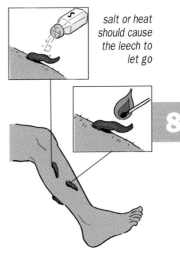

salt or heat should cause the leech to let go

1 Begin ESM—do a scene survey (see page 2-3).

2 Detach the leech by applying salt, heat from a match or hot cigarette, a drop of kerosene, turpentine or oil to its body. The leech should detach itself from the skin and fall off in one piece. Do not pull or scrape the leech off the skin.

3 Clean the area with a paste of baking soda and water or a weak solution of ammonia. This will also relieve irritation.

4 If the site of the bite shows any sign of infection in the next week, the casualty should get medical help.

FOCUS ON SAFETY

How to prevent poisoning

● ●

Preventing poisoning

Most poisonings can be prevented if the risk of poison is recognized and proper care is taken in their use and storage. The average household has as many as 250 poisonous substances in the form of medicines, cleaning products, plant care products, and products used in hobbies and crafts. Take the following precautions to prevent poisoning:

◆ keep household and drug products in their original containers for identification, so that instructions will be available each time they are used, and so that label information will be at hand in case of poisoning

◆ read label instructions on containers before using, and follow the directions

◆ do not put harmful products in food or drink containers

◆ destroy foods which you believe may be contaminated

◆ ventilate areas where toxic chemicals are used—open windows and doors so that fumes do not become concentrated

◆ operate gas combustion engines where there is good ventilation, preferably outdoors

◆ prevent medication errors by carefully checking the **five rights** for giving medicines—the **right medicine**, the **right person**, the **right amount**, the **right time**, the **right method**

◆ teach young children to recognize warning labels on products, and to stay away from these products

◆ many houseplants are poisonous—if you have children in the house, discard all poisonous plants. Keep a tag in every plant so it can be identified quickly

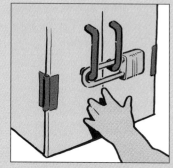

harmful products should be locked up and out-of-reach of children

◆ do not leave medications in a purse or on a night table where children can get at them

◆ do not take medications in front of children, because they may imitate you

◆ flush unused portions of medicines down the toilet and throw out empty containers

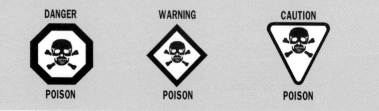

DANGER   WARNING   CAUTION

POISON   POISON   POISON

FOCUS ON SAFETY

How to prevent bites and stings

· ·

> The best way to prevent being bitten or stung is to avoid exposure to the insect or animal, but this is not always practical. Insects and animals will usually bite or sting only if they feel threatened. By giving creatures plenty of room, and by not startling them, you will reduce the risk of being bitten or stung. Follow the precautions below to further reduce your risk.

Preventing animal bites

◆ when travelling in the bush, make lots of noise as you go—animals in your path will hear you coming and get out of your way

◆ when camping, use the proper precautions for storing food, washing dishes, etc.—get more information on this from books on wilderness travel

◆ do not feed wild animals

◆ stay away from any animal that seems unusually friendly or fearless

Preventing snakebite

Snakes do not attack or "hunt" people to bite—they only bite when they feel threatened. If you are in "snake country":

◆ learn more about snakes' habits so you can better avoid them

◆ never put your hands or feet where you can't see what is there first:

– if climbing rocks, don't reach up and put your hand on a ledge where a snake may be sunning itself

– don't kick under a dead tree to loosen it, there could be snake under the tree—use a stick to loosen the tree

◆ if you do see a poisonous snake, and avoid it, remember that snakes don't travel very far, so the snake will probably be in the same area when you return

Preventing insect bites and stings

◆ avoid using or wearing products that stinging insects are attracted to, for example:

– certain perfumes and other scents

– particularly aromatic hair shampoos

◆ if you discover a nest of stinging insects near your home, have it safely destroyed as soon as possible—delaying this will only result in a larger nest with more insects

◆ teach children not to panic when a bee or wasp comes near them—panicking will only agitate the insect. Teach children to calmly wait for the insect to leave, or to gently swat it away

Preventing tick bites

◆ wear a long-sleeve shirt with a tight collar and cuffs, and tuck your pants into your socks, when walking through grassy or wooded areas

◆ after a walk in a grassy or wooded area, check your body for ticks—they are very small and may look like a moving freckle

◆ if you find one tick, check very carefully for others

8

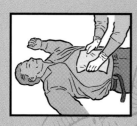

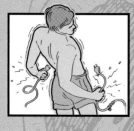

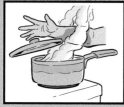

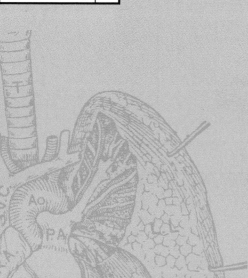

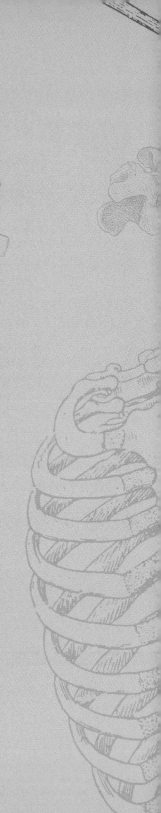

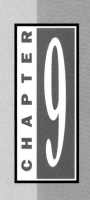

CHAPTER 9

Burns

• •

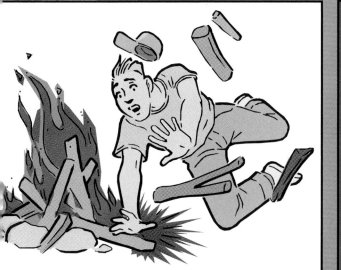

- ◆ Types of burns
- ◆ Severity of a burn
- ◆ Rule of nines
- ◆ Complications of burns
- ◆ Inhalation injuries
- ◆ Precautions for first aid for burns
- ◆ Heat burns
- ◆ Chemical burns
- ◆ Electrical burns
- ◆ Radiation burns
- ◆ How to put out a fire on your clothes
- ◆ How to prevent burns

Burns are injuries to the skin and other tissues caused by heat, radiation or chemicals. They are a leading cause of injury in the home. Young children and elderly people are especially at risk of being burned, and at these ages, burn injuries are more serious. Many burns in the home are preventable—see page 9-15 for information on preventing burns.

Types of burns

Based on the mechanism of injury, there are four types of burns.

Heat burns (also called "thermal" burns)

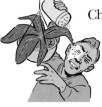

Burns from too much heat applied to the body are the most familiar kind of burns. Common heat sources include open flames, like candles or fire, and hot objects like stoves or car engines. A scald is a heat burn caused by hot liquid or steam. Heat burns can also be caused by friction.

Chemical burns

Chemical burns are often serious because the chemicals continue to burn as long as they remain on the skin. Examples of industrial chemicals that can burn include acids, alkalies, phenols and phosphorus. Chemicals kept in the home that can burn include paint stripper, oven cleaner, drain cleaner and rust remover.

Electrical burns

Electrical burns result from contact with an electric current. Although it is heat that causes these burns, electrical burns are considered separately because of the complications caused by the electricity.

Radiation burns

Most people have experienced a radiation burn in the form of a sunburn, where the sun is the source of radiant energy. Other types of radiant energy that can cause burns include X-rays, arc welder's flash and radiation from radioactive material.

Severity of a burn

The severity of a burn is determined according to the characteristics listed below. Burns are classified as **critical**, **moderate** or **mild**. This is important when there is more than one casualty and you have to decide who to send to medical help first.

◆ the depth of the burn—this is called the **degree** of the burn

◆ the amount of body surface that is burned

◆ the part(s) of the body that is burned

◆ the age and physical condition of the casualty

Burn depth

The skin has two layers, a top layer and a second layer. Underneath the second layer is fat tissue and below that is muscle tissue. The skin protects the body from bacteria, helps control body temperature and keeps body fluid in the body. When the skin is damaged by a burn, it cannot do these functions properly, or at all.

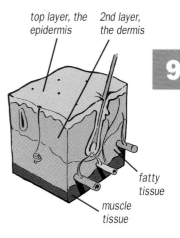

top layer, the epidermis   2nd layer, the dermis

fatty tissue

muscle tissue

The degree of a burn depends on the depth of the tissue damage. The deeper the burn, the more serious it is. In first aid, there are three degrees of burns—first, second and third-degree. Third-degree burns are the most serious.

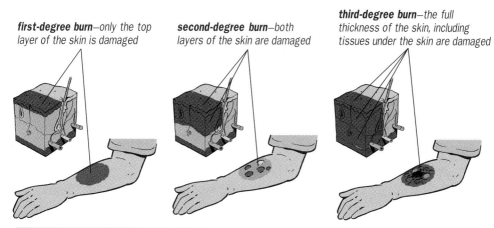

first-degree burn—only the top layer of the skin is damaged

second-degree burn—both layers of the skin are damaged

third-degree burn—the full thickness of the skin, including tissues under the skin are damaged

Estimating the burned area—the rule of nines

A first aider can quickly estimate how much body surface area has been burned using the **rule of nines**. The body is divided up into areas of either nine or eighteen percent of total body area. Add these areas to quickly calculate the percentage of the body that is affected. The percentages change slightly for a child's body.

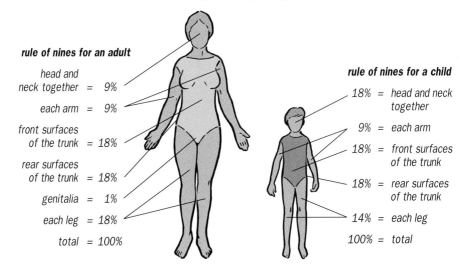

rule of nines for an adult

head and neck together	=	9%
each arm	=	9%
front surfaces of the trunk	=	18%
rear surfaces of the trunk	=	18%
genitalia	=	1%
each leg	=	18%
total	=	100%

rule of nines for a child

18%	=	head and neck together
9%	=	each arm
18%	=	front surfaces of the trunk
18%	=	rear surfaces of the trunk
14%	=	each leg
100%	=	total

Critical, moderate and mild burns

The burns listed below are critical, meaning they may be life threatening or can cause serious, life-long disability or disfigurement.

◆ any burn that interferes with breathing, including burns to the face and throat and inhalation injuries (see page 4-12)

◆ any burn where there is also a serious soft tissue injury or fracture

◆ all burns to areas where the skin bends, including the elbows, neck, knees, etc.

◆ all electrical burns

◆ most chemical burns

◆ burns to casualties under two or over fifty years old—these people don't tolerate burns very well

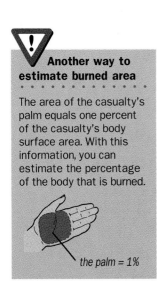

⚠ Another way to estimate burned area

The area of the casualty's palm equals one percent of the casualty's body surface area. With this information, you can estimate the percentage of the body that is burned.

the palm = 1%

◆ burns to casualties who have serious underlying medical
conditions including diabetes, seizure disorders, hypertension, respiratory difficulties, or mental illness

The table below shows the severity of burns based on the degree
of the burn, the percentage of the body burned, and the part of
the body burned.

Severity of burns			
	Percentage of body with burns of the:		
Severity	**3rd degree**	**2nd degree**	**1st degree**
critical burn	> 10% (>2% in a child) or any part of the face, hands, feet or genitals	> 30% (>20% in a child)	> 70%
moderate burn	2 – 10% face, hands or feet not burned	15 – 30% (10–20% in a child)	50 – 70%
minor burn	< 2%	< 15% (<10% in a child)	< 20% face, hands, feet or genitals **not** burned

9

Complications of burns

Burn injuries often affect much more than just the burned tissue.
In critical burns, all the major systems of the body can be affected.
For this reason, burn casualties need medical help immediately so
the extent of the injuries can be properly assessed. Common
complications of burns include:

◆ **shock** caused by the loss of blood or blood plasma to the
surrounding tissues. Shock can be aggravated by the pain of
the burn

◆ **infection** because burned skin isn't a good barrier to bacteria,
and the injured area may provide a place for bacteria to breed

◆ **breathing problems** if the face or throat is burned, or the
casualty has inhaled smoke, fumes or steam

◆ **swelling** because tight clothing and jewellery will cut off
circulation when the area swells

Inhalation injuries

Inhalation injuries are often associated with burns. These occur when the casualty breathes steam, smoke or fumes. The signs of an inhalation injury may appear quickly, or may become apparent hours after the incident. For this reason, keep checking the casualty and asking if her breathing is alright. If the casualty begins to cough or wheeze, you should suspect an inhalation injury. The signs, symptoms and first aid for an inhalation injury are given on page 4-12.

Recognizing burns

Use the signs and symptoms of burns to recognize them and determine the degree of the burn (sometimes this is difficult to do). The mechanism of injury will also give you clues as to the severity of the burn and whether the injury is critical.

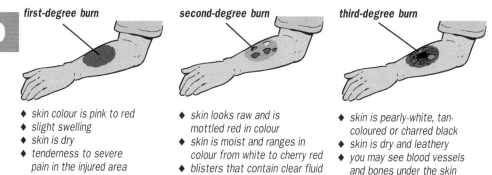

first-degree burn

- skin colour is pink to red
- slight swelling
- skin is dry
- tenderness to severe pain in the injured area

second-degree burn

- skin looks raw and is mottled red in colour
- skin is moist and ranges in colour from white to cherry red
- blisters that contain clear fluid
- extreme pain

third-degree burn

- skin is pearly-white, tan-coloured or charred black
- skin is dry and leathery
- you may see blood vessels and bones under the skin
- little or no pain (nerves are destroyed)

Precautions for first aid for burns

- Do not breathe on, cough over or touch the burned area.
- Do not break blisters.
- Do not remove clothing that is stuck to the burned area.
- Do not use butter, lotions*, ointments* or oily dressings on a burn.

- Do not cover a burn with cotton wool or other fluffy material.
- Do not use adhesive dressings.
- Do not cool the casualty too much. Once the area is cooled, take action to keep the casualty warm.

  * sunburn lotions and ointments can be used on minor sunburn

First aid for heat burns

1 Begin ESM—do the scene survey (see page 2-3). Do a primary survey (see page 2-5).

2 Cool the burn right away—immerse it in cool water. If you can't do this, pour cool water on the area or cover it with a clean, wet cloth.

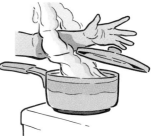

immerse the burned area in cool water

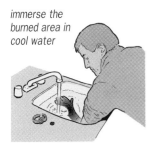

pour cool water on the burn

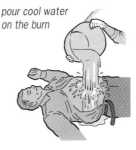

cover the burned area with cloths soaked with cool water

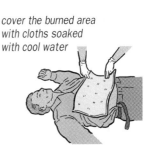

Cool the burn until the pain has lessened. This will reduce the temperature of the burned area, and reduce tissue damage, swelling, blistering and relieve the pain.

3 Loosen or remove anything on the burned area that is tight—this means jewellery and tight clothing. Do this as soon as you can, before the injury swells. Don't remove anything that is stuck.

4 When the pain has lessened, loosely cover the burn with a clean, lint-free dressing. If the area is large, use a sheet. Secure the dressing with tape, making sure there is no tape on the burned area.

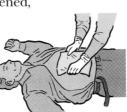

use a sterile dressing if you have one

5 Give ongoing casualty care including arranging for medical help, first aid for shock and monitoring the casualty.

Burn dressings

A good burn dressing is sterile, lint-free and won't stick to the injury when it is removed. If you don't have something like this, use something clean and lint-free, like a linen sheet.

A new type of burn dressing is the "gelled water" burn dressing, e.g. Water-Jel®. These sterile dressings are coated with a jelly-like substance that is mostly water. As such, the dressings are effective in cooling the burn, keeping it clean and providing pain relief. Use these dressings according to the instructions on the package.

9

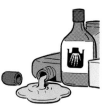

First aid for chemical burns

A corrosive chemical will keep burning as long as it is on the skin. The faster you get the chemical off the skin, the less tissue damage there will be.

1 Begin ESM—do a scene survey (see page 2-3). Do a primary survey (see page 2-5).

2 Remove the chemical from the body by flushing the area with large amounts of cool water. If the chemical is a dry powder, quickly brush off any loose chemical with a cloth before flushing.

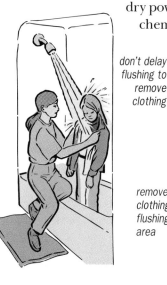

don't delay flushing to remove clothing

remove the clothing while flushing the area

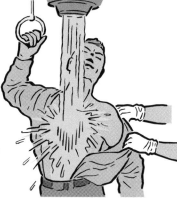

Using chemical neutralizers

Do not use chemical neutralizers such as vinegar, soda or alcohol, to treat any chemical burn, unless advised to do so by a medical doctor.

If you work with chemicals, make sure you know the specific first aid for the chemicals in your workplace. The MSDS* for each chemical contains this information.

* material safety data sheet—see page 15-7

3 Continue flushing the area with water for 15 to 20 minutes.

4 When the area has been flushed, loosely cover the burn with a clean, lint-free, preferably sterile dressing. If the area is large, use a sheet. Secure the dressing with tape, making sure no tape touches the burned area.

5 Give ongoing casualty care including arranging for medical help, first aid for shock and monitoring the casualty. If the casualty begins to feel an increased sensation of burning in the injured area, flush the area again for at least 10 minutes.

First aid for chemical burns to the eye

The eyes can be permanently injured by corrosive chemicals in either solid or liquid form. Casualties normally suffer intense pain and are very sensitive to light. Give first aid as follows:

1 Begin ESM—do a scene survey (see page 2-3). If you can, put gloves on or wash your hands.

2 Sit or lay the casualty down. Tilt the head back and turn it slightly to the injured side. If only one eye is injured, protect the uninjured eye.

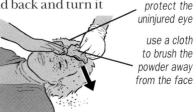

protect the uninjured eye

use a cloth to brush the powder away from the face

3 If the chemical is a dry powder, brush away whatever is on the skin.

4 Flush the injured eye with cool water. Since pain may make it hard for the casualty to keep the eye open, gently open the eye with your fingers. Flush the eye for at least 15 minutes.

when there is a risk of eye injury from chemicals, proper eye-wash equipment should be kept nearby

9

use gently running water to flush the eye

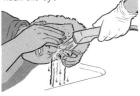

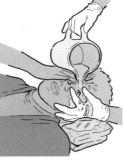

commercial eye-wash bottle

5 Cover the injured eye with dressings. If both eyes are injured, cover the more seriously injured eye. Only cover both eyes if the casualty is more comfortable that way. Covering both eyes, so the casualty can't see, adds to the stress of the scene. If you do cover both eyes, reassure the casualty by explaining what is being done and why.

6 Get medical help right away and give ongoing casualty care.

⚠ If the casualty is wearing contact lenses

Don't waste time trying to remove contact lenses. Flush the eyes for 15 minutes—this may wash the lenses out. If not, have the casualty remove them. Lenses exposed to chemicals should be thrown away (so it doesn't matter if they are washed away during flushing).

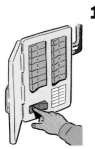

First aid for electrical burns

An electrical burn may be more serious than it appears. An electrical current going through the body can cause breathing to stop and/or the heart to stop. Also, an electric shock can violently throw the casualty. Head/spinal injuries, fractures or dislocations may be present. There is also the danger of electrical injury to the first aider.

1   Begin ESM—do a scene survey (see page 2-3). Make sure there is no further danger from electricity. If you are not sure, don't put yourself in danger—call the power company or other officials to make the scene safe. Only turn electricity off at the source—never try to cut or move live wires. If high voltages are involved, all you can do is keep others out of the area until the power is shut off.

Examine the scene carefully. Does it look like the casualty was thrown? If so, suspect a head or spinal injury.

shut off power at the source before entering the scene

2   Do a primary survey (see page 2-5) and give first aid for life-threatening injuries.

3   Do a secondary survey to locate burns and any fractures, dislocations, etc. Look for both entry and exit burns.

Two kinds of electrical burns

Electrical burns can be either **flash burns** or **contact burns**. Although you may not be able to tell the type of burn at an emergency scene, knowing the two types helps to understand electrical burn injuries.

A **flash burn** results when electricity arcs (jumps) from the electric source to the casualty. When electricity arcs, it produces intense heat for a very short time. This heat causes flash burn, which can be a very deep third-degree burn. In some cases the tissue is completely burned away, leaving a hole. The electricity does not travel through the body in flash burn, so tissue damage inside the body is usually not severe.

In a **contact burn**, electricity travels through the body. Here, the body conducts the electricity from one place to another, and the electricity travels along a path through the body. The body may be burned at both the point where the electricity entered the body and where it exited. There may also be severe tissue damage inside the body, along the path the electricity followed.

entry burn

exit burn

4   Give first aid for the entry and exit burns by covering them with clean, dry dressings. Tape these in place, making sure the tape doesn't touch damaged skin.

5   Give first aid for any fractures or dislocations—see Chapter 7.

6   Give ongoing casualty care including getting medical help, giving first aid for shock and monitoring the casualty.

Emergency scene management when there are downed power lines

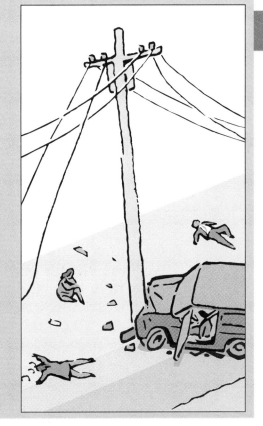

◆ Inspect the emergency scene as you arrive. If there is a possibility of a downed power line or a weakened pole, go no further. Don't leave your vehicle until you have inspected the surrounding area, looking for downed power lines.

◆ Stay inside your vehicle if it is touching power lines. Wait for authorities to arrive, than follow their instructions.

◆ If you suspect or see any downed power lines, don't let anyone enter the area. When you are sure no one will enter the area, notify the power company.

◆ With high voltages, electricity can travel through the ground, energizing the area around the power lines. If the soles of your feet tingle as you enter an area, you've gone too far—get back.

◆ Assume all downed power lines are live unless the power company crew says otherwise. A high voltage wire may be unpredictable—it may jump to an object for a better ground. Stay well away from any wires.

◆ Remember that vehicles, guardrails, metal fences, etc., conduct electricity.

9

First aid for radiation burns

Radiation burns are caused by radiant energy—energy that radiates from a source. Sunburn and snowblindness are radiation burns caused by sunlight. Sunlamps at tanning parlours can also cause radiation burns to the skin and eyes. Other causes of radiation burns include X-rays and the flash of arc welding.

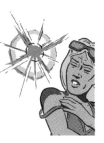

First aid for sunburn

Sunburns can range in severity from those that are mildly uncomfortable to those that are serious, cover a large portion of the body, and are complicated by heatstroke. For minor sunburn, give first aid as follows:

1   Begin ESM—do a scene survey (see page 2-3) and a primary survey (see page 2-5). Get out of the sun. Gently sponge the area with cool water or cover with a wet towel, to relieve the pain. Repeat this step as needed to relieve pain.

2   Pat the skin dry and put on a medicated sunburn ointment or lotion (these can cause an allergic reaction in some people). Apply the lotion according to directions on the package.

3   Protect burned areas from further exposure to the sun.

4   Don't break any blisters—doing so may promote infection. If large areas of the skin begin to blister, get medical help.

5   If the casualty begins to vomit, or develops a fever, give first aid for heatstroke (see page 10-13) and get medical help.

First aid for burns from X-rays and nuclear radiation

There is no specific first aid for radiation burns from X-rays or radioactive material. Give first aid following the guidelines for first aid for heat burns. In an environment where there is radioactive material, protect yourself accordingly.

First aid for intense light burns to the eye(s)

Burns to the eyes may be caused by intense light such as direct or reflected sunlight and arc welder's flash. Snowblindness is a common injury of this kind. As with a sunburn, the casualty may not feel the tissue damage happening but will develop symptoms several hours after exposure. Signs and symptoms include:

◆ sensitivity to light

◆ pain

◆ a gritty feeling in the eyes

Give first aid as follows:

1   Begin ESM—do a scene survey (see page 2-3) and a primary survey. Wash your hands or put gloves on if available.

2   Cover the eyes to cool them and keep the light out.

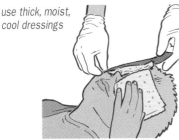

use thick, moist, cool dressings

secure dressings in place with either tape or a narrow triangular bandage

The casualty will be temporarily blinded, so you must reassure her often and explain what you are doing. If the casualty doesn't want both eyes covered, even after an explanation and reassurance, than cover only one eye.

3   Get medical help and give ongoing casualty care.

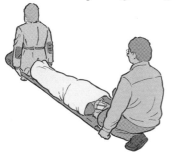

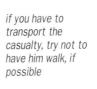

if you have to transport the casualty, try not to have him walk, if possible

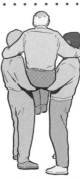

9

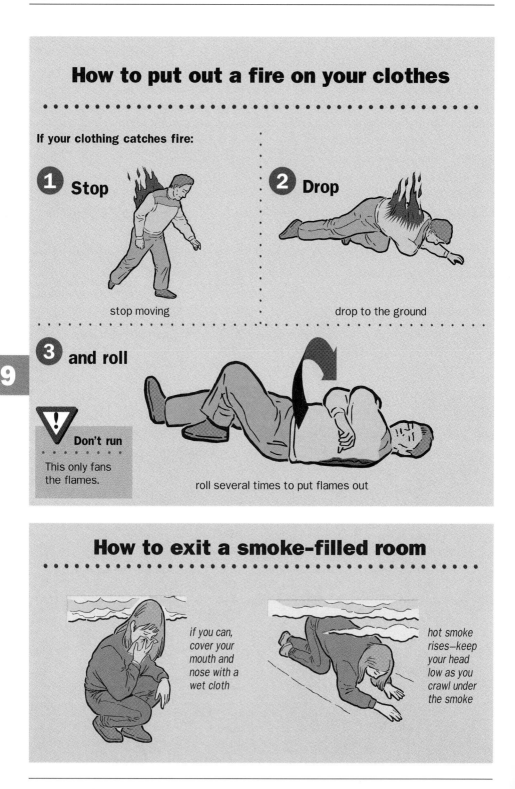

How to put out a fire on your clothes

If your clothing catches fire:

1 Stop

stop moving

2 Drop

drop to the ground

3 and roll

⚠️ **Don't run**
This only fans the flames.

roll several times to put flames out

How to exit a smoke-filled room

if you can, cover your mouth and nose with a wet cloth

hot smoke rises—keep your head low as you crawl under the smoke

FOCUS ON SAFETY

How to prevent burns

● ●

Prevent thermal (heat) burns

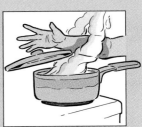

◆ set water tank thermostats not higher than 54°C (130°F)

◆ prepare a child's bath with cold water, then add hot water to reach the desired temperature, and finish with cold to cool the taps

◆ keep hot liquids (e.g. coffee, tea) out of the reach of children

◆ teach children the dangers of heat from stoves, ovens, fireplaces, candles and matches

◆ ensure clothing is not flammable (especially for small children and the elderly). Workers in high-risk jobs should wear flame-resistant clothing

◆ guard children and the elderly from stoves and open flames, especially when wearing loose clothing, nightgowns, etc.

◆ supervise the use of stoves, fires and smoking materials —keep matches, lighters, and all smoking materials out of the reach of children

Prevent chemical burns

◆ wear eye protection when working with chemicals

◆ store chemicals in locked cupboards to keep children safe

◆ store chemicals in lower cupboards to prevent spillage when taking containers off shelves

Prevent electrical burns

◆ prevent children from chewing on electric cords, which can result in severe burns of the mouth

◆ secure electrical cords attached to hot irons, kettles etc. out of the reach of children to prevent them pulling on the cords

◆ always check that electricity is turned off before you disassemble or repair electrical equipment/tools

Prevent radiation burns

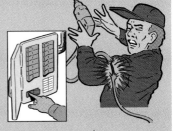

◆ protect all family members from sunburn with protective clothing and sunscreen lotions

◆ wear sunglasses that block the harmful rays of the sun

◆ beware of medications that make your skin more sensitive to the sun—ask your pharmacist about this

9

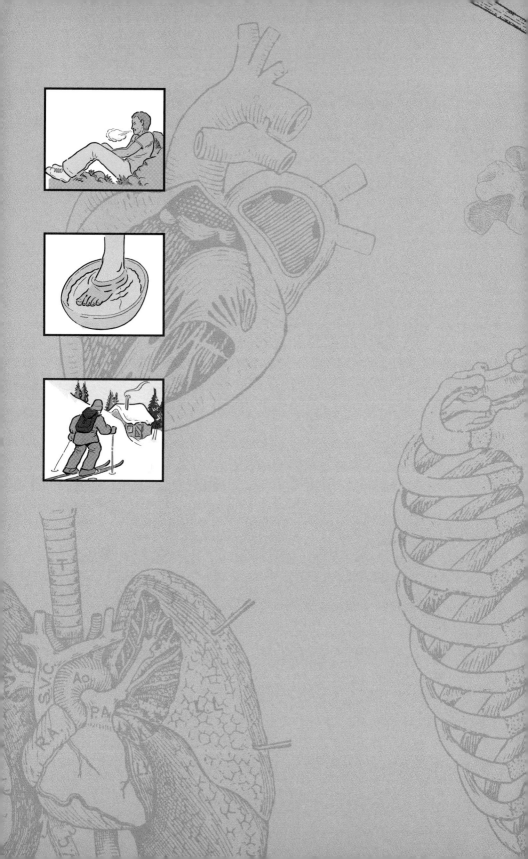

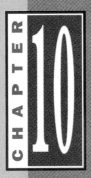

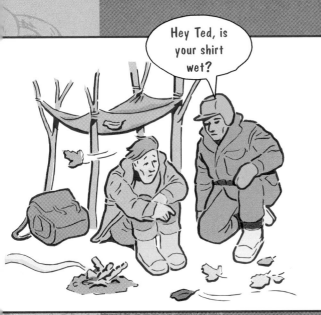

- *How the body loss heat*

- *Who gets hypothermia*

- *Recognizing hypothermia*

- *About rewarming a casualty*

- *First aid for hypothermia*

- *Frostbite*

- *First aid for deep frostbite*

- *Heat exposure and illnesses*

- *Lightning injuries*

- *Five ways to prevent cold injuries*

Hypothermia

The normal temperature of the body's core is 37°C (98.6°F). If the body core temperature drops more than two degrees, the body's tissues cannot function properly. This state of generalized cooling is called **hypothermia**. Hypothermia, often called **exposure**, kills many Canadians each year—but it is a condition that can be detected and corrected by a first aider if recognized early.

the body's core

How the body loses heat

Core body temperature drops when the body loses more heat than it produces. There are five ways the body loses heat. The table below explains each of these. In an outdoor emergency, heat loss by conduction and convection (wet and wind) are often the main contributors to hypothermia. But when trying to prevent heat loss, you must look for all the ways the body is losing heat.

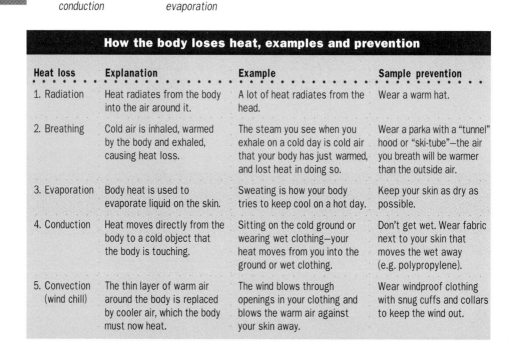

radiation   breathing   convection
conduction   evaporation

How the body loses heat, examples and prevention			
Heat loss	**Explanation**	**Example**	**Sample prevention**
1. Radiation	Heat radiates from the body into the air around it.	A lot of heat radiates from the head.	Wear a warm hat.
2. Breathing	Cold air is inhaled, warmed by the body and exhaled, causing heat loss.	The steam you see when you exhale on a cold day is cold air that your body has just warmed, and lost heat in doing so.	Wear a parka with a "tunnel" hood or "ski-tube"—the air you breath will be warmer than the outside air.
3. Evaporation	Body heat is used to evaporate liquid on the skin.	Sweating is how your body tries to keep cool on a hot day.	Keep your skin as dry as possible.
4. Conduction	Heat moves directly from the body to a cold object that the body is touching.	Sitting on the cold ground or wearing wet clothing—your heat moves from you into the ground or wet clothing.	Don't get wet. Wear fabric next to your skin that moves the wet away (e.g. polypropylene).
5. Convection (wind chill)	The thin layer of warm air around the body is replaced by cooler air, which the body must now heat.	The wind blows through openings in your clothing and blows the warm air against your skin away.	Wear windproof clothing with snug cuffs and collars to keep the wind out.

How the body adapts to heat loss

The body has a number of ways to minimize heat loss and keep the body core warm. One of the first things the body does when it is losing heat is start shivering. The muscle action of shivering generates heat. By shivering, the body is trying to warm itself. If the body keeps getting colder, the blood vessels in the arms, legs and at the skin surface get smaller. This keeps the blood in the core, where it is warmest. By doing this, the body core uses the surface tissues to insulate itself from the cold.

If heat loss continues, the body processes get slower. This includes thinking, muscular action and the senses. Shivering will slow down and then stop. The muscles get stiff and movements become jerky. Thinking is confused, speech difficult and the senses dulled. The heart and breathing rates slow down and the person eventually loses consciousness. At this point, the condition is very serious. The heartbeat becomes unsteady and faint, and finally the heart stops beating.

When the heart stops beating, the person is considered dead. However, when body tissues are cold, they aren't damaged as easily by a lack of oxygen. For this reason, there is often a chance of resuscitating a hypothermic person who doesn't show any signs of life. This means that as long as you aren't putting yourself or others at risk, you should continue your rescue efforts to get a hypothermic casualty to medical help.

In hypothermia, a person isn't dead until he is warm and dead.

Who gets hypothermia?

Anyone can become hypothermic, but the following groups are especially prone:

◆ elderly people, because they often have poor circulation, less ability to sense the cold, and may be on medication that promotes heat loss

◆ babies have less ability to recover from mild and moderate hypothermia because they lose heat more quickly and their bodies don't control body heat as well

◆ people who are already weakened due to illness, injury, lack of food, fatigue or through the use of alcohol or drugs

◆ teenagers, because they often underdress for the weather conditions

Signs of hypothermia

There are three stages of hypothermia: mild, moderate and severe.
The table below lists the signs for each stage, but it may be hard to
tell exactly when one stage ends and another begins. Body
temperatures are not listed here because the first aider has no
practical way to take the temperature of the body's core.

Signs of hypothermia			
Sign	**Mild**	**Moderate**	**Severe**
pulse	normal	slow and weak	weak, irregular or absent
breathing	normal	slow and shallow	slow or absent
appearance	shivering, slurred speech	shivering violently or stopped, clumsy, stumbling, pupils dilated, skin bluish	shivering has stopped
mental state	conscious but withdrawn or disinterested	confused, sleepy irrational	unconscious

Recognizing hypothermia

The key to successful first aid for hypothermia is recognizing the
casualty's condition as soon as possible, and than preventing
hypothermia from getting worse. Hypothermia is the obvious
thing to look for at the end of a cold winter day, but it is less obvious when the temperature is above zero. Be on the lookout for
hypothermia whenever the temperature is below 20°C, the weather is
windy, wet or both, or the casualty is in one of the groups at risk for
hypothermia.

Sometimes hypothermia is mistaken for other conditions. Hypothermia has been mistaken for drunkenness, stroke and drug abuse.
This often happens in the city, where a warm environment doesn't
seem far away. For example, an elderly person's home may not feel
cold to you since you are warmly dressed, but in fact the room
temperature is 15°C, the elderly person is underdressed, and is
hypothermic.

And don't forget yourself—as soon as you begin to shiver, think
"I've got to prevent further heat loss." If you don't, hypothermia
will soon affect your mind, and you won't be able to think clearly
enough to take the right actions.

First aid for hypothermia aims to prevent further heat loss and get medical help.

1　Begin ESM—do a scene survey (see page 2-3). If the temperature is lower than 15°C, suspect hypothermia either as the casualty's main problem or as a complication of another injury. Do a primary survey (see page 2-5).

2　Take measures to prevent further heat loss:

◆ cover exposed skin with suitable clothing or covers; make sure the head is well insulated

◆ adjust the casualty's clothing to keep wind or drafts out. Wrap the casualty in something windproof—reflective "space blankets" and plastic garbage bags are good for this

◆ if possible, move the casualty out of the cool or cold environment. If you cannot move indoors, protect the casualty from the wind

◆ loosen or remove tight clothing

◆ wet clothing causes severe heat loss. If you are in a shelter and have a dry change of clothes, gently replace wet clothes with dry ones. If you are not sheltered, put the dry clothes over the wet clothes. If you don't have dry clothes, press as much water out of the wet clothes as possible and wrap the casualty with something windproof

◆ insulate the casualty from cold objects— have him sit on a rolled-up jacket or lie on a blanket

3　Get medical help. If you have to transport the casualty, transport in the recovery position.

4　Give ongoing casualty care, monitoring the ABCs. If breathing is ineffective, give assisted breathing—see page 4-33. If there is no pulse, give CPR, but don't delay transporting the casualty.

Cautions in first aid for hypothermia

◆ Handle the casualty **very gently** and keep him horizontal if possible. Cold affects the electrical impulses that make the heart beat. As a result, the hypothermic casualty's heart beat is very delicate. The heart can stop with rough handling of the casualty.

◆ When checking for a pulse in a casualty who may be hypothermic, continue checking **for one to two minutes.** The heart may be beating very slowly or very faintly—you have to take longer to find the pulse.

◆ Don't give the casualty any alcohol, coffee, or other drinks with caffeine, or let him smoke —these can increase heat loss.

◆ Don't rub the casualty's body to improve circulation—this will cause cold blood to flow back to the body core and cool the body further.

10

Immersion hypothermia

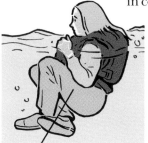

Immersion hypothermia refers to hypothermia caused by being in cold water. A person loses heat 25-30 times faster in water than in air of the same temperature. Immersion hypothermia can happen very quickly, within minutes, if a person falls into cold water. Suspect hypothermia whenever someone falls into water by mistake even in the summer. Immersion hypothermia can also happen more slowly, for instance while swimming or scuba diving in a lake. In these cases, hypothermia creeps up on the casualty, and may not be suspected right away.

if possible, use the "heat escape lessening position" (HELP)

Do the following when a hypothermic casualty is in the water:

◆ tell the casualty not to take off any clothing—clothing helps keep heat in

◆ tell the casualty to move as little as possible—moving around causes more heat loss (by convection)

When taking a casualty out of the water, keep him in a horizontal position, and handle him as gently as possible. Give first aid for hypothermia as outlined on page 10-5, to prevent further heat loss, and get medical help.

Frozen state

When the temperature is below zero, it is possible to discover someone who is completely frozen—this is a **frozen state**. Recognize a frozen state when:

◆ the casualty is found in a cold location and is unresponsive

◆ the joints of the jaw and neck are rigid when you try to open the airway

◆ the skin and deeper tissues are cold and cannot be depressed

◆ the entire body moves as a solid unit

If the casualty is in a frozen state, do not attempt first aid for the ABCs. Transport the casualty to medical help if this doesn't pose a risk to the rescuers. Otherwise, get yourself to safety and advise the police of the location of the frozen person.

Hypothermia scenarios

Below are three hypothermia scenarios—mild hypothermia, moderate hypothermia and severe hypothermia. The first aid you give in an emergency depends on the situation, and a variety of factors, including: the casualty's condition, the resources you have, your own condition, the distance to medical help, etc.

Scenario 1: Mild hypothermia

Early recognition is the key to preventing hypothermia from getting worse.

I'll get out of the wind and dry out my shirt at the ski shack. . . should have a snack too.

Recognition	Action

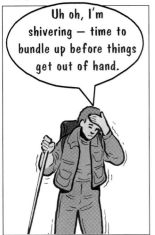

Uh oh, I'm shivering — time to bundle up before things get out of hand.

- *put on a hat to prevent radiant heat loss*

- *put on a windproof shell to prevent heat loss by convection*

- *put on a scarf or "ski tube" to reduce heat loss by breathing*

- *get into a warm environment as quickly as possible*

- *the muscular activity of skiing will generate heat to help warm the body, as long as there is water and food energy in the body*

- *make sure the body is fully rewarmed before continuing activity*

10

About rewarming a casualty

Types of rewarming

There are two types of rewarming: passive rewarming and active rewarming. **Passive rewarming** means preventing further heat loss and letting the casualty's body rewarm itself—this usually works well for mild and moderate hypothermia. **Active rewarming** means adding heat to the casualty's body to warm it up. Active rewarming can cause complications and should only be done at a hospital—but active rewarming is what a casualty in severe hypothermia needs. This is why in severe hypothermia the first aid is to prevent further heat loss and safely transport the casualty to medical help.

Active rewarming by the first aider

In mild hypothermia, you can give the fully conscious casualty something warm and sweet to drink. Although it probably won't add much heat to the casualty's body, it will help him to feel better. Don't give a casualty in moderate hypothermia anything to drink. His muscles for swallowing may not work well and he could choke. The effectiveness of rewarming a person by skin-to-skin contact has not been proved, and neither has the use of hot water bottles, etc. Also, these can cause complications. The best first aid is to prevent further heat loss and get medical help.

Scenario 2: Moderate hypothermia

Look for how heat is being lost and take action to stop further heat loss. If possible, get the casualty into a sheltered, warm place.

Recognition

Action

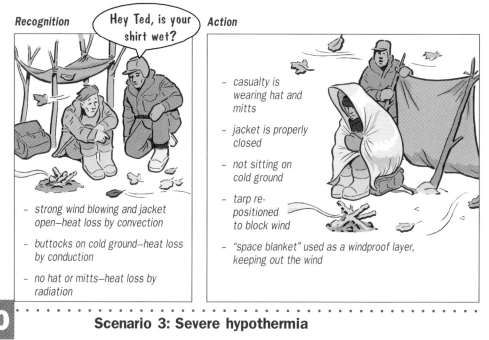

- casualty is wearing hat and mitts

- jacket is properly closed

- not sitting on cold ground

- tarp re-positioned to block wind

- "space blanket" used as a windproof layer, keeping out the wind

- strong wind blowing and jacket open–heat loss by convection

- buttocks on cold ground–heat loss by conduction

- no hat or mitts–heat loss by radiation

10

Scenario 3: Severe hypothermia

Preventing further heat loss is important, but getting medical help is the priority.

Recognition

Action

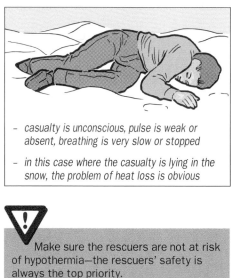

- casualty is unconscious, pulse is weak or absent, breathing is very slow or stopped

- in this case where the casualty is lying in the snow, the problem of heat loss is obvious

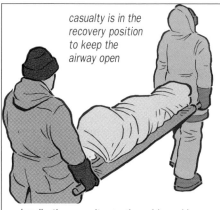

casualty is in the recovery position to keep the airway open

Make sure the rescuers are not at risk of hypothermia–the rescuers' safety is always the top priority.

- handle the casualty gently and keep him horizontal–use a blanket lift to place the casualty on the stretcher and wrap him to reduce heat loss

- transport to medical help

Frostbite

Frostbite refers to the freezing of tissues when exposed to temperatures below zero. It is a progressive injury with two stages: frostnip, superficial frostbite and deep frostbite.

Stages of frostbite and their signs and symptoms

Stage	Description		Signs & symptoms
superficial frostbite	The full thickness of the skin is frozen. This follows frostnip when further heat loss isn't prevented and freezing continues.		– white, waxy-looking skin – skin is firm to touch, but tissue underneath is soft – may feel pain at first, followed by numbness
deep frostbite	The skin, and the tissues underneath the skin, are frozen, sometimes to the bone. A serious condition, often involving an entire hand or foot.		– white, waxy-looking skin that turns greyish-blue as frostbite progresses – skin feels cold and hard – there is no feeling in the area

First aid for superficial frostbite

1 Begin ESM—do a scene survey (see page 2-3). Gradually rewarm the frostbitten part with body heat.

◆ cover frostbitten toes, ears, etc. with warm hands

◆ warm up frostbitten fingers by breathing on them or placing them in a warm area of the body like the armpit, abdomen or groin

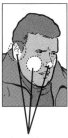

frostbitten skin looks white and waxy

2 Take measures to prevent these areas from freezing again—either stop the activity or dress more appropriately.

First aid for deep frostbite

How much tissue is permanently damaged by deep frostbite depends on how long the part was frozen, how much the part was used while frozen and how the part was thawed. Deep frostbite needs medical help as soon as possible.

1 Begin ESM—do a scene survey (see page 2-3). Prevent further heat loss from the frozen part and the rest of the body. Handle the frozen tissue very gently to prevent further tissue damage.

2 Do not rub the arms and legs. Keep the casualty as still as possible.

3 Get medical help. If the feet or legs are frozen, don't let the casualty walk (if possible)—transport using a rescue carry or stretcher, see Chapter 14.

If medical help is not available, you are in a safe, warm place and there is no danger of the part refreezing, then thaw the frozen part according to the instructions below.

If the casualty must walk, do not thaw the frozen part—there will be less tissue damage and pain if the part is left frozen. Make sure the rest of the body is well protected from the cold and the casualty has plenty of food and water during the journey to safety.

4 Make the casualty warm and as comfortable as possible. Gently remove the clothing from the affected part. Find a container that is large enough to hold the entire frozen part. Fill this with water that feels warm when you put your elbow in it (about 40°C). Make sure you have more water at this temperature available.

5 Remove any jewellery and put the whole frozen part in the water. Keep adding warm water to keep the water in the container at a constant temperature. Keep the part in the water until it is pink or does not improve any more—this can take up to 40 minutes, and may be painful.

6 Gently dry the affected part. Put sterile dressings over wounds and between fingers or toes.

7 Keep the part elevated and warm. Do not break any blisters that form.

8 Get medical help. Give ongoing casualty care.

Cautions in first aid for frostbite

♦ **Do not** rub the area—the tiny ice crystals in the tissues may cause more tissue damage.

♦ **Do not** rub snow on the area—this may cause further freezing and tissue damage from the rubbing.

♦ **Do not** apply direct heat; this may rewarm the area too quickly.

Heat exposure and illnesses

Prolonged exposure to extreme heat or heavy exertion in a hot environment can cause heat illnesses.

in a dry environment, the casualty may not seem to be sweating because the sweat evaporates quickly

Heat cramps

Heat cramps are painful muscle cramps, usually in the legs and abdomen, caused by losing too much water and salt through sweating. Heat cramps are usually caused by heavy exercise or physical work in a hot environment. They are not serious and may be reversed by first aid. The casualty will complain of cramps and show signs of excessive sweating.

First aid for heat cramps

1 Begin ESM—do a scene survey (see page 2-3). Place the casualty at rest in a cool place.

2 Give the conscious casualty water to drink. She can have as much as she wants.

3 If the cramps don't go away, get medical help.

Heat exhaustion

Heat exhaustion is more serious than heat cramps. The casualty has lost fluid through sweating. Circulation is affected because the blood flows away from the major organs and pools in the blood vessels just below the skin.

Signs and symptoms of heat exhaustion

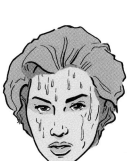

◆ excessive sweating and dilated pupils

◆ casualty may complain of dizziness, blurred vision, headache or cramps

◆ signs of shock, including: cold, clammy skin; weak, rapid pulse; rapid, shallow breathing; vomiting and unconsciousness

First aid for heat exhaustion

First aid for heat exhaustion combines the first aid for heat cramps with the first aid for shock.

1   Begin ESM—do a scene survey (see page 2-3) and a primary survey (see page 2-5). Send for medical help.

2   If the casualty is **conscious**:

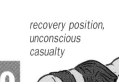

shock position, conscious casualty

- ◆ place her at rest in a cool place with the feet and legs elevated (shock position)

- ◆ remove excessive clothing and loosen tight clothing at the neck and waist

- ◆ give her water to drink, as much as she will take. If the casualty vomits, don't give anything by mouth and get medical help right away

If the casualty is **unconscious**:

recovery position, unconscious casualty

- ◆ place her in the recovery position

- ◆ get medical help right away

- ◆ monitor breathing and pulse and give life-saving first aid as needed

3   Give ongoing casualty care until medical help takes over

Heatstroke (sunstroke)

Heatstroke is a life-threatening condition where the body's temperature rises far above normal. It is caused by prolonged exposure in a hot, humid, and perhaps poorly ventilated environment. In **classic heatstroke,** the body's temperature control mechanism fails, sweating stops and the body temperature rises rapidly. In **exertional heatstroke**, the body temperature rises rapidly due to heavy physical exertion in high temperatures, even though sweating continues. Elderly people and those in poor health are more likely to suffer from heatstroke. Without immediate first aid heatstroke can result in permanent brain damage or death .

Signs and symptoms of heatstroke

- ◆ body temperature rapidly rises to 40ºC or higher—the casualty is hot to the touch

◆ the pulse is rapid and full but gets weaker in later stages

◆ breathing is noisy

◆ skin is flushed, hot and dry in classic heatstroke, and flushed, hot and sweaty in exertional heatstroke

◆ casualty is restless and may complain of headache, fatigue, dizziness and nausea

◆ vomiting, convulsions, unconsciousness

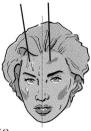

skin is flushed and hot, and may be wet or dry

You can tell the difference between heat exhaustion and heatstroke by the condition of the skin. In heat exhaustion, the skin is moist and cold. In heatstroke, the skin is hot, flushed and may be dry or wet.

First aid for heatstroke

1 Begin ESM—do a scene survey (see page 2-3). Lowering body temperature is the most urgent first aid for heatstroke. The casualty's life depends on how quickly this can be done.

10

◆ move the casualty to a cool, shaded place

◆ cool the casualty—remove outer clothing and either:

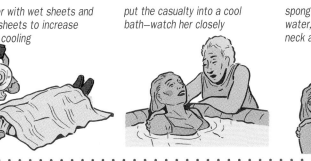

cover her with wet sheets and fan the sheets to increase cooling

put the casualty into a cool bath—watch her closely

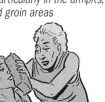

sponge the casualty with cool water, particularly in the armpits, neck and groin areas

2 When her body feels cool to touch, cover her with a dry sheet. Put the conscious casualty into the shock position and the unconscious casualty into the recovery position. Monitor the casualty closely. If her temperature begins to rise again, repeat the cooling process.

3 Give ongoing casualty care until handover to medical help.

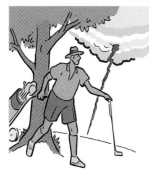

Lightning injuries

Electrical storms occur throughout most of Canada. Although people generally think that the chance of being struck by lightning is very low, there are many injuries each year from lightning strikes.

The sidebar lists some of the injuries that a lightning strike can cause. Give first aid at the scene of a lightning strike as you would any other emergency scene, keeping the following in mind:

Seventy to eighty percent of the people struck by lightning do not die.

- ◆ a person struck by lightning does not hold an electrical charge—you can touch the casualty without fear of electric shock

- ◆ the casualty has probably been thrown—suspect a head or spinal injury

- ◆ lightning **does** strike the same place twice— assess the risk of another strike, and move to a safer location if needed

- ◆ if more than one person is injured, the princi- ples of multiple casualty management are reversed—**give first aid to casualties without breathing and/or pulse** since the casualties still breathing are on the road to recovery

- ◆ advise all casualties of a lightning strike to seek medical help to ensure a full evaluation of any injuries

10

Injuries caused by lightning
• • • • • • • • • • • • • •

Injuries
from the electricity:
- ◆ burns—1st, 2nd & 3rd degree
- ◆ stopped breathing
- ◆ stopped heart
- ◆ injured nervous system

Injuries
from being thrown:
- ◆ head and/or spinal injury
- ◆ sprains, strains & fractures

Injuries
from the light & thunder:
- ◆ injured cornea and/or retina
- ◆ injured optic nerve
- ◆ ruptured eardrums
- ◆ loss of hearing

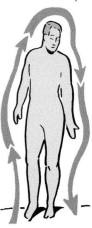

in a lightning strike, the lightning often travels around the person rather than through him

FOCUS ON SAFETY

Five ways to prevent cold injuries

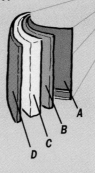

wear several layers of loose-fitting clothing made of fabric that breathes, and keeps you warm even when it is wet

1 Dress for the weather and your activity

Before you go into the cold, know the weather forecast and be prepared for the worst possible conditions.

Physical activity makes you sweat, which makes you wet and causes heat loss. Learn how to dress for your specific activity, and avoid over-activity. The illustration at the right is a guideline for dressing in cold weather.

2 Stay dry

Being wet is a leading cause of heat loss and hypothermia. If there is rain or snow in the forecast, bring a waterproof layer of clothing. If you're not prepared for wet weather, take shelter **before** it turns wet. Stop physical activity **before** sweating dampens your clothing. Change your socks as they get damp and **before** your feet get cold.

3 Stay safe

When weather conditions are extreme, shorten the time you'll be outside. Use the "buddy" system and check on each other often for signs of cold injuries.

A. *wicking layer against the skin to "wick" moisture off the skin and to the next layer*

B. *light insulating layer that insulates even when wet—wool and polyester are good choices, cotton is a poor choice*

C. *heavy insulating layer(s) to keep you warm in the specific conditions—wool sweater, synthetic fleece are good choices*

D. *windproof/waterproof layer to protect you from the elements—choose a fabric appropriate for your activity*

10

4 Nourish yourself

Bring high-energy foods with you—raisins, dried fruits, nuts and candy bars are good choices. Also bring plenty of liquids for drinking to prevent dehydration. Hot sweet drinks, weak tea and herbal teas without caffeine are best. Cool water is also a good choice. Avoid eating snow as this contributes to heat loss. Never drink alcohol (or use tobacco)—these add to heat loss.

5 Keep your furnace running

The best way to make your body generate more heat is to use your big muscles—the muscles in your legs, buttocks and arms. Jog on the spot, do knee bends or swing your arms to generate heat. When exercising to warm up, tighten your collar and cuffs to prevent the warm air inside your clothing from escaping. And remember that to exercise, your body needs fuel—don't forget to eat and drink.

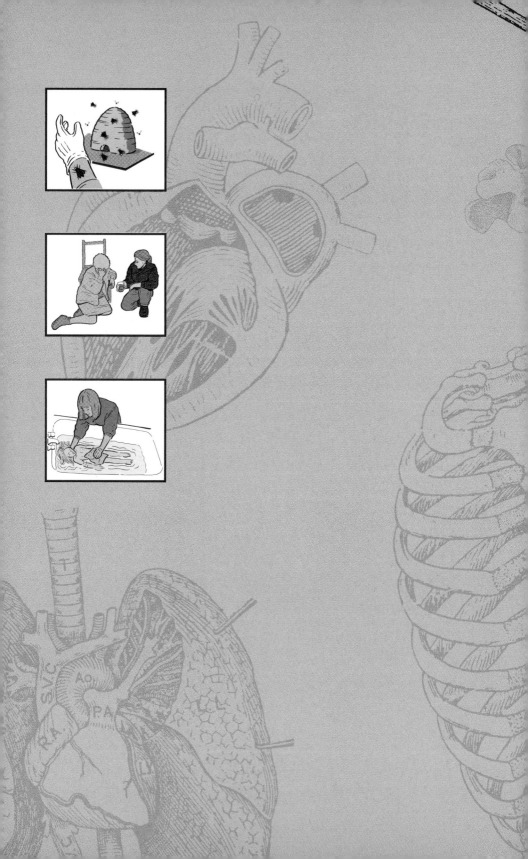

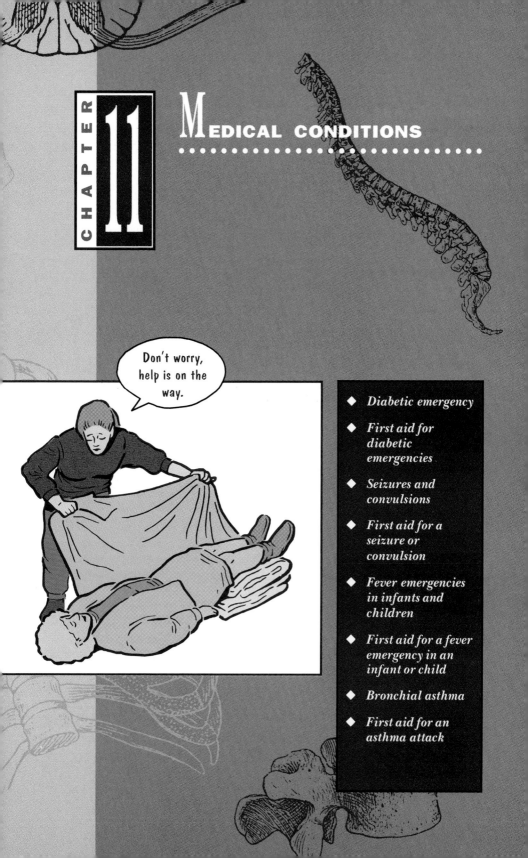

- *Diabetic emergency*
- *First aid for diabetic emergencies*
- *Seizures and convulsions*
- *First aid for a seizure or convulsion*
- *Fever emergencies in infants and children*
- *First aid for a fever emergency in an infant or child*
- *Bronchial asthma*
- *First aid for an asthma attack*

Diabetic emergency

In a healthy person, the body produces the **insulin** needed to convert sugar in the blood into energy for the body's cells to use. **Diabetes** is a condition in which there is not enough insulin in the blood, so sugar isn't converted into energy. As a result, sugar builds up in the blood, and the cells don't get the energy they need. A person with diabetes takes medication by mouth or injection, and carefully controls what he eats (the source of energy) and her level of exercise (the use of energy). A diabetic emergency occurs when there is too much or too little insulin in the blood.

insulin shock—
not enough
sugar, too
much insulin

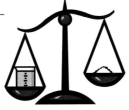

diabetic coma—
too much sugar,
not enough
insulin

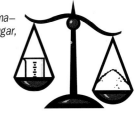

There are two kinds of diabetic emergency—**insulin shock** (hypoglycemia) and **diabetic coma** (hyperglycemia). The signs and symptoms for each are listed in the table below, along with the possible causes. As a first aider, it is not important to know the type of diabetic emergency—follow the first aid on the next page. What is important is that you recognize the casualty's condition as an emergency and get medical help quickly.

Causes, signs and symptoms of diabetic emergencies		
	Insulin shock (needs sugar)	**Diabetic coma (needs insulin)**
time to develop	develops very quickly	develops over hours or days
possible cause	– took too much insulin – not eaten enough, or vomited – more exercise than usual	– did not take enough insulin – eating too much food – less exercise than usual – casualty has an ongoing illness and her body needs more insulin
pulse/breathing	strong and rapid/shallow	weak and rapid/deep and sighing
skin condition	sweaty, pale and cold	flushed, dry and warm
level of consc.	faintness to unconscious	drowsy, becoming unconscious
other signs and symptoms	– headache – confused, irritable and aggressive – trembling, staggering – difficulty speaking	– thirsty, then nausea and vomiting – frequent urination – breath has a nail polish smell

First aid for diabetic emergencies

The aim of first aid in a diabetic emergency is to keep the casualty's condition from getting worse while you get medical help.

1   Begin ESM—do a scene survey (see page 2-3). If the casualty is unresponsive, get medical help immediately. If you are alone—see page 1-18.

2   Do a primary survey and give first aid for the ABCs.

3   If the casualty is unconscious, place her into the recovery position and monitor the ABCs until medical help takes over. The casualty may be wearing a medical alert device that will give you more information about her condition.

look for a medical alert device at the neck or wrist

If the casualty is conscious, ask what is wrong. She may be able to tell you, or she may be confused.

◆ if the casualty can tell you what she needs, or if you can tell by the signs and symptoms, help her take what is needed—sugar or her prescribed medication

◆ if the casualty is confused about what is needed, give her something sweet to eat or drink—sugar may help, and if it doesn't, it won't make the casualty any worse

sweeten a drink with 30 ml (2 tablespoons) of sugar or something else sweet, like orange juice

> I know you're not sure what's wrong, but drinking this may help and it won't hurt.

11

4   Give ongoing casualty care. Send for medical help if you have not done so already.

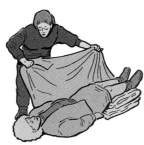

if the casualty is conscious and very weak, place her in the position of most comfort, which may be the shock position

Warning

Don't confuse a diabetic emergency with drunkenness. Many of the behavioural signs are the same, but a person having a diabetic emergency needs immediate medical help. Check the signs and look for a medical alert device.

Seizures and convulsions

A **seizure** is caused by abnormal electrical activity in the brain. In a **partial seizure**, only part of the brain is affected. The person may experience a tingling or twitching in one area of the body. In a **generalized seizure**, the whole brain is affected—the person loses consciousness and may have convulsions. A **convulsion** is an abnormal muscle contraction, or series of muscle contractions, that the person cannot control.

Epilepsy is a disorder of the nervous system characterized by seizures. Many people with seizure disorders like epilepsy take medication to control the condition. Other causes of seizures include:

◆ head injury

◆ stroke

◆ brain infection

◆ drug overdose

◆ a high fever in infants and children

11

A typical generalized seizure . . .

. . . has two phases:
The **"tonic"** phase:

◆ a sudden loss of consciousness causing the person to fall. The person's body becomes rigid for up to a minute during which the face and neck may turn bluish.

The **"clonic"** phase:

◆ convulsions occur, breathing is noisy, frothy saliva may appear around the mouth and the teeth may grind.

When the seizure is over, the muscles gradually relax and the person regains consciousness.

With epilepsy, the person may feel that a seizure is about to occur because of a brief sensation she experiences, called an **aura**. The aura, which may be a hallucinated sound, smell, or a feeling of movement in the body, is felt just before the seizure. A major seizure can come on very suddenly, but seldom lasts longer than three minutes. After the seizure, the person may not remember what happened. She may appear dazed and confused, and feel exhausted and sleepy.

Signs and symptoms of a generalized seizure

◆ a sudden cry, stiffening of the body and loss of consciousness causing the person to fall

◆ noisy breathing and frothy saliva at the mouth

◆ the body jerks

◆ breathing may stop or be irregular for a minute—the casualty may turn blue

◆ loss of bladder and bowel control

First aid for a seizure or convulsion

First aid for a seizure aims to protect the casualty from injury during convulsions and to keep the airway open while the casualty is unconscious.

1   Begin ESM—do a scene survey (see page 2-3). Make the area safe—clear away hard or sharp objects that could cause injury. Clear onlookers away to ensure the casualty's privacy.

turning the casualty to the side allows for drainage of fluids, and keeps the tongue from falling back and blocking the airway

2   During convulsions:

- don't restrict the casualty's movements. Gently guide them, if necessary, to protect from injury

- carefully loosen tight clothing, especially around the neck

- place something soft under the head

- **do not** try to put anything in the mouth, between the teeth or to hold the tongue

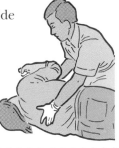

3   After convulsions:

after convulsions, place the unconscious casualty into the recovery position

- assess responsiveness and do a primary survey (see page 2-5). Place the unconscious casualty into the recovery position—wipe away any fluids from the mouth and nose

- do a secondary survey to see if the casualty was injured during the seizure (although it is rare, injury is possible)—give first aid for any injuries

- give ongoing casualty care, monitoring breathing, keeping the casualty warm and allowing her to rest (she may need up to an hour)

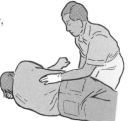

- don't give the casualty any liquids during or immediately after a seizure

Call for medical help if:

- the casualty is unconscious for more than five minutes, or has a second major seizure within a few minutes

- this is the person's first seizure or the cause of the seizure is unknown (ask the casualty when she regains consciousness)

Fever emergencies in infants and children

A rapid rise in temperature to 40°C (104°F) or higher can cause convulsions in infants and children. A fever emergency is when the temperature, taken in the armpit, is:

◆ 38°C (100.5°F) or higher for an infant

◆ 40°C (104°F) or higher for a child

First aid for a fever emergency in an infant or child

1 Begin ESM—do a scene survey (see page 2-3).

2 Advise the parent/caregiver to call the doctor immediately and follow her advice. If the doctor can't be reached, advise the parent/caregiver to give acetaminophen (e.g. Tempra® or Tylenol®, not ASA—see warning below) according to the directions on the label. This should bring down the child's temperature.

sponge the child with lukewarm water for 20 minutes

3 Encourage the child to drink fluids.

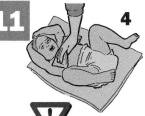

4 If the temperature doesn't go down, sponge the child with lukewarm water for about 20 minutes. Don't immerse the child or infant in a tub—the temperature will go down more quickly if the wet skin is exposed to air currents.

5 Dry and dress the child in comfortable but not overly warm clothing. Monitor the child's temperature and repeat steps 3 to 5, as necessary, until medical help is reached.

6 If the child has a convulsion:

◆ don't restrain the child, but protect her from injury by removing hard objects and gently guiding movements

◆ loosen constrictive clothing

◆ when the convulsions stop, place the child into the best recovery position for her age—see page 1-32.

Bronchial asthma

Bronchial asthma (often called, simply, "asthma") is an illness in which the person has repeated attacks (asthmatic attacks) of shortness of breath. These usually include wheezing and coughing. More children have asthma than adults. In half of these children, the condition goes away by the time they are adults.

Asthmatic attacks are often caused by certain common **triggers**, such as having a cold. Other common triggers are shown at the right. People with asthma can avoid the things that trigger an asthmatic attack, but even with this precaution, an asthmatic attack can occur unexpectedly.

In an asthmatic attack, air flow to the lungs is reduced. How much it is reduced determines whether the attack is mild or severe. A mild asthmatic attack can simply be annoying; a severe asthmatic attack can be fatal.

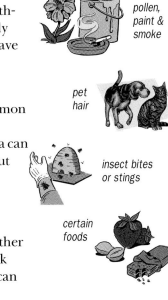

common asthma triggers

pollen, paint & smoke

pet hair

insect bites or stings

certain foods

healthy air passageway in the lungs

during an asthmatic attack, airflow in the lungs is reduced three ways:
– the muscles around the air passages tighten

– the inner linings of the air passages swell

– the amount and thickness of mucus increases

11

First aid for an asthma attack

As a first aider, your help will only be needed when an asthmatic attack is severe. The signs and symptoms and first aid for a severe asthma attack are given on page 4-15 under *Breathing emergencies caused by illnesses.* In a mild asthmatic attack, the casualty will be able to manage on her own.

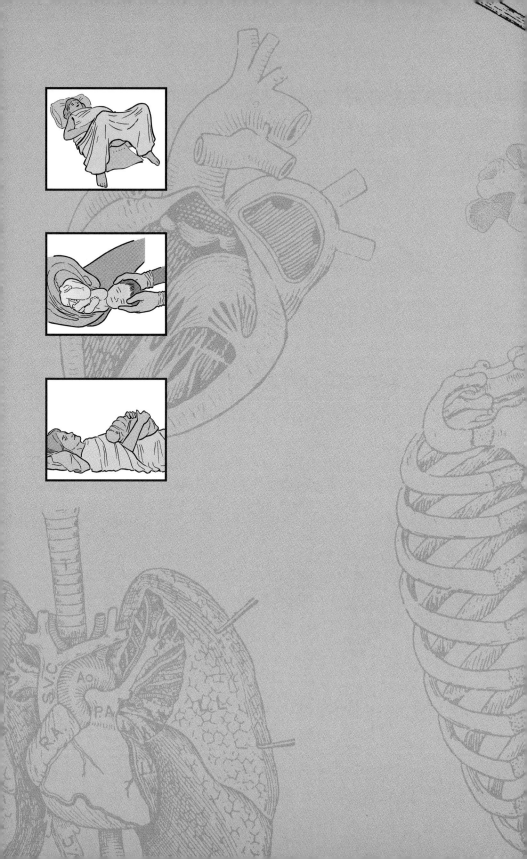

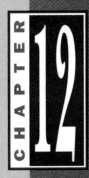
EMERGENCY CHILDBIRTH AND MISCARRIAGE

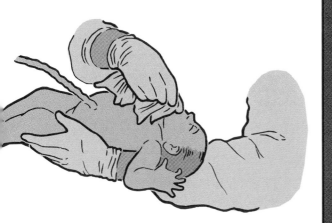

◆ *Anatomy*

◆ *Pregnancy and childbirth*

◆ *Early labour*

◆ *Birth of the baby*

◆ *Delivery of the placenta*

◆ *Emergency childbirth*

◆ *Assessing the stage of labour*

◆ *Vaginal bleeding and miscarriage*

◆ *First aid for miscarriage*

Emergency childbirth occurs when a child is born at an unplanned time or at an unplanned place. This may happen when there is a sudden, premature delivery or when the mother cannot get to the hospital for a full-term delivery. Miscarriage, also called **spontaneous abortion**, occurs when the fetus is "born" before it is developed enough to survive. This is before the 20th week of pregnancy.

Anatomy

A basic knowledge of the female reproductive system during pregnancy will help you to give the needed care and protection during an emergency delivery.

mother's back

mother's front

uterus–the hollow, muscular structure, also called the **womb**, that holds the developing baby

placenta–a large, flat, spongy organ that is attached to the inside wall of the uterus, that supplies the fetus with nutrients and oxygen from the mother

umbilical cord–a rope-like structure that carries blood between the mother and the fetus

fetus–what the baby is called until it is born

amniotic sac–the bag that the fetus develops in; it is full of fluid called **amniotic fluid**

amniotic fluid–liquid that surrounds and protects the fetus in the amniotic sac

cervix–the neck of the uterus that opens during labour so the fetus can be born

vagina–the muscular passageway through which the baby is born, also called the **birth canal**

Pregnancy and childbirth

A normal pregnancy is 40 weeks. If the baby is born before the 38th week, it is considered premature. If the baby is born between the 38th and 42nd week, it is full term. Most babies born are full term, but it is not uncommon for a baby to be born prematurely.

A baby is born in a three-stage process called **labour**. It can be hard to tell when labour has started, but it has probably begun when one of the following happens:

◆ the uterus contracts at regular intervals of ten to twenty minutes, with contractions getting increasingly stronger and closer together

◆ amniotic fluid comes out of the vagina, which means the amniotic sac has broken—this may be called the "water breaking." There may be a trickle or a rush of fluid

◆ blood and mucus come from the vagina—this "bloody show" means that the mucus plug that had sealed the cervix has come out because the cervix has started to open

Stage 1: Early labour—opening of the cervix

The first stage of labour, called **early labour**, can take up to eighteen hours for a first child, but may be much shorter for second or subsequent children. Usually there is enough time to get the mother to a medical facility. **Early labour** involves muscular contractions that may begin as an aching feeling in the lower back. As contractions get stronger, they feel like cramps in the lower abdomen. Contractions cause the cervix to open, or dilate. The cervix has to dilate until the opening is about 10 cm across before the fetus can be pushed down the birth canal, which is the second stage of labour.

Stage 2: Birth of the baby

The second stage of labour usually takes about one hour. It begins when the cervix is fully dilated and the contractions start to push the fetus out of the uterus and through the vagina. When the baby's head is close to the vaginal opening, the mother may feel a tremendous urge to push the fetus out. Usually, the fetus' head is born first, then one shoulder, then the other shoulder, and then the rest of the body is pushed out quite quickly. The second stage of labour ends when the baby is born. The baby is still connected to the mother by the umbilical cord. The cord is attached to the placenta, still in the uterus.

Stage 3: Delivery of the placenta

The third stage of labour is the delivery of the placenta after the baby is born. The uterus gets smaller and pushes the placenta out. This stage usually takes between ten and twenty minutes. Labour is finished when the placenta is delivered.

Emergency childbirth

Your role as a first aider in emergency childbirth is to help the mother deliver the baby, to protect the mother and baby, and to save all parts of the placenta and amniotic sac until medical help takes over.

Assessing the stage of labour

If the mother is still in early labour, you probably still have time to get her to a hospital—if you are not sure, call for medical help and stay where you are. If labour is in the second stage, the baby will be born quite soon. Recognize the second stage of labour by:

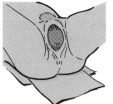

when you can see the baby, it will be born very soon

♦ longer and stronger contractions, less than two minutes apart

♦ the mother's previous experience—if she says the baby is coming, believe her

♦ bulging of the vaginal opening and seeing the baby's head (called **crowning**)

♦ the mother is straining and pushing down, and feels like she has to have a bowel movement

What you'll need

. . . .

♦ clean towels or sheets, and a baby blanket

♦ gloves (preferably sterile), or soap, water and towels to wash your hands

♦ sterile tape or a narrow roller bandage to tie off the umbilical cord, if necessary

♦ absorbent material to absorb vaginal bleeding after the delivery

♦ container or plastic bag for the placenta

When you see these signs, you will not have time to get the mother to medical help. Call medical help to the scene, if possible, and get ready to deliver the baby.

Emergency delivery

1   Begin ESM—do the scene survey (see page 2-3). Locate someone to help you, preferably a woman. Get the materials you will need to deliver the baby and the placenta. You may find some of these things in a bag the mother has packed for the hospital.

2 During early labour, let the mother find the position of most comfort—usually on her left side. Put a folded towel under her right hip if she wants to lie on her back.

Encourage the mother to empty her bladder and bowels as often as possible to avoid complications later. It is also important at this stage that the mother does not push or strain with the contractions. She should try to breathe and relax through them.

3 During the second stage of labour, when the baby will be born very soon, place the mother on her back with knees bent and head supported, unless she prefers another position. Cover her with sheets so you can easily lift them to check on the progress of labour.

Prevent infection

You need to do what you can to prevent infection:

◆ keep anyone who has a cold or other infectious condition away

◆ wear gloves if available—don't let the gloves touch anything except the baby

◆ if no gloves, wash your hands, forearms and fingernails for at least 5 minutes

◆ there should be no need to put your fingers inside the mother's vagina; keep them away from the anus

◆ protect yourself from infectious conditions the mother may have—minimize your contact with her blood, and wash carefully after the delivery

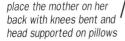

place the mother on her back with knees bent and head supported on pillows

place a clean sheet or towel under her buttocks extending between her thighs

cover the mother with sheets or towels so that she is not exposed unnecessarily

place clean towels between the mother's legs on which to lay the baby when it is born (keep some clean towels for wrapping the baby)

12

Reassure the mother and try to appear calm and unhurried. When the mother is in position, put on your gloves, or wash your hands, arms and fingernails.

4 Tell your assistant to help the mother through the contractions. When you can see the baby's head, the mother can push with the contractions. Tell her to wait until the contraction peaks, then take a deep breath, put her chin on her chest and push down as hard and as long as she can, while she is holding her breath. She may be able to push like this twice for each contraction. Position yourself to watch for the baby.

5 When you see the baby, get ready to deliver it. Usually the head is born first and if it comes out too quickly, the baby could be injured. As the head comes out, tell the mother to control her pushing. One way for her to do this is to breathe in fast, shallow breaths (panting).

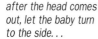
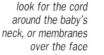
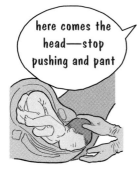

here comes the head—stop pushing and pant

Use your hand to gently control the head, making sure it comes out slowly.

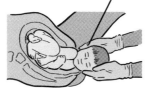

look for the cord around the baby's neck, or membranes over the face

When the head is delivered, tell the mother to stop pushing. Check the baby's face and neck.

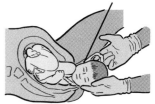

if the umbilical cord is around the baby's neck, gently remove it

If there are membranes over the baby's mouth and nose, pull them away.

Do not...

...pull or exert any force on the umbilical cord, it is delicate and still supplying the baby with blood.

12

If the neck and face are clear, tell the mother to push during the contractions again. Support the baby as it is born, but be careful. A newborn baby has a very slippery whitish coating—handle the baby gently, firmly and carefully.

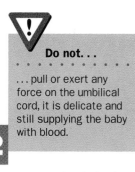

after the head comes out, let the baby turn to the side...

Don't put your hands or fingers into the vagina, and don't touch the mother's anus.

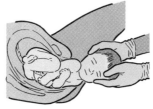

...so the shoulders can come out

Once the shoulders are out, the baby will come out very quickly.

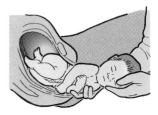

gently support the baby—don't pull

Until the baby begins to breathe, it will look blue-white with a waxy coating.

6 Clear the baby's airway—all babies have fluid in the nose and throat. Hold the baby with the head lower than the body to help drainage.

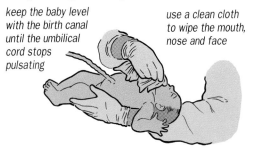

keep the baby level with the birth canal until the umbilical cord stops pulsating

use a clean cloth to wipe the mouth, nose and face

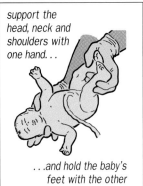

support the head, neck and shoulders with one hand...

...and hold the baby's feet with the other

Most babies will cry right away. When they do, they become pink as they start breathing. If the baby doesn't start to breathe and remains pale and limp, try stimulating him. If the baby still doesn't breathe, start mouth-to-mouth-and-nose AR—see page 4-30. If there is no pulse, start infant CPR—see page 5-26.

Do not...

...hold the baby upside down by the heels and slap him on the back or buttocks to make him cry.

if the baby doesn't breathe, try stimulating him by rubbing his back or gently tapping the soles of his feet

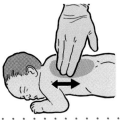

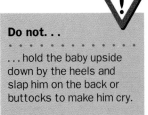

12

7 Once the baby is breathing, pat him dry with a towel, being careful not to remove the slippery coating. Wrap the baby in a dry towel or blanket to keep him warm. Check the umbilical cord. If the cord is still pulsating, keep the baby at the level of the vagina. If the cord has stopped pulsating, place the baby on his side in the mother's arms with his head low to assist drainage. The baby may want to nurse at the mother's breast.

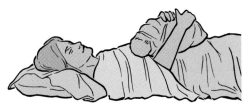

note and record the time the baby was born

8 Check the vagina for bleeding. If there is little or no bleeding, there is no need to tie or cut the umbilical cord. If bleeding from the vagina is severe—act quickly. The umbilical cord must be tied because the baby's blood may be bleeding through the cord and out of the placenta. Tie the umbilical cord and keep the baby at the same level as the vagina.

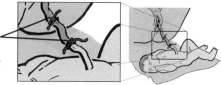

tie the cord in two places about 7 cm (3 in) apart, 15 to 30 cm (6-12 in) from the baby's body— use clean tape or heavy string— ordinary string or thread may cut the cord and should not be used

9 Wait for the placenta to be delivered. This usually happens within twenty minutes of the baby's birth, but don't be surprised if it takes longer. Gently massaging the mother's lower abdomen will quicken the delivery of the placenta.

! Do not. . .

... pull on the umbilical cord and make sure there is no tension or pressure on it.

let the placenta be delivered into a clean towel or container. Make sure that all parts of the placenta are saved and taken to the hospital with the mother and baby

10 There may be some bleeding from the vagina after the delivery of the placenta. This is normal, and can usually be controlled by firmly massaging the uterus. The uterus can be felt as a hard, round mass in the lower abdomen. Massaging it every few minutes will help it to contract which helps control any bleeding. The baby's nursing at the mother's breast also helps to contract the uterus. Use sanitary pads to absorb any bleeding. If the bleeding cannot be controlled, elevate the legs and feet and transport to medical help as soon as possible.

Examine the skin between the anus and the vagina for lacerations and apply pressure with sterile dressings to any bleeding tears of the skin.

12

If medical help will be delayed more than 12 hours and the mother and baby are well, the umbilical cord can be tied and cut. First, check the cord for a pulse. If there is a pulse, don't cut the cord. When pulsations have stopped, tie the cord as shown in step 8 above. Cut the cord between the two ties with a pair of sterilized scissors or a knife that has been sterilized. Periodically check the end of the cord for bleeding and control any bleeding that occurs.

11 Give ongoing casualty care to the mother and infant. Keep them warm and comfortable and transport them to medical help as soon as possible.

Vaginal bleeding and miscarriage

Miscarriage is the loss of the fetus before the 20th week of pregnancy. Most miscarriages happen because the fetus was not developing properly and was not able to survive. The medical term for a miscarriage is **spontaneous abortion**.

Signs and symptoms

◆ vaginal bleeding that could be severe

◆ signs of shock

◆ cramp-like pains in the lower abdomen

◆ aching in the lower back

◆ passage of tissue

First aid for miscarriage

use a pillow under the head if bleeding is not severe

Your main concern in first aid for miscarriage is shock caused by severe bleeding. The woman may be very distressed.

1 Begin ESM—do a scene survey (see page 2-3). Do a primary survey (see page 2-5). Give first aid for shock—place the woman in the shock position, or on her left side.

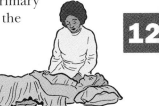

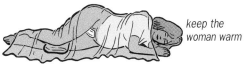

keep the woman warm

2 Call for medical help immediately.

3 Ensure the woman's privacy. Reassure her and give her emotional support. If the woman is upset over losing the baby, explain that the miscarriage was not her fault and was not caused by anything she did.

4 Keep any evidence of tissue and blood loss (bloody sheets, clothing, etc.). Send this with the woman to medical help for examination by the doctor.

5 Give ongoing casualty care.

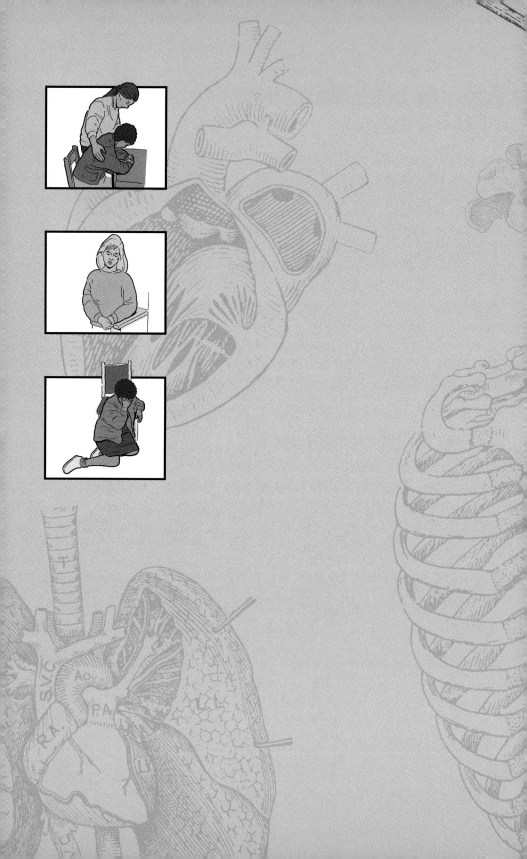

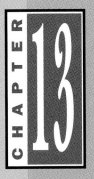

PSYCHOLOGICAL EMERGENCIES

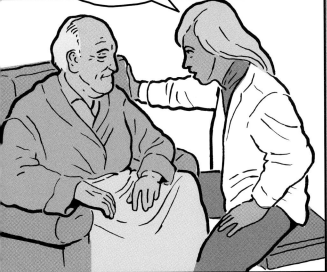

It's O.K. to feel like that—make sure you tell the doctor what you told me.

◆ *Introduction*

◆ *General first aid for psychological emergencies*

◆ *Hysteria*

◆ *Anxiety (panic) attack*

◆ *Physical and sexual assault*

◆ *General first aid for assault*

◆ *Drugs, including alcohol*

◆ *First aid for a casualty on drugs or alcohol*

◆ *Mental illness and suicide gestures*

Introduction

A psychological emergency occurs when a person's state of mind makes it difficult for her to cope with the situation at hand. Your role as a first aider is to help the casualty cope, while protecting her, and others at the scene, until medical help arrives.

There are many causes of psychological emergencies. Knowing the cause of a person's behaviour helps you to decide the best first aid. Some psychological emergencies you may encounter include:

◆ hysteria

◆ anxiety and panic attacks

◆ emotional reaction to assault

◆ alcohol and drug-induced behaviour

◆ mental illness and suicide gestures

General first aid for psychological emergencies

1   Begin ESM—do a scene survey (see page 2-3). In a psychological emergency:

◆ always approach the casualty from the front

◆ identify yourself as a first aider and offer to help. The casualty may refuse your help. If you suspect the casualty isn't able to make a responsible decision about needing help, consider helping anyway

Ensure your safety
. . . .
If the casualty is violent, or you think she may become violent, keep your distance and be very careful. Don't stop the casualty from leaving the area—especially don't block the casualty's exit. Let the casualty go and call the police.

2   Do a primary survey (see page 2-5) and give first aid for life-threatening emergencies—these are always the priority.

Note the casualty's vital signs. Be alert to any changes in the casualty's condition since there may be "unseen" reasons for the behavioural emergency like a head injury or medical condition.

3 Find out the history of the emergency by questioning the casualty and others at the scene. It may take some time before the casualty will talk about the situation.

4 Provide quiet, supportive, reassuring care while arranging for medical help. If the casualty shows any signs of aggressive behaviour, or if you think a crime has taken place, call the police to the scene.

Give first aid for a psychological emergency in a warm, sensitive and compassionate manner. Remember to:

◆ control your own emotions at the scene. Don't overreact to the casualty's behaviour or to emotional attacks directed at you

◆ only get involved to the level you feel comfortable—don't put yourself at risk

◆ only make promises you can keep, and don't lie to the person in any way

◆ include the casualty's friends and/or family in giving care— these people may be able to reassure and help the casualty

◆ be careful whenever there is aggressive behaviour—avoid restraining the casualty—only use restraint to ensure the safety of others

Hysteria

Hysteria is a psychological emergency that causes violent fits of laughing and/or crying, imagined illnesses and a general lack of self-control.

Signs and symptoms of hysteria

◆ loss of control of behaviour that may show as shouting, rolling on the ground, and beating the chest. Behaviour is often made worse by the presence of an audience

◆ hyperventilation that may be severe, causing muscle spasms, especially in the wrists and hands

◆ obvious tremors or "paralysis." The casualty is apparently unable to move

13

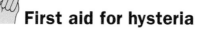

First aid for hysteria

1   Begin ESM—do a scene survey (see page 2-3) and a primary survey (2-5).

2   Lead the casualty to a quiet place, away from onlookers, and try to help the casualty calm down and regain self-control.

3   Be firm and positive. Do not over-sympathize. Listen calmly as the casualty talks. Do not question or contradict the casualty.

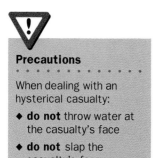

Precautions

When dealing with an hysterical casualty:

◆ **do not** throw water at the casualty's face

◆ **do not** slap the casualty's face

◆ **do not** use force to restrain the casualty

4   It may help to "give the casualty permission" to start feeling better. A hysterical casualty may be very "suggestible" this way. For example, say, "I see your legs aren't working now, but I'm sure they will feel better in a couple of minutes."

5   Stay with the casualty until medical help takes over.

Anxiety (panic) attack

During an anxiety attack, the casualty shows the normal response of a person faced with a life-threatening situation, but there is no threatening situation at hand. Anxiety attacks are quite common.

Signs and symptoms of an anxiety attack

◆ a feeling of fear or a sense that something terrible will happen

◆ the casualty may say:

  ❖ "I can feel my heart pounding!"

  ❖ "I feel like I'm smothering. . . I just can't get enough air!"

  ❖ "I'm having trouble swallowing."

◆ trembling and sweating

◆ hyperventilation, tingling hands and feet

◆ nausea or vomiting

First aid for an anxiety attack

1   Give the same first aid as for hysteria —see previous page.

2   If the casualty is hyperventilating, give first aid for hyperventilation—see page 4-17.

3   Give first aid for any signs and symptoms.

4   Get medical help. Stay with the casualty until medical help takes over.

Physical and sexual assault

Being assaulted is a devastating life crisis because it involves both emotional and physical violence. Along with physical injuries, sexual assault casualties often go into severe emotional shock during or shortly after the attack. Signs and symptoms of this emotional state include:

◆ choking, gagging, nausea, vomiting

◆ hyperventilation

◆ casualty seems dazed

◆ seizures or loss of consciousness

> For related information, see child abuse on page 1-11 and first aid in a violent situation, page 1-9.

General first aid for assault

1   Begin ESM—do a scene survey (see page 2-3). If you suspect an assault, don't disturb evidence by removing, washing, or disposing of clothing.

2   Do a primary survey (see page 2-5). Give first aid for life-threatening injuries.

3   Give general first aid for psychological emergencies (see page 13-2). Tell the casualty not to wash, and if possible, not to use the toilet until told to do so by a trained health professional.

4   Give ongoing casualty care and get medical help.

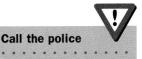

Call the police

In cases of assault, contact the police immediately and stay at the scene until police arrive—you may have information that is helpful.

13

Drugs, including alcohol

Drugs are defined as any substance that can produce a physical or mental effect on the body. They include alcohol, prescription drugs and illegal substances. The effects of drugs are wide-ranging and can be unpredictable. Dosages and combinations of drugs (including alcohol) will affect the casualty's condition. Be prepared for behaviour which can change quickly and range from quiet and disoriented to aggressive.

First aid for a casualty on drugs or alcohol

1 Begin ESM—do a scene survey (see page 2-3). Approach the casualty in a calm, professional, sympathetic manner and try to gain her confidence.

2 Be aware of the possibility of infectious hepatitis or AIDS caused by using contaminated needles—follow the universal precautions to avoid infection (see page 1-8 and 1-9).

3 Try to find out the type and amount of the drug consumed.

4 Monitor all vital signs frequently. If the casualty has convulsions, vomiting or unconsciousness, be sure to maintain an open airway and effective breathing.

5 Check for possible fractures or other injuries and give appropriate first aid.

6 Do not leave the casualty.

7 Give ongoing casualty care as appropriate and get medical help.

- ◆ Do not overlook a serious injury or medical condition as a result of the casualty's behaviour or because signs and symptoms are masked by the effects of alcohol or drugs. The signs of a diabetic emergency can look like drunkenness.

- ◆ Be aware that the behaviour of someone under the influence of alcohol or drugs may interfere with attempts to give first aid.

- ◆ Get help if necessary to calm and reassure the casualty.

- ◆ If the casualty does not become calm, get help.

13

Mental illness and suicidal gestures

When there are no other obvious causes, you can assume that persistent abnormal behaviour results from some form of mental illness. Give general first aid for psychological emergencies (see page 13-2) and get medical help.

Any threats of suicide must be taken very seriously. A person who threatens to commit suicide is usually severely disturbed and suffers some underlying emotional illness. Give the first aid required for any injuries. Use a calm, professional approach at all times and work to establish trust and confidence. Never lie to the casualty. Do not leave the casualty alone. Keep the casualty from harm by whatever means possible.

Call the police and give ongoing casualty care until help arrives.

13

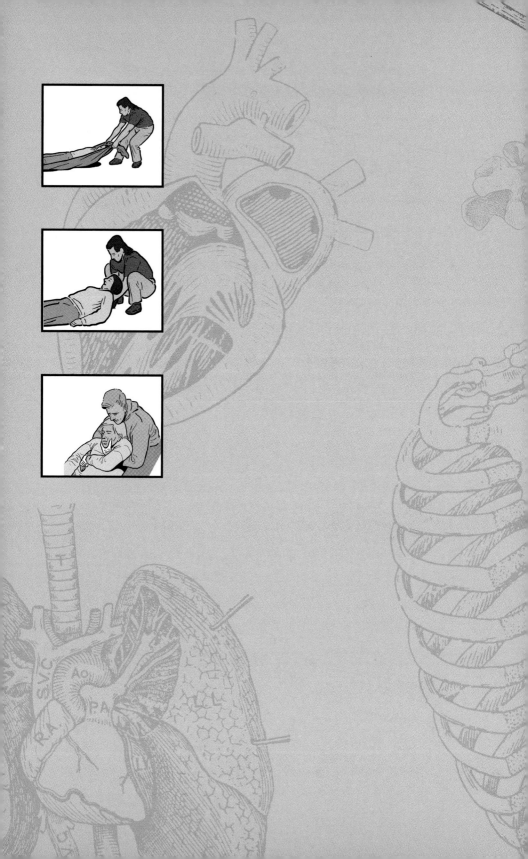

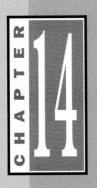

CHAPTER

14

LIFTING TECHNIQUES AND TRANSPORTATION

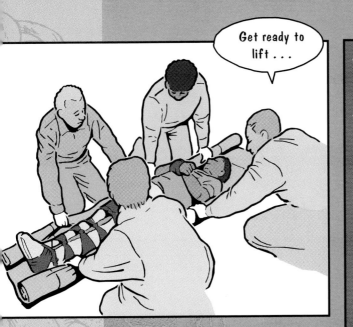

Get ready to lift . . .

◆ Principles of safety for moving a casualty

◆ Lifting techniques and proper body mechanics

◆ Rescue carries

◆ One-rescuer carries

◆ Carries with two or more rescuers

◆ Stretchers

◆ Placing a casualty on a stretcher

◆ Carrying a stretcher

◆ Extrication

◆ Using a short spine board

Principles of safety for moving a casualty

Always try to give necessary first aid where the casualty is found, and wait for the ambulance officers to move the person. However, there are times when this is not possible.

You may have to move a casualty when:

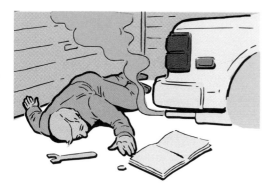

◆ there are life-threatening hazards to yourself or the casualty e.g. danger from fire, explosion, gas or water

◆ essential first aid for wounds or other conditions cannot be given in the casualty's present position or location

◆ the casualty must be transported to a medical facility

If life-threatening hazards make moving a casualty right away necessary, you may need to use a rescue carry.

In urgent and dangerous situations where casualties are moved with less than ideal support for injuries, the casualty's injuries may be made worse by improper movement and handling. The chance of further injury can be reduced with proper rescue carry techniques.

Always move the casualty the shortest possible distance for safety and/or for essential first aid. Use any bystanders available to help you and support any injuries the best you can during the move. Keep the risks to the casualty, yourself, and others to a minimum.

Pick the best method

Moving any casualty from an emergency scene poses dangers to the rescuer as well as the casualty. If the casualty must be moved, select the method that will pose the least risk to the casualty and to yourself. You can be of little help to a casualty if you injure yourself in the rescue.

14

Lifting techniques and proper body mechanics

Using incorrect body mechanics in lifting or moving a casualty may leave the rescuer suffering muscle strain. Use the following lifting guidelines:

1 Stand close to the object to be lifted.

2 Bend your knees, not your waist.

3 Tilt the object so that you can put one hand under the edge or corner closest to you.

4 Place your other hand under the opposite side or corner, getting a good grip on the object.

5 Use your leg muscles to lift, and keep your back straight.

6 When turning, turn your feet first; don't twist your body.

When lowering the object, reverse the procedure.

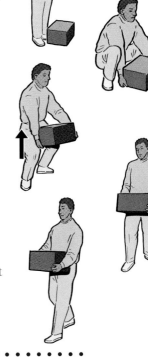

Rescue carries

A rescue carry is an emergency method of moving a casualty over a short distance to safety, shelter, or a better means of transportation. One-rescuer carries can be used depending on the circumstances, the weight of the casualty and the strength of the rescuer. Whenever possible, ask a bystander to help you. When help is available, remember that you:

◆ remain responsible for the casualty

◆ give instructions to the bystander about what to do and what safety precautions to take

◆ fully coordinate the rescue activities

Types of rescue carries

One-rescuer   Page
◆ drag carry 14-4
◆ pick-a-back carry ... 14-4
◆ cradle carry 14-5
◆ human crutch 14-5
◆ fire fighter's carry 14-6

Two or more rescuers
◆ two-hand seat 14-6
◆ four-hand seat 14-7
◆ chair carry 14-7
◆ extremities carry .. 14-8
◆ blanket lift 14-8

14

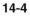

Because of the risk of aggravating any injuries, only use drag carries in the most extreme cases when there is an immediate threat to life.

Drag carry

This carry is used by the single rescuer to drag a casualty who is either lying on his back or in a sitting position. The drag carry provides maximum protection to the head and neck.

If time permits, tie the casualty's wrists together across her chest before dragging.

1   Stand at the casualty's head facing her feet.

2   Crouch down and ease your hands under the casualty's shoulders. Grasp the clothing on each side. Support the casualty's head between your forearms to stop movement.

3   Drag the casualty backward only as far as necessary for her safety.

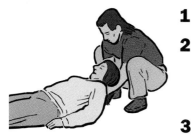
as an alternate method, the first aider can use a blanket to support the casualty, or...

...straddle the casualty, slip the casualty's tied wrists around your neck and drag the casualty to safety

Pick-a-back

This carry is used for a conscious casualty with lower limb injuries, provided he can use his arms. The casualty must be able to help get into position on your back or be already seated at chair or table height.

If the casualty is to be carried pick-a-back for a long distance, make a carrying seat.

♦ make a large adjustable loop from a strap or belts. Put your arms through the loop, arranging it behind your neck and down the front of your shoulders. Leave the bottom half of the loop free at the back about the level of your buttocks

♦ pass the casualty's legs through the bottom of the loop; one on each side. Position the loop under the casualty's buttocks, adjusting it for a good carrying position and proper weight distribution

14

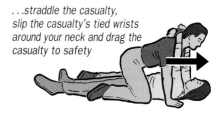

1   Crouch with your back between the casualty's knees.

2   Have the casualty hold on around your neck.

3   Support the casualty's legs and lift. Use your leg muscles to stand up, keeping your back straight.

Cradle carry

Use the cradle carry to lift children and lightweight adults.

1 Kneel on one knee at the casualty's side.

2 Place the casualty's arm around your neck as you support the back and shoulders.

3 Pass your other arm under the knees to grasp the thighs.

4 Ensure a solid footing and place the feet apart for good balance.

5 Lift using your legs, keep your back straight, and your abdominal muscles tense.

If the casualty is on the ground, lift her in two stages:

♦ kneel on one knee at the casualty's side near the head and shoulders

♦ place one arm under the armpits and the other under the casualty's legs at the knees and lift to rest on your raised knee

♦ using the muscles of both legs, stand up in one smooth motion

Human crutch

If a leg or foot is injured, help the casualty to walk on his good leg while you give support to the injured side.

1 Take the weight of the casualty's injured side on your shoulders by placing the casualty's arm on the injured side around your neck and grasp the wrist firmly.

2 Reach around the casualty's back with your free hand, and grasp his clothing at the waist.

3 Tell the casualty to step off with you, each using the inside foot. This lets you, the rescuer, take the casualty's weight on the injured side.

rescuer is on the injured side

14

the casualty can use a walking stick on the uninjured side for additional support

step off with the inside foot

Fire fighter's carry

The fire fighter's carry is used for casualties who are helpless and are not too heavy for the rescuer.

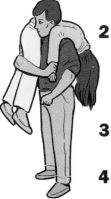

1 With the casualty lying face up in front of you, stand with your toes against the casualty's toes. Grasp her wrists and pull her upward and forward.

2 Maintain a grip on one wrist as you turn and bend to catch the casualty's upper body across your shoulder. The lifting manoeuvre is a continuous, smooth motion to bring the casualty through a sitting position to an upright position, finishing with the casualty draped over your shoulder.

3 Adjust the weight across your shoulders, with the casualty's legs straddling your shoulder.

4 Pass your arm between the casualty's legs and grasp her wrist. This will stabilize the casualty on your shoulders and leave your other hand free.

Two-hand seat

A casualty, who is unable to support his upper body, can be carried by two rescuers, using the two-hand seat.

1 The rescuers crouch on either side of the casualty.

2 Each rescuer reaches across the casualty's back to grasp his clothing at the waist on the opposite side.

3 Each rescuer passes his other hand under the thighs, keeping his fingers bent and holding padding to protect against the fingernails. Hook the bent fingers together to form a rigid seat. Alternatively, the rescuers can hold each other's wrists.

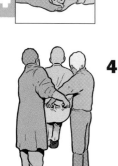

4 The rescuers lift with their legs, keeping their backs straight. Once in the standing position, the rescuers adjust their hands and arms for comfort. When the casualty is securely positioned, the bearers step off together, each using the inside foot.

Four-hand seat

A conscious casualty who can use his hands and arms can be carried on a four-hand seat by two rescuers.

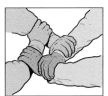

four-hand seat

1 Each rescuer grasps his own left wrist with his right hand, then grasps the right wrist of the other rescuer with his left hand to form a square.

2 Tell the casualty to put his arms around the rescuers' shoulders and hoist himself up to permit the bearers to pass their hands under the buttocks to position them under the thighs at a point of balance.

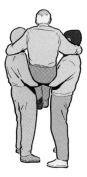

3 Instruct the casualty to hold onto the rescuers' shoulders to keep his balance and support his upper body.

4 The bearers step off together, each using the inside foot.

Chair carry

The chair carry enables two rescuers to carry a conscious or unconscious casualty through narrow passages and up and down stairs. Do not use this carry for casualties with suspected neck or back injuries.

1 Two rescuers carry the chair, one at the front and one at the back. The rescuer at the back crouches and grasps the back of the chair, while the rescuer at the front crouches between the casualty's knees and grasps the front chair legs near the floor.

2 The rescuers walk out-of-step.

14

going downstairs

the casualty faces forward

the front rescuer faces the casualty

a third person should act as a guide and support the front rescuer in case he loses his footing

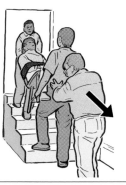

if the casualty is unconscious or helpless

place an unconscious casualty on a chair by sliding the back of the chair under his legs and buttocks, and along the lower back

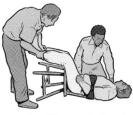

strap his upper body and arms to the back of the chair

Extremities carry

Use the extremities carry when you don't have a chair and you don't suspect fractures of the trunk, head or spine.

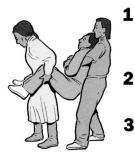

1   One rescuer passes his hands under the casualty's armpits and grasps the casualty's wrists, crossing them over his chest.

2   The second rescuer crouches with her back between the casualty's knees and grasps each leg just above the knee.

3   The rescuers step off on opposite feet—walking out-of-step is smoother for the casualty.

Blanket lift with four bearers

place the rolled edge along the casualty's injured side

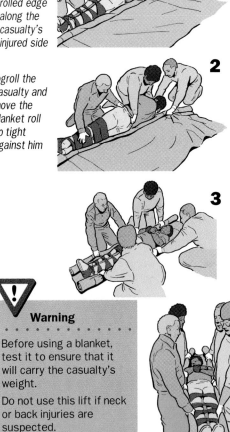

logroll the casualty and move the blanket roll up tight against him

1   Roll the blanket or rug lengthwise for half its width. Position bearers at the head and feet to keep the head, neck and body in line.

2   Kneel at the casualty's shoulder and position another bearer at the waist to help logroll the casualty onto the uninjured side. Turn the casualty as a unit so the casualty's body is not twisted during the logroll—see page 7-17 for more on the logroll.

3   Roll the casualty back over the blanket roll to lay face up on the blanket. Unroll the blanket and then roll the edges of the blanket to each side of the casualty. Get ready to lift the casualty—have the bearers grip the rolls at the head and shoulders, and at the hip and legs.

4   Keep the blanket tight as the casualty is lifted and placed on the stretcher.

14

⚠️ **Warning**

Before using a blanket, test it to ensure that it will carry the casualty's weight.

Do not use this lift if neck or back injuries are suspected.

Stretchers

There may be times when medical help cannot be contacted, or for other reasons, cannot come to the scene. When this happens, transport the casualty to medical help. If the casualty can't walk, or if the injury or illness allows only the most gentle movement, a stretcher should be used.

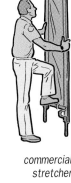

Commercial stretchers

The most common of the commercial stretchers is the rigid-pole, canvas stretcher. It has hinged bracing bars at right angles between the rigid poles at either end that must be locked in the extended position before the stretcher is used.

commercial stretcher

Improvised stretchers

If a commercially prepared stretcher is not available, you can improvise one by using a tabletop, door, or two rigid poles and a blanket, clothing or grain sacks. Don't use non-rigid stretchers like this for casualties with suspected head or spinal injuries.

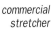

Warning
. . . .

Test an improvised stretcher with someone equal to or heavier than the casualty to ensure that it will hold.

Check the clearance of an improvised stretcher to ensure that it will pass through hallways, doors and stairways without harm to the casualty.

Improvised blanket stretcher

1 Place the blanket flat on the ground and place a pole one-third of the way from one end. Fold the one-third length of blanket over the pole.

2 Place the second pole parallel to the first so that it is on the doubled part of the blanket, about 15 cm (6 in) from the doubled edge.

3 Fold the remaining blanket over the two poles. The casualty's weight on the blanket holds the folds in place.

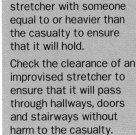

Improvised jacket stretcher

A non-rigid stretcher can also be improvised from two jackets and two or four poles.

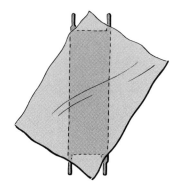

sleeves are pulled inside the jackets

1   Button and zipper the jackets closed and pull the sleeves inside out so that the sleeves are inside. Lay the jackets on the ground so that the top edge of one jacket meets the bottom edge of the other.

2   Pass the poles through the sleeves of the two jackets on either side to complete the stretcher.

3   If the casualty is tall, prepare another jacket as before and add it to the stretcher with the head of the jacket towards the middle.

Using a blanket with a stretcher

A casualty can be wrapped on a stretcher so that a blanket provides maximum warmth with minimum weight on the casualty. It will also allow easy access to the casualty's wounds if that is necessary during transportation.

1   Place a blanket on the stretcher under the casualty with diagonally opposite corners at the head and feet.

2   Place padding at appropriate places on the blanket to fill the natural hollows at the casualty's neck and back. Centre the casualty on the blanket.

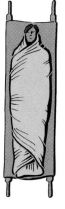

3   Cover the feet with the bottom corner and bring the corner at the head around the neck to the chest. Wrap the legs and lower body with one side. Tuck in the last corner on the opposite side.

Placing a casualty on a stretcher

Complete all essential first aid and immobilization before moving the casualty onto a stretcher.

1   Bring the blanketed and padded stretcher to the casualty, rather than moving the casualty to the stretcher.

2   As the first aider in charge, take the position that permits you to watch and control the most sensitive area of the body, usually at the head and shoulders, or the injured part.

3   Tell the bearers what each is expected to do. If the move is difficult, and time permits, it's a good idea to practise with a simulated casualty. This reduces risks and reassures the conscious casualty.

4   Use clear commands to ensure smooth, coordinated movements.

Four-bearer method—no blanket

1   All bearers kneel on their left knees, three on one side of the casualty and one on the other, as shown below. Bearer 4 helps in lifting and lowering the casualty, and also places the stretcher under the casualty.

2   When you are assured that each bearer has a firm hold on the casualty, direct the bearers to "Get ready to lift" and then give the command "Lift." Lift the casualty smoothly to the height of the raised knees.

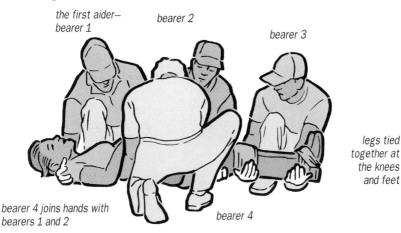

the first aider—
bearer 1

bearer 2

bearer 3

14

legs tied together at the knees and feet

bearer 4 joins hands with bearers 1 and 2

bearer 4

3   On your command "Rest," the casualty is gently laid on your knee and the raised knees of bearers 2 and 3. Tell bearer 4 to position the stretcher. Bearer 4 than resumes his position supporting the casualty by linking his hands with one of yours and one of bearer 2's.

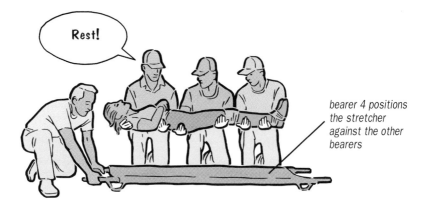

Rest!

bearer 4 positions the stretcher against the other bearers

4   When all are ready, give the commands "Get ready to lift" and then "Lift," lifting the casualty from the knees.

5   Follow this command with, "Get ready to lower" and then "Lower." The casualty is gently laid on the stretcher.

Three-bearer method, no blanket

The three-bearer method is essentially the same as the four-bearer method, except the first aider and one bearer share the weight on one side of the casualty. The third bearer links hands with the first aider from the opposite side to take up the weight of the head and trunk. The casualty is lifted and rested on the bearers' knees while the stretcher is positioned and bearer 3 links hands again with the first aider to help lower the casualty to the stretcher.

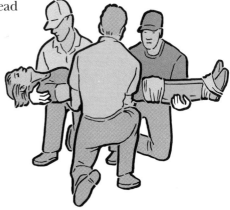

Carrying a stretcher

A stretcher may be carried by two or four bearers. As the first aider in charge, decide on the carrying method and give clear instructions to the bearers. After the casualty has been strapped to the stretcher, position yourself so you can watch the casualty and at the same time give direction to the other bearers.

Assign the remaining bearers (depending whether you are two or four) to respective corners or ends of the stretcher. Bearers crouch by the carrying handles of the stretcher, facing in the direction of travel.

◆ When the bearers have a firm footing and a good grip on the stretcher, give the command, "Get ready to lift," and then, "Lift."

◆ Ask the bearers if they are ready. When they are, give the command, "Go forward."

◆ When it is necessary to stop, give the commands "Stop," Get ready to lower," and then, "Lower."

To ensure the smoothest carry for the casualty:

◆ four bearers carrying a stretcher step off together on the foot nearest the stretcher and keep in step

◆ two bearers step off on opposite feet and walk out-of-step

Although stretcher casualties are usually carried feet first, certain conditions call for a head-first carry:

◆ leg injuries during a long downhill carry or when descending stairs, a head-first carry decreases pressure on the lower limbs and minimizes discomfort

◆ uphill carries and going up stairs if there are no injuries to the legs—a head- first carry decreases blood flow to the casualty's head and is more comfortable

◆ loading an ambulance or transferring the casualty to a bed—it is safer to do this head first, and easier to watch the casualty

14

if

If there are enough bearers to carry the stretcher, walk beside the stretcher to watch the casualty and the route.

Obstacles

When crossing uneven ground, a stretcher should be carried by four bearers and kept as level as possible. Bearers must adjust the height of the stretcher to compensate for dips and rises in the terrain.

Crossing a wall

Avoid crossing a wall, even if it means a longer carry. Where a wall must be crossed, follow these steps:

1 Lift the stretcher onto the wall so that the front handles are just over it. The rear bearers hold the stretcher level while the front bearers cross the wall. All lift together and the stretcher is moved forward until the rear handles rest on the wall.

2 The front bearers hold the stretcher level until the rear bearers have crossed the wall and resumed their positions at the rear of the stretcher.

3 The stretcher is then lowered to continue the journey.

Extrication

Extrication is the process of freeing casualties who are trapped or entangled in a vehicle or collapsed structure and cannot free themselves. Provide as much support as possible to the casualty during extrication. Whenever possible, give essential first aid and immobilize the injuries before the casualty is moved.

Urgent extrication

When there is an immediate danger and you are alone and must move a casualty from a sitting position, proceed as follows:

1 Disentangle the person's feet from the wreckage and bring the feet toward the exit. Ease your forearm under the person's armpit on the exit side, extending your hand to support the chin.

2 Ease the person's head gently backward to rest on your shoulder while keeping the neck as rigid as possible.

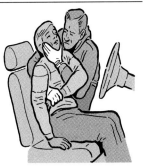

3 Ease your other forearm under the armpit on the opposite side and hold the wrist of the casualty's arm which is nearest the exit.

4 Establish a firm footing and swing around with the person, keeping as much rigidity in the neck as possible. Drag the casualty from the vehicle to a safe distance, with as little twisting as possible.

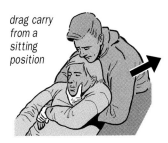

drag carry from a sitting position

Using a short spine board

A short spine board is used to immobilize the head, neck and upper spine while the casualty is in a sitting position. They are especially useful for removing a casualty with a suspected head and/or spinal injury from a motor vehicle following a crash.

Two rescuers are needed to use a short spine board. The first rescuer, who can be a bystander, supports the casualty, holding the head and neck in a rigid position as shown by the first aider. The second rescuer, the first aider, completes the immobilization onto the short spine board.

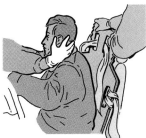

putting a short spine board into position

◆ Position the short spine board along the back of the casualty with the bottom edge below the pelvis and the headpiece at least level with the top of the head. All natural hollows of the body must be padded. Pad both sides of the head to prevent rotation.

◆ Secure the casualty's head to the board and the casualty's arms to the sides. Secure the chest and lower trunk to the board.

Commercial spine boards and extrication devices are available. If you have access to these materials, be sure you are properly trained in their use. Always follow the manufacturer's instructions.

Warning

A short spine board is better than no spine board, but to fully immobilize the head and neck, use a hard cervical collar—see page 7-16.

When the casualty is removed from a sitting position on a short spine board, immobilize him and the short spine board onto a long spine board, then transport.

14

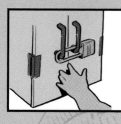

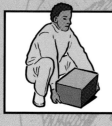

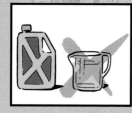

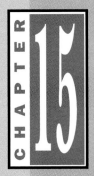

CHAPTER 15

Be safe, be prepared

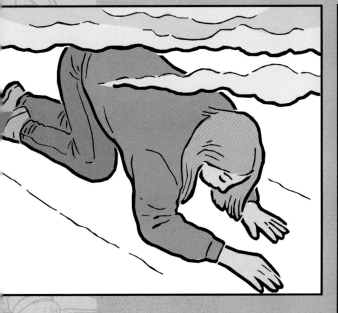

◆ *Safety tips about coming home alone*

◆ *Familiarize members of family with safety routes in case of fire*

◆ *Tips on childproofing your home*

◆ *Safety tips for seniors*

◆ *Workplace safety*

◆ *Road safety*

◆ *Be prepared!*

You can't make all things safe all of the time, but you can make most things safe most of the time. And when things aren't safe, you can recognize them and avoid the hazards. It's usually more than one factor that contributes to an injury. For instance, consider the combination of an unsafe situation, a tired person and poor lighting conditions. Individually, the chance of injury is low. But together, it's almost a sure thing.

Learn to recognize combinations of factors that can lead to injury—this is your safety sense. It goes beyond simply doing this and that in the name of safety—it means thinking on your feet all of the time, recognizing potential injury situations and doing something about them. Taking a first aid course will help to develop your safety sense. Research has shown that people with first aid training have fewer injuries. Make safety a habit. Once you've got it, it'll rub off on those around you.

Safety at home

If safety isn't a regular topic of conversation in your home, now is a great time to make it one. Talk about how to deal with possible emergencies. This prepares everyone. Talk with children about how to recognize an emergency and what to do. Talk about the people in your community who are trustworthy and can help, including block parents, store clerks and teachers.

Personal safety

15

Safety when leaving home

Make a plan of where you are going. Tell someone your plan, where you can be reached and when you expect to return. Tell her what to do, and when, if you don't return by your expected time.

Safety when coming home

If you are coming home and suspect you are being followed:

◆ do not go into your house if noone is home

◆ go to a busy area, like a shopping mall or restaurant, where there are other people to help you if needed. If you are not near a public place, go to a home where lights are on and it looks as if someone is home. Telephone someone you know. Explain the situation and have them meet you

◆ call the police immediately if you continue to be concerned

Don't take risks regarding your personal safety. If you are in an unfamiliar neighbourhood or city, play it safe.

Fire safety

Many, many homes and lives are lost to fires each year. Take the time today to look for, and eliminate, fire hazards in your home. Start with the following:

◆ do you have rules about smoking in
your house? _____ Yes _____ No

◆ do you have smoke detectors between the living areas and sleeping areas of your home. Do you test them once a month and change the batteries once a year? _____ Yes _____ No

◆ is the electrical wiring in good repair? _____ Yes _____ No

◆ are matches and lighters kept in a safe place, out of reach of children? _____ Yes _____ No

◆ are flammable materials safely stored? _____ Yes _____ No

Replace old smoke detectors with new ones every 10 years.

Prepare—even with the finest prevention program, your family must always be ready for a fire. Everyone should know what to do in case of a fire. This includes knowing where fire extinguishers are and how to use them.

Plan—make an escape plan of what to do if there is a fire. Include a meeting place where everyone is to go if there is a fire, such as a tree in the neighbour's yard.

Protect—in case of fire do the following:

◆ remain calm and stop whatever you are doing

◆ use your escape plan to get out quickly and safely—close doors and windows behind you to help stop the fire from spreading

◆ go immediately to your meeting place

◆ send one person to call for help

◆ don't go back inside for anything— possessions aren't worth the cost of a life and many lives have been lost this way

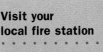

Visit your local fire station

Your local fire station can provide you with all you need to take action to prevent fires in your home. They are in the business of fire prevention and are happy to help you.

15

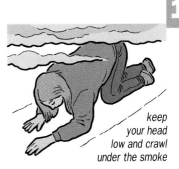

keep
your head
low and crawl
under the smoke

Safety for young children

Here (at home)

The easiest and most effective way to make your home safe for young children is to get down on your hands and knees and have a good look around from your child's perspective. Use your child's point of view—be curious and search for new and exciting adventures. Especially beware of everyday items that could be fatal to a child (window blind cords, electrical cords, appliances and poisonous houseplants).

There (when you aren't there to help)

Teach youngsters skills that are important in an emergency. As early as possible teach your children:

- ◆ their address and telephone number

- ◆ your proper names ("mommy" and "daddy" don't help in an emergency)

- ◆ how to use the local emergency phone numbers—make sure they know how to use them properly

- ◆ how to use a pay telephone—remember that you don't need money to call emergency services

9-1-1

911 is the emergency phone number in many communities

What is an emergency?

Talk to your children about emergencies and discuss specific examples. Explain that there are many different types of emergencies. Talk about what to do if:

- ◆ they lose a favourite toy
- ◆ the cat gets stuck in a neighbour's tree
- ◆ a friend falls and cuts his knee
- ◆ mommy or daddy falls down and can't get up
- ◆ they see a fire in the house

Teach your children basic safety rules. Very young children can learn to recognize dangerous situations. They can also understand what they should do in an emergency. As children grow, give them more and more responsibility. Get them involved in your regular safety check-ups.

15

Safety for seniors

Falls

Falls are a common cause of injury for seniors, often resulting in serious emergencies. This is partly because bones become more fragile as we get older. Relatively minor injuries can become serious and perhaps life threatening. Take action to prevent falls—see the sidebar on the right.

Medications

Medications present many potential hazards. Dispose of unused prescriptions and expired over-the-counter medications by flushing them down the toilet. This is an acceptable way to dispose of them. Remember the following tips when taking medications:

◆ do not take prescription medication intended for someone else

◆ always keep medications in their original containers with the dosage and the instructions clearly indicated

◆ write down when prescription medicines are taken, so you can refer back, if required, at a later time

◆ if you have any questions about your medication, call your doctor or pharmacist right away—they're there to help

Prevent falls

◆ secure all rugs and carpets

◆ use secure foot stools to reach high places (cupboards, shelves)

◆ use non-slip mats in the bathtub or shower

◆ use handrails when climbing and descending stairs

◆ don't take risks—don't use a stool when you know you should use a ladder; don't carry too many parcels at a time—better safe than sorry!

Safety when living alone

Seniors often live alone. If you live alone, make sure you have a plan in place in case something happens. If you fell and were injured this evening, how long would it be before someone came to look for you?

If you have a routine activity such as work or school, someone may notice your absence. But if you don't have a regular routine, arrange to speak to a certain person every day. The contact can be with anyone, and it can be short and simple. Two people, each living alone, can check in on each other. If one does not hear from the other at the right time, she gets help right away.

15

Safety at work

Safety in the workplace is the responsibility of everyone involved. Take time to assess your situation. Recognize that the specific hazards, and what you can do about them, depend on the nature of your work.

Management should. . .

◆ meet and exceed the occupational health and safety regulations for all aspects of the workplace

◆ actively promote a safe attitude

◆ establish procedures to encourage employees to report safety concerns

◆ have, and practise, an emergency evacuation plan

Employees should. . .

◆ know the occupational health and safety regulations that affect your jobs

◆ collaborate with employers in improving workplace safety

◆ encourage safety among the people you work with, and discourage unsafe acts

◆ use the personal protective equipment provided to you

◆ report unsafe conditions

◆ learn about, and use, safe and healthy work practices, including: following safety rules, using proper procedures for lifting heavy items, working at ergonomic workstations and using equipment designed to help with potentially dangerous activities, like using a cart or dolly to move a heavy item.

lift heavy items properly

Make the place safe

Develop a workplace floor plan including location of:

◆ emergency exits

◆ sprinkler systems

◆ hazardous materials/ chemicals

◆ valuable equipment (computer systems etc)

◆ information on key personnel to contact in case of emergency

15

WHMIS

The Workplace Hazardous Materials Information System (WHMIS) is used to identify hazardous materials and to help workers protect themselves from real dangers. WHMIS includes labelling products with supplier labels and workplace labels, and having a material safety data sheet (MSDS) available for each hazardous product in the workplace.

Know how

If there are hazardous materials in your workplace, make sure you know how to use WHMIS.

supplier label—these are put on by the supplier of the product. They include:

- *product identifier*

- *risk phrases*

- *precautionary measures*

- *first aid measures*

- *supplier identifiers*

- *class symbol(s)*

- *reference to MSDS being available*

- *English and French information*

- *a distinct hatchmark border in a contrasting colour to the container to which it is being applied*

GASOLINE

workplace label—these are put on at the workplace. They include:

- *product identifier*

- *safe handling procedures*

- *reference to MSDS being available*

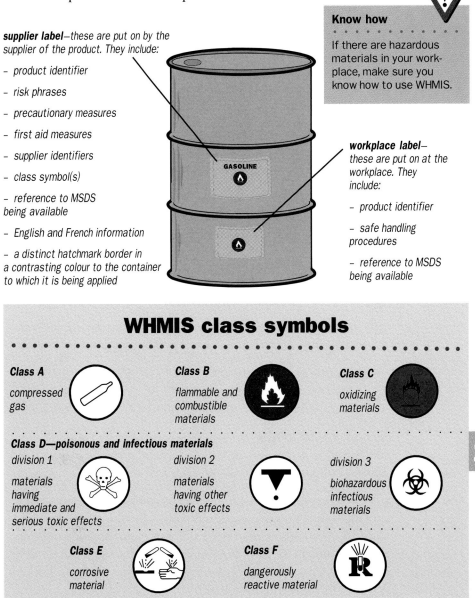

WHMIS class symbols

Class A
compressed gas

Class B
flammable and combustible materials

Class C
oxidizing materials

Class D—poisonous and infectious materials

division 1
materials having immediate and serious toxic effects

division 2
materials having other toxic effects

division 3
biohazardous infectious materials

Class E
corrosive material

Class F
dangerously reactive material

15

Safety at play

Canadians are active people, and sometimes it's when we're playing that we put ourselves at the greatest risk for injury. When you're out playing, know the risks and play it safe.

SMARTRISK Foundation (formerly the Canadian Injury Prevention Foundation) encourages teenagers to reduce their risk of injury by making smart choices—they do this through a program called **HEROES**™. **HEROES**™ is sponsored by Royal Insurance, General Motors of Canada, Canadian Forces Air Command, Bell Canada and Bell Mobility. The program has been adapted for a military audience and is available in both official languages. We can all use the messages from **HEROES**™ to help us make smart choices too. Here they are:

It's not what you don't do, but what you do do that's impor- tant.

◆ **buckle up**—wear your seat belt… it greatly reduces the likelihood of being injured in a collision

◆ **drive sober**—this means more than choosing to not drink and drive… it means 100% concentration on driving all the time, no matter what you're driving

◆ **get trained**—virtually everything we do at work and at play we can do better, and more safely, with training… learn how to do it right by taking a lesson—this includes first aid training too

◆ **look first**—whatever it is, look before you leap… whether it's diving, mountain biking or jumping into the future, look first

◆ **wear the gear**—whatever you do, have a look at the gear the pros wear—they dress for safety. By wearing the gear for the way you play, you'll reduce the chance of injuring yourself

By using the **HEROES**™ messages, you can reduce your risk of injury during an activity. But there is also the choice you have to make on whether or not to do an activity.

Just about everything we do involves some element of risk—risk ranging from what seems insignificant, like walking down a sidewalk, to risks none of us would take, like jumping in front of a moving train. In the middle, however, are risks that we can choose to take, or not take. Risk is personal—always make your own choice on how much risk you want to take.

15

Be a hero

Heroes are people who put themselves on the line to save a life—
any life—even their own. Injuries can and will happen if you don't
take steps to prevent them. It's your choice to take those steps, and
your call on what your personal level of risk is.

Choose to use the HEROES™ messages – you can reduce your risk of injury

HEROES™ messages	Activity			
	Driving	**Hiking**	**Cycling**	**Water sports**
Drive Sober	means more than "no alcohol and no drugs"—it means driving with 100% of your attention on what you're doing all the time—no distractions, whether you're driving a car, bike, snowmobile, etc.	avoid using alcohol and keep your mind on what you're doing—only do one thing at a time	avoid using alcohol and keep your mind on what you're doing—wearing a personal stereo means your attention is not 100% on your riding—leave the tunes at home	water sports and alcohol is a well-known deadly combination
Get Trained	take a defensive driving course, or whatever training there is for the driving you're doing	take a wilderness first aid course and an orienteering course	know your bike and how it works (e.g., gear changes, distance required for braking) before you go riding	learn basic water safety skills as well as how to swim
Wear the Gear	wear the safety gear available for whatever you're doing—it's there for a reason—this is as simple as putting on sunglasses when the sun is so bright you can't see effectively	dress properly for the weather and the terrain—use the proper footwear	look at what the pros wear—proper cycling clothing, gloves (hand protection during falls), eye protection and a helmet (see buckle up below)	wear an approved life jacket (personal floatation device or PFD) when boating
Look First	know what you're driving into—be sure you can see what's coming before you get there—don't over-drive your headlights	watch where you're walking—step-for-step—it only takes one miss to be injured	know what you're riding into, especially when mountain biking or riding in heavy traffic	know what you're jumping or diving into before you jump
Buckle Up	seat belts save thousands of lives each year—choose to wear yours	hike with a buddy	always wear an approved helmet	swim with a buddy

St. John Ambulance thanks SMARTRISK Foundation for helping prepare these pages.

15

Safety on the road

Take a defensive driving course

A defensive driving course is a good way to safety check your driving. With professional training, your chances of driving collision-free are much improved. If you drive as part of your job, take a refresher course for professional drivers every few years. We can all use reminders to keep the bad habits away, and it's a great way to learn of any changes to the rules of the road.

Are you ready?

There are many conditions that will affect your next trip. If you are driving, you will have to contend with variable conditions of the road, light, weather, traffic, not to mention the other drivers and vehicles. But the most important condition is the condition of the driver—you! If you are properly prepared to begin your journey (even a short one) you will be able to compensate for other conditions that are less than perfect.

Be prepared to drive before you get into the vehicle

Are you overtired or preoccupied? Is your ability to react quickly impaired by alcohol or drugs? What effect does your prescription or over-the-counter medication have on your abilities? Plan your trip before your leave the house and check expected weather conditions. Review the plan with your passengers so you won't have to consult the map while driving.

Helping other motorists

If someone else is stopped on the side of the road and you think they need help, pull over. Don't get out of your car—open your window just enough to talk.

Get information about the problem and offer to go and get help. Send police or a service vehicle to the scene.

15

Be sure your vehicle is well maintained

This includes both regular service and appropriate daily maintenance. Walk around your car before you get in it. Look for any signs of potential trouble. Are there lights that need replacing? Do the windshield wipers work properly and are all fluids topped up? Are there any fluids leaking underneath? Are all windows clean and completely clear of obstructions (ice, snow or mud)? Make sure all your lights are clear too.

Use seat belts and appropriate infant and child restraints

Your seat belt gives you your best protection in a collision—wear it all the time. It must be worn over your hips and adjusted so it feels snug. Infants and children must be properly fastened into "car seats" fitted to their size and weight. Until an infant is about nine kilograms (20 pounds), she should be in a rear-facing car seat. Forward-facing child car seats need to be anchored by both the seat belt and the tether strap—check to make sure your child seats are properly anchored. Always fasten your infant or child into her car seat according to the directions that came with the car seat—if you don't, the car seat won't protect your child the way it's designed to.

Keep your mind on the job

- ◆ use a cellular phone only when you are stopped and pulled over to the side of the road

- ◆ pull off the road to a safe place before tending to children or other situations in your car

- ◆ if you get drowsy, do the right thing—stop and rest or have someone else drive

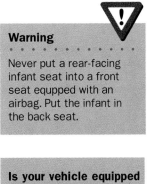

Warning

Never put a rear-facing infant seat into a front seat equpped with an airbag. Put the infant in the back seat.

Is your vehicle equipped for an emergency?

- ◆ an appropriate first aid kit
- ◆ booster cables
- ◆ flares or other warning devices
- ◆ candles with water-proof matches
- ◆ warm blankets
- ◆ extra clothing, including hats, mitts or gloves and warm boots
- ◆ high energy snacks

In case of a collision

- ◆ stay calm
- ◆ stay with your vehicle
- ◆ check yourself and anyone travelling with you—is anyone hurt?
- ◆ give first aid if required
- ◆ call police, if required
- ◆ exchange insurance information with other drivers involved
- ◆ before you leave the scene, be sure to write down the names, addresses and telephone numbers of any other drivers involved as well as witnesses to the collision

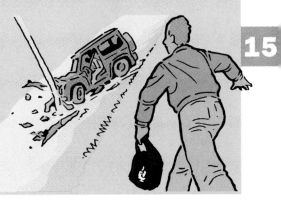

15

Be prepared

An emergency can happen any place, any time. With a little advance planning, you can be prepared for the unexpected. First, know what to do in an emergency—this means being trained in first aid. Second, make sure you have the materials you're going to need in an emergency—this means having first aid kits.

Call the St. John Ambulance office nearest you for detailed course information.

First aid training

As discussed on page 1-2, a good first aid course is the only way to learn the skills of first aid—and it is the skills that matter the most in an emergency. St. John Ambulance offers a wide variety of first aid courses—many of them are listed below. Why take a course from St. John Ambulance? St. John Ambulance first aid courses offer many advantages, including:

◆ highly trained instructors—St. John Ambulance instructors must be certified through our *National Instructor Training and Development Programme*

◆ proven training techniques—our emergency and standard first aid courses, for example, are presented through a careful mix of workbook exercises, video demonstrations, instructor demonstrations and practice sessions

◆ flexible course content—many of our courses are based on the modular concept, so you can choose the topics most suited to your needs

◆ national certification—a St. John Ambulance first aid certificate is recognized across Canada

Selected St. John Ambulance courses

First aid courses
- *We can help*—first aid training for kids
- *The Lifesaver*—a 3½-hour course for busy people
- *Emergency First Aid*—a 1-day course
- *Standard First Aid*—a 2-day course
- *Advanced First Aid*—Level I and Level II
- *National Instructor Development Training Programme*—Phase I and Phase II

CPR courses
- *Level A* – Heart Saver
- *Level C* – Basic Rescuer
- *Level D* – Child and Infant CPR

15

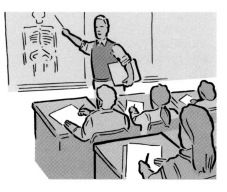

First aid kits

Good first aiders take pride in their ability to improvise in an emergency, but it is always best to have the materials you need with you in a first aid kit. Make sure that wherever you are, you have a first aid kit nearby. When buying a first aid kit, ask yourself:

- ◆ how many kits do I need—you should have at least one at each residence and in each vehicle, carry smaller ones with you when you are away from the house and car

- ◆ what kind of emergencies are likely? Are there special items you should add? For instance, if you spend a lot of time outdoors, add lotion for mild sunburn to your kit

St. John Ambulance first aid kits

St. John Ambulance first aid kits add a feeling of security to travel, work, home and play. Each of the kits below has been carefully designed and contains only quality items.

Family kit—this modular kit is well organized and easy to use. It has what you need to give first aid to small, medium and large wounds, as well as burns.

Personal kit—light and compact enough to be tucked into a backpack or worn on a belt, this kit contains the materials to deal with small and medium wounds.

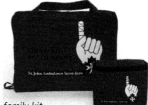
family kit

personal kit

Compact kit—this kit is designed for people on the go. Tucked into your luggage or worn on a belt, it has what you need to give first aid to small and medium wounds.

Fanny pack—prevents minor injuries from becoming major problems. The "fanny pack" design keeps it out of your way until you need it.

15

These first aid kits are available from your local St. John Ambulance office, or from National Headquarters—see the beginning of the book for the address and phone number. And remember to restock your first aid kit after you use it.

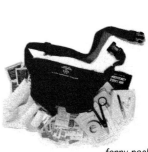
fanny pack

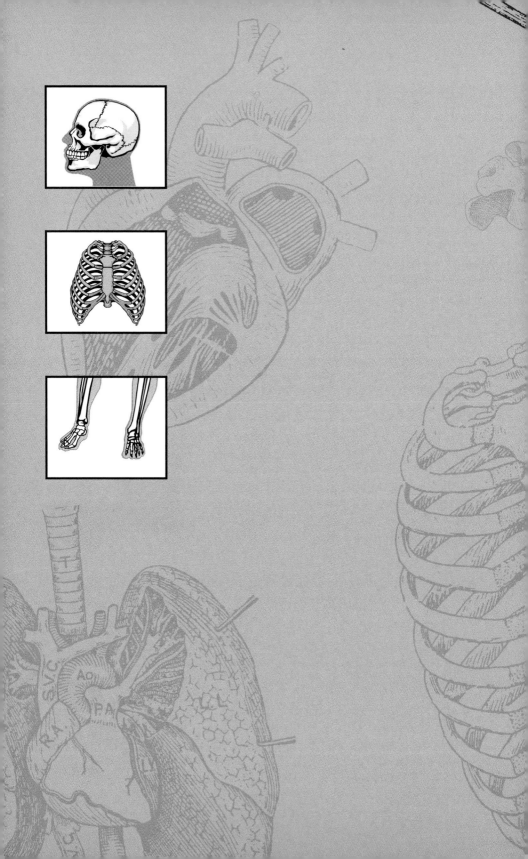

THE BODY
AND HOW IT WORKS

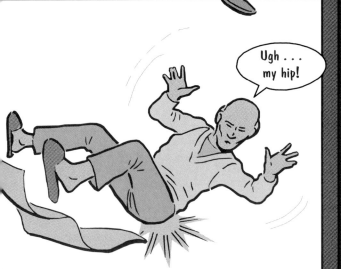

Ugh . . .
my hip!

◆ Introduction to anatomy and physiology

◆ Anatomical terms

◆ The skin

◆ Musculoskeletal system

◆ Joints

◆ Nervous system

◆ Brain

◆ Eyes

◆ Digestive and urinary systems

◆ Circulatory system

◆ Blood pressure

◆ Respiratory system

Introduction to anatomy and physiology

As a first aider, you don't need a full knowledge of anatomy and physiology. However, you should know the basic structure of the human body and how it functions normally. This chapter describes the terms used in anatomy so that you can be more precise when giving information about a person's condition. It gives a short description of the major organs and functions of the skin, musculoskeletal system, nervous system including the eye, digestive and urinary, circulatory and respiratory systems.

Anatomical terms

These are the words used to describe where things are on the body and how they relate to each other.

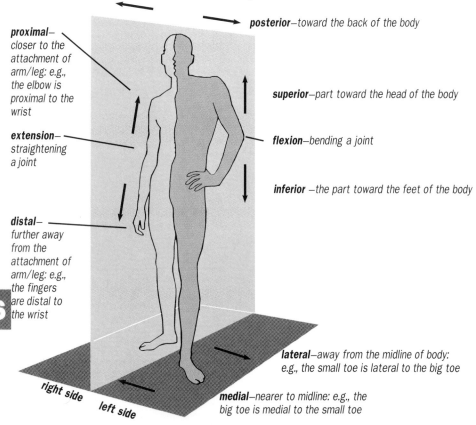

anterior–toward the front of the body

posterior–toward the back of the body

proximal–closer to the attachment of arm/leg: e.g., the elbow is proximal to the wrist

superior–part toward the head of the body

extension–straightening a joint

flexion–bending a joint

inferior –the part toward the feet of the body

distal–further away from the attachment of arm/leg: e.g., the fingers are distal to the wrist

lateral–away from the midline of body: e.g., the small toe is lateral to the big toe

medial–nearer to midline: e.g., the big toe is medial to the small toe

right side

left side

16

The skin

The skin is an important organ of the body. Its primary functions are to protect the body from environmental hazards and infection, eliminate waste in the form of sweat, help maintain normal body temperature and tell the brain of environmental temperature changes.

Environmental control

A rich supply of nerves in the skin keeps the brain aware of environmental changes. These nerves are sensitive to heat, cold, pain and touch, and they transmit these sensations to the brain. The skin helps the body adjust to its environment and protects it from extreme temperatures. In cold temperatures, blood vessels constrict to reduce blood flow near the surface of the skin. This helps prevent loss of heat from the body core. The fatty layers under the skin insulate the body to keep in body heat. In hot temperatures, the blood vessels near the skin surface dilate (get larger), allowing more blood flow near the skin. This cools the body by moving heat from the core to the surface, where it either radiates from the body, or is used to evaporate perspiration, having a cooling effect.

Functions of the skin

- to protect the body from bacterial invasion
- to help control body temperature
- to retain body fluids
- to help eliminate waste products through perspiration
- to insulate the body

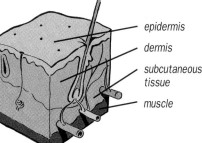

epidermis

dermis

subcutaneous tissue

muscle

Musculoskeletal system

The musculoskeletal system is the framework of the body within which organs and body systems function. This framework includes bones, muscles, tendons and ligaments. Bones act as levers for muscle action; muscles shorten to produce movement; tendons attach muscles to bones; ligaments attach bones to bones at the joints. The musculoskeletal system protects organs, supports the body, and provides for its movement.

16

Muscles

Muscles are made of a special kind of tissue that contracts (shortens) when stimulated by nerve impulses. Generally, body movement is caused by several muscles working in combination—as some are contracting, others are relaxing. The nerves in the muscles carry impulses to and from the brain.

Muscles are classified as either voluntary or involuntary. Voluntary muscles are consciously controlled by the person, meaning they can be contracted or relaxed as the individual wishes. The muscles that move the skeleton are voluntary.

Involuntary muscles contract and relax rhythmically without any conscious effort on the part of the person. The heart, which has its own regulating system, is a good example of an involuntary muscle.

The diaphragm, a large dome-shaped muscle that separates the chest and abdominal cavities and is used in breathing, has characteristics of both voluntary and involuntary muscles. The contraction of this muscle, and thus the rate of breathing, can be changed at will for short periods of time.

diaphragm

Skeleton

The skeleton, made up of bones, forms the supporting structure that gives the body its shape. It also protects many of the organs—for example, the brain is protected by the skull, the heart and lungs by the ribs, and the spinal cord by the vertebrae.

The joints

The bones allow body movement by serving as rigid levers for tendons and muscles. The joints are formed where two or more bones come together. Immovable joints allow no movement, as in the bones of the adult skull. Slightly movable joints allow only limited movement and are found between the vertebrae and between the pelvis and the spine. Freely moving joints are covered with smooth **cartilage** to minimize friction, and are held together by bands of strong tissue called **ligaments**.

bone

ligaments—hold bones together

cartilage—cushions the bone ends

lubricating membrane—nourishes and lubricates the joint structure

capsule—tough covering over the joint

16

Spine

The spine is divided into five parts as shown in the diagram. There are 33 bones in the spine, called **vertebrae**. The vertebrae stack on top of each other with **discs** between them. The discs are made of a tough flexible material and serve as shock absorbers in the spine. All the discs and vertebrae have an opening in the centre such that, when they stack together, there is a long channel that runs from the top to the bottom of the spine. The spinal cord, which carries all nerve impulses to and from the brain, runs through this channel. The spine protects the spinal cord, but if the spine is fractured, broken bones, displaced tissue and swelling can damage the spinal cord, possibly causing lifelong disability.

Parts of the spine

cervical
7 vertebrae

thoracic
12 vertebrae

lumbar
5 vertebrae

sacral
5 fused vertebrae

coccygeal
4 fused vertebrae form the tailbone

Thorax

The thorax is made up of the ribs, the 12 thoracic vertebrae and the sternum (breastbone). The thorax protects the organs in the chest, mainly the heart and lungs. It also provides some protection for the upper abdominal organs, including the liver at the front and the kidneys at the back. Injuries to the bones of the thorax threaten the organs they protect, and can therefore be life threatening.

ribs *—12 pairs are attached to the vertebrae in back and either to the sternum, or to each other, in front. The lowest ribs attach to the vertebrae only, and are called "floating ribs"*

sternum—*a dagger-shaped bone with the point downward*

xiphoid process *(tip of sternum)—a strong piece of cartilage. Pressure on this cartilage can damage underlying organs*

Skull

All the bones of the head make up the skull. The skull gives the head its shape and also protects the brain. When the skull is fractured, the brain may also be injured.

cranium—*the plate-like bones fuse together during childhood to form a rigid case for the brain*

facial bones *join with bones of the cranium to form the eye and nose cavities which protect the eyes and nose*

upper jaw *(maxilla)*

lower jaw *(mandible)*

Main bones of the skeleton

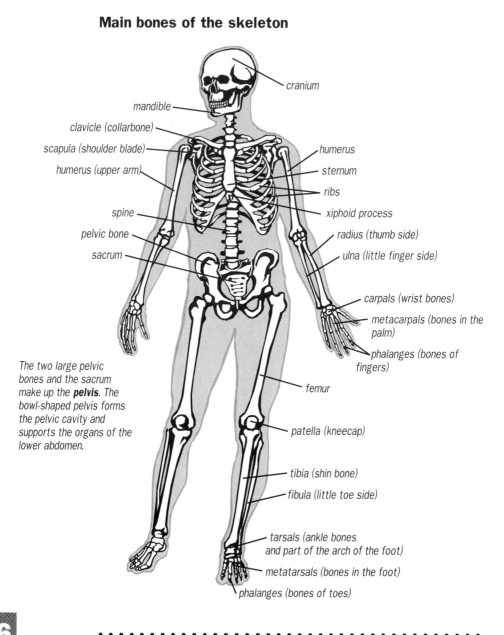

cranium

mandible

clavicle (collarbone)

scapula (shoulder blade)

humerus (upper arm)

spine

pelvic bone

sacrum

humerus

sternum

ribs

xiphoid process

radius (thumb side)

ulna (little finger side)

carpals (wrist bones)

metacarpals (bones in the palm)

phalanges (bones of fingers)

femur

patella (kneecap)

tibia (shin bone)

fibula (little toe side)

tarsals (ankle bones and part of the arch of the foot)

metatarsals (bones in the foot)

phalanges (bones of toes)

*The two large pelvic bones and the sacrum make up the **pelvis**. The bowl-shaped pelvis forms the pelvic cavity and supports the organs of the lower abdomen.*

16

Nervous System

The nervous system is composed of the brain, spinal cord and nerves. The brain and spinal cord together are called the **central nervous system.** The nerves that spread out to all parts of the body are called **peripheral nerves**. The nervous system is subdivided into the **voluntary nervous system** and the **autonomic nervous system**. The voluntary nervous system controls functions at the will of the individual. The autonomic nervous system controls functions without the conscious effort of the individual—e.g. heartbeat, breathing, blood pressure, digestion and glandular secretions such as hormones.

The peripheral nerves that extend from the spinal cord to all parts of the body are of two kinds—motor nerves and sensory nerves. Motor nerves control movement. Sensory nerves transmit sensations of touch, taste, heat, cold and pain to the brain.

Brain

The brain, the controlling organ of the body, occupies almost all the space in the cranium. It is the centre of consciousness, memory and thought. It receives information and transmits impulses to all parts of the body for voluntary and involuntary activities.

Eyes

The eye is the organ of sight. Any injury to the eye is potentially serious and may result in impaired vision or blindness. The quick response of the first aider and the correct first aid may help prevent permanent damage to the eye.

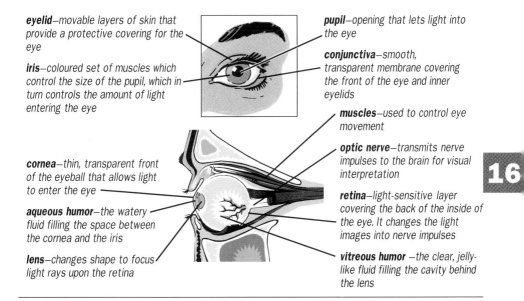

eyelid–movable layers of skin that provide a protective covering for the eye

iris–coloured set of muscles which control the size of the pupil, which in turn controls the amount of light entering the eye

cornea–thin, transparent front of the eyeball that allows light to enter the eye

aqueous humor–the watery fluid filling the space between the cornea and the iris

lens–changes shape to focus light rays upon the retina

pupil–opening that lets light into the eye

conjunctiva–smooth, transparent membrane covering the front of the eye and inner eyelids

muscles–used to control eye movement

optic nerve–transmits nerve impulses to the brain for visual interpretation

retina–light-sensitive layer covering the back of the inside of the eye. It changes the light images into nerve impulses

vitreous humor –the clear, jelly-like fluid filling the cavity behind the lens

16

Digestive and urinary systems

The digestive and urinary systems convert food and drink into nutrients for the cells and collect and dispose of solid and fluid waste. The organs of these systems are classified as hollow or solid. The hollow, tubular organs carry digestive and urinary materials. The solid organs are tissue masses with a rich blood supply.

Injury to hollow organs may allow the contents to spill out into the abdominal or pelvic cavities, causing infection. Injury to the solid organs can result in severe internal bleeding.

Digestive system

liver–contains many blood vessels–a very important organ for production of plasma (blood), energy and bile (for fat digestion)

stomach–digests and stores food until it is ready to move on to the intestine

pancreas– produces digestive juices, and makes insulin to help control blood sugar levels (located behind the stomach)

intestines–a tube made up of the small and large intestines that function to absorb nutrients from digestion, and to collect solid wastes for excretion

small intestine

large intestine

gall bladder– stores and releases bile (located under the liver)

rectum (exit for wastes)

Urinary system

The urinary system removes and collects waste products from the blood and eliminates them from the body in the form of urine. It is made up of the kidneys, ureters, bladder and urethra.

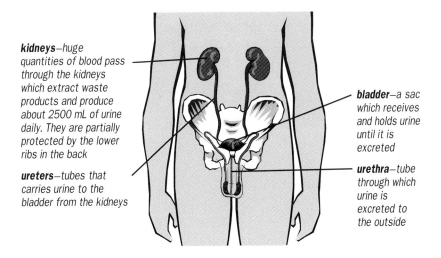

kidneys–*huge quantities of blood pass through the kidneys which extract waste products and produce about 2500 mL of urine daily. They are partially protected by the lower ribs in the back*

ureters–*tubes that carries urine to the bladder from the kidneys*

bladder–*a sac which receives and holds urine until it is excreted*

urethra–*tube through which urine is excreted to the outside*

Circulatory system

The circulatory system is a complex closed circuit consisting of the heart and blood that circulates blood throughout the body. Blood circulation is essential for distributing oxygen and nutrients to cells, and for collecting waste products from cells for excretion from the body.

Heart

The heart is a hollow, muscular organ about the size of a fist. It is located in the chest cavity behind the sternum. The heart functions as a two-sided pump, continuously pumping blood to the lungs and throughout the body. It pumps by first relaxing and filling up with blood, then contracting to squeeze or pump the blood out into the blood vessels. To make the heart beat effectively, it has a complex system of nerves. These nerves carry electrical impulses that control the beating of the heart.

16

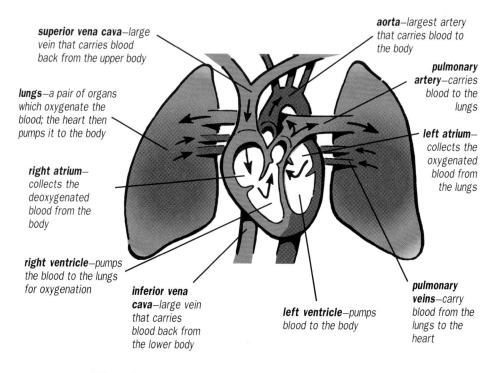

superior vena cava–*large vein that carries blood back from the upper body*

aorta–*largest artery that carries blood to the body*

pulmonary artery–*carries blood to the lungs*

lungs–*a pair of organs which oxygenate the blood; the heart then pumps it to the body*

left atrium–*collects the oxygenated blood from the lungs*

right atrium–*collects the deoxygenated blood from the body*

right ventricle–*pumps the blood to the lungs for oxygenation*

inferior vena cava–*large vein that carries blood back from the lower body*

left ventricle–*pumps blood to the body*

pulmonary veins–*carry blood from the lungs to the heart*

Blood vessels

The blood travels through blood vessels. There are three main types of blood vessels: arteries, capillaries and veins. The **arteries** are the strongest blood vessels. They carry blood, under pressure, from the heart to all parts of the body. The arteries expand according to the volume of blood being forced through them by the pumping action of the heart, and return to normal size as the heart refills for the next contraction. This pressure wave can be felt as a pulse.

The largest artery, the aorta, emerges from the top of the heart. The coronary arteries branch off from the top of the aorta to supply the heart with blood. The smallest arteries are called arterioles and eventually form **capillaries**. Capillaries are the tiny blood vessels that reach every living cell to deliver oxygen, food, etc. and collect waste products. They have very thin walls to allow for the exchange of fluids and gases. Capillaries eventually join to form tiny venules, which in turn form veins. The **veins** take the blood back to the heart. Veins have thinner walls than arteries and most have cuplike valves that allow blood to flow only toward the heart.

Blood

Blood is the fluid that circulates through the heart and blood vessels. It transports oxygen and nutrients to the cells and carries away carbon dioxide and other waste products. Blood is composed of plasma, red cells, white cells and platelets—see sidebar.

Blood circulation

The blood circulation system is a closed loop beginning and ending at the heart. It consists of:

> **Blood components**
>
> - **plasma**—pale yellow liquid that carries cells, platelets, nutrients and hormones
> - **red blood cells**—carry oxygen
> - **white blood cells**—protect the body against microbes
> - **platelets**—help form blood clots to stop bleeding

- **pulmonary circulation**—starting at the right side of the heart, blood is pumped to the lungs, where it drops off carbon dioxide and picks up oxygen, and then moves it back to the left side of the heart

- **systemic circulation**—starting at the left side of the heart, blood is pumped to the body, where it delivers oxygen and picks up carbon dioxide, and then moves it back to the right side of the heart

Blood pressure

Blood pressure is the pressure of the blood pushing against the inside walls of the blood vessels. With each heartbeat, there is a wave of pressure that travels throughout the circulatory system. The pressure wave is strong enough to be felt as a pulse at various points in the body, including the wrist (radial pulse), the neck (carotid pulse), and the upper arm (brachial pulse). Three factors control blood pressure:

- blood volume (how much blood is in the body)

- the capacity and elasticity of the blood vessels

- the strength of the heartbeat

If blood pressure is too low, the body's tissues don't get enough oxygen. This results in shock. Severe bleeding reduces the blood volume, which affects blood pressure. The body tries to compensate for blood loss by contracting the blood vessels and reducing the capacity of the circulatory system. With continued blood loss, however, the body cannot compensate and blood pressure drops. The casualty then starts showing signs of shock.

16

Respiratory system

The respiratory system causes air to be drawn into, and pushed out of, the lungs. The fresh air we breathe contains about 21% oxygen. In the lungs, blood picks up some of the oxygen and releases carbon dioxide. The air we breathe out has less oxygen (about 16%) and more carbon dioxide.

The respiratory system has three main parts: the airway, the lungs and the diaphragm. The airway is the passage which air follows to get from the nose and mouth to the lungs. In the lungs, blood drops off carbon dioxide and picks up oxygen. This process is called **gas exchange**. The diaphragm, a smooth, flat muscle just below the lungs, is used in breathing.

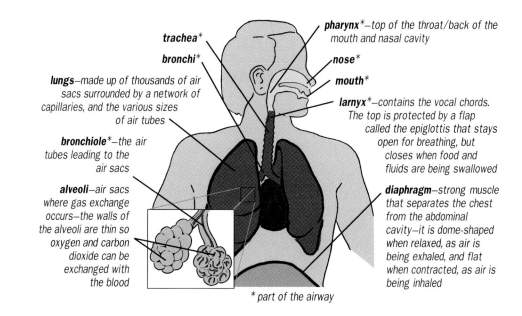

trachea*

bronchi*

lungs–made up of thousands of air sacs surrounded by a network of capillaries, and the various sizes of air tubes

bronchiole*–the air tubes leading to the air sacs

alveoli–air sacs where gas exchange occurs–the walls of the alveoli are thin so oxygen and carbon dioxide can be exchanged with the blood

pharynx*–top of the throat/back of the mouth and nasal cavity

nose*

mouth*

larynx*–contains the vocal chords. The top is protected by a flap called the epiglottis that stays open for breathing, but closes when food and fluids are being swallowed

diaphragm–strong muscle that separates the chest from the abdominal cavity–it is dome-shaped when relaxed, as air is being exhaled, and flat when contracted, as air is being inhaled

* part of the airway

Respiratory control

Breathing is controlled by the respiratory centre in the brain, located near the base of the neck. It monitors the amount of oxygen and carbon dioxide in the blood. As the levels of oxygen and carbon dioxide change, the respiratory centre responds by changing the rate and depth of breathing.

How much oxygen is used, and how much carbon dioxide is given off, is related to the level of physical activity of the person. As physical activity goes up, more oxygen is used and more carbon dioxide is given off, so the respiratory centre increases the rate and depth of breathing to compensate (the heart rate also goes up). Breathing slows down when less oxygen is needed and less carbon dioxide is being produced.

Mechanism of breathing

The lungs have no way of drawing air into themselves. Instead, the diaphragm and the muscles between the ribs work together to expand the chest, which in turn expands the lungs. This causes air to be pulled into the lungs. As the breathing muscles relax, the chest returns to its smaller size and air is forced out of the lungs.

The lungs are covered with a smooth, slippery tissue called the pleural membrane. It is a continuous, double-layered tissue, one layer attached to the lungs and the other to the inside of the chest wall. The **pleura** acts as a lubricating layer to allow easy movement between the chest wall and the lungs, and to ensure that the lungs expand with the action of the chest wall.

16

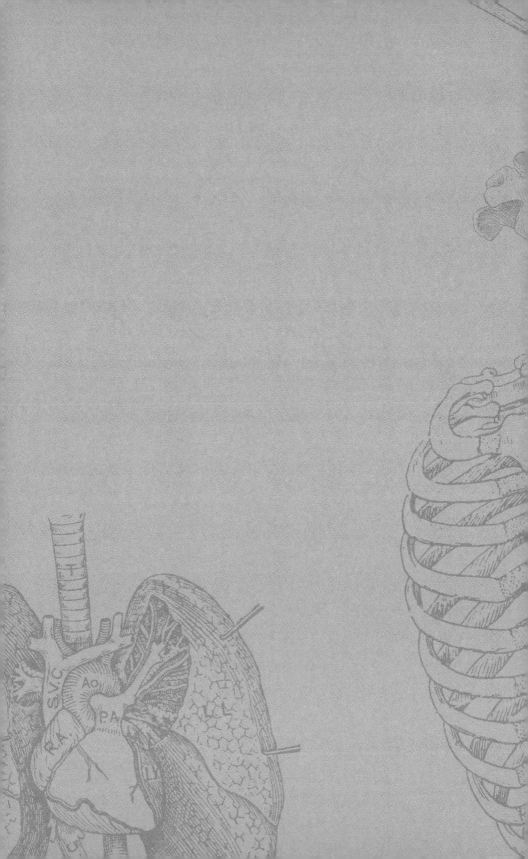

Glossary

A

Abandonment: a first aider leaves the casualty without consent and without the care of a responsible person.

Abdominal thrust: the Heimlich manoeuvre; the manual thrusts to create pressure to expel an airway obstruction.

ABC's: Acronym meaning A= airway; B = breathing; C= circulation.

Abortion: the premature expulsion from the uterus of the products of conception.

Abrasion: a scraped or scratched skin wound.

Acute: a condition that comes on quickly, has severe symptoms and lasts a relatively short time.

Adam's apple: the bump on the front surface of the neck formed by part of the larynx (voice-box).

A.I.D.S.:   *acquired immunodeficiency syndrome*; a fatal disease spread through the HIV (human immunodefiency virus).

Airway: the route for air in and out of the lungs.

Allergens: substances which trigger an allergic reaction in the body.

Allergic reaction: a hypersensitive response to normally harmless substances.

Alveoli: air sacs of the lungs.

Amniotic sac :   a sac holding fluid surrounding a fetus in the uterus.

Amputation: complete removal of an appendage (leg, arm, finger, etc.).

Anaphylaxis: an exaggerated allergic reaction; may be rapidly fatal.

Anatomy: the structure of the body.

Angina (pectoris):   a spasmodic pain in the chest due to a lack of blood supply to the heart.

Aorta: the largest artery in the body; originates at the left ventricle.

Aqueous humor: the watery fluid produced in the eye and located between the lens and the cornea.

Arteries: blood vessels that carry blood away from the heart.

Arteriosclerosis: a name for several conditions that cause the walls of the arteries to become thick, hard and inelastic.

ASA: acetylsalicylic acid—a medication available without prescription used to relieve pain, reduce swelling, reduce fever, etc.

Asthma: attacks of difficult breathing with wheezing/ coughing, often due to allergens.

Atherosclerosis: a form of arteriosclerosis caused by fat deposits in the arterial walls.

Aura: a sensation of an impending seizure; may be a smell, taste, etc.

Autonomic nervous system: part of the nervous system that regulates involuntary functions (not controlled by conscious thought), such as pulse, breathing, digestion, hormone secretion, etc.

Avulsion: an injury where a piece of tissue is partially or completely torn away.

B

Back blows: sharp blows to the back, done to relieve an airway obstruction in an infant.

Bacteria: germs which can cause disease.

Bandage: material which holds a dressing in place.

Basic life support (BLS):   maintaining the ABC's without equipment (excluding barrier devices)

Blood clot: a semi-solid mass of blood products used by the body to stop bleeding.

Blood pressure: the pressure of blood against the walls of arterial blood vessels.

Blood volume: the total amount of blood in the heart and the blood vessels.

Bloody show: the mucous and bloody discharge signalling the beginning of labour.

Brachial pulse: pulse felt on the inner upper arm, normally taken on infants.

Breech birth: the delivery of a baby's buttocks or a foot first, instead of the head.

Bronchi: the main branches of the trachea carrying air into the lungs. Smaller branches called bronchioles.

Bronchospasm: severe tightening of the bronchi/ bronchioles.

Bruise: broken blood vessels under the skin.

C

Capillaries: very small blood vessels that link the arteries and the veins; allow gases and nutrients to move into and out of the tissues.

G

Carbon dioxide (CO$_2$): a waste gas produced by the cells; an important stimulant for control of breathing.

Carbon monoxide (CO): a dangerous, colourless, odourless gas which displaces the carrying of oxygen by the red blood cells.

Cardiovascular disease: refers to disorders of the heart and blood vessels; e.g. high blood pressure and arteriosclerosis.

Cardiac arrest: the sudden stopping of cardiac function with no pulse, and unresponsiveness. In first aid, also means no breathing.

Carotid artery: the main artery of the neck; used to assess the carotid pulse.

Carpals: small bones of the wrist.

Cartilage: a tough, elastic tissue covering the surfaces where bones meet, also forms part of the nose, and ears.

Central nervous system: part of the nervous system consisting of the brain and the spinal cord.

Cerebrovascular accident (CVA): stroke; sudden stopping of circulation to a part of the brain.

Cervical collar: a device used to immobilize and support the neck.

Cervix: the lowest portion, or neck, of the uterus.

Chest thrusts: a series of manual thrusts to the chest to relieve an airway obstruction.

Cholesterol: a fatty substance found in animal tissue or products; also produced by the body; thought to contribute to arteriosclerosis.

Chronic: a condition with a long and/or frequent occurrence.

Chronic obstructive pulmonary disease (COPD): a term describing a group of lung diseases that cause obstructive problems in the airways: usually consists of chronic bronchitis, emphysema.

Circulatory system: the heart and blood vessels.

Clavicles: the collarbones.

Clonic phase: describes a convulsion where tightness and relaxation follow one another.

Closed wound: wound where the skin is intact.

Compression: is a condition of excess pressure on some part of the brain, usually caused by a buildup of fluids inside the skull.

Concussion: a temporary disturbance of brain function usually caused by a blow to the head or neck.

Congestive Heart Failure: failure of the heart to pump effectively, causing a back-up of fluid in the lungs and body tissues.

Conjunctiva: the transparent membrane covering the front of the eyeball (cornea) and the inner eyelids.

Contamination: contact with dirt, microbes , etc.

Contract: to shorten; usually refers to a muscle which exerts a pull when it shortens.

Convection: the loss of heat caused by the movement of air over the body.

COPD: Chronic obstructive pulmonary disease (see above).

Cornea: the transparent front part of the eyeball.

Coronary artery: vessel which feeds the heart muscle.

Cranium: the part of the skull covering the brain.

Crepitus: the grating noise made when fractured bone ends rub together.

Croup: a group of viral infections that cause swelling of the inner throat.

Cyanosis: a bluish or gray colour of the skin due to insufficient oxygen in the blood.

D

Decapitation: the traumatic removal of the head.

Defibrillation: applying an electrical shock to a fibrillating heart.

Deoxygenated blood: blood containing a low level of oxygen.

Dermis: the inner layer of the skin containing hair germinating cells, sweat glands, nerves and blood vessels.

Diabetes: a disease caused by insufficient insulin in the blood; causes excessive blood sugar.

Diaphragm: a large dome-shaped muscle separating the chest and abdominal cavities.

Diarrhea: excessive watery bowel movements.

Direct pressure: force applied directly on a wound to help stop bleeding.

Dislocation: when the bone surfaces at a joint are no longer in proper contact.

Distal: refers to a part that is farther away from the attachment of a leg/arm/finger/toe.

Dressing: a covering over a wound, used to stop bleeding and prevent contamination of the wound.

G

E

Embedded object: an object stuck onto the surface (usually on the eye) or impaled into tissues.

Embolus: any foreign matter such as a blood clot, fat clump or air bubble carried in the blood stream.

Emetic: a substance used to cause vomiting.

E.M.S.: Emergency Medical Services system—a community's group of services which respond to emergencies.

Emphysema: a chronic lung disease characterized by overstretched alveolar walls. See COPD.

Epidermis: The outermost layer of the skin.

Epiglottis: a lid-like piece of tissue which protects the entrance to the larynx (voice-box).

Epiglottitis: an infection usually in children resulting in a swelling of the epiglottis —may cause an airway obstruction.

Epilepsy: a chronic brain disorder characterized by recurrent convulsions.

E.S.M.: Emergency Scene Management—the sequence of actions a first aider should follow to give safe and appropriate first aid.

Exhalation: expiration; breathing out.

Extrication: freeing from being trapped (usually a car collision).

F

Femur: the thigh bone.

Fibrillation: uncoordinated contractions of the heart muscle, so that the blood out-flow is almost nil.

Fibula: the bone of the lower leg on the little toe side.

Flail chest: a condition in which several ribs are broken in at least two places, allowing a free-floating segment.

Flexion: bending a joint.

First aid: the help given to an injured or suddenly ill person using readily available materials.

First aider: someone who takes charge of an emergency scene and gives first aid.

First responders: people such as police, fire fighters, ambulance attendants, etc. who are called first to an emergency scene.

Fracture: a broken or cracked bone

Frostbite: tissue damage due to exposure to cold.

G

Gallbladder: a sac under the liver that concentrates and stores bile; used for fat digestion.

Gastric distention: a swelling of the stomach usually with air, due to ventilating with excessive volume or force during artifical respiration .

Gauze: an open mesh material used for dressings.

Glasgow Coma Scale (modified):   a method of estimating the casualty's level of consciousness.

Guarding: a tightening of the abdominal muscles when the casualty has abdominal pain and is touched there.

H

Head-tilt chin-lift manoeuvre: opening the casualty's airway by tilting the head backward and lifting the chin forward.

Heart attack: chest pain due to a death of a part of the heart muscle; a myocardial infarction.

Heart failure: a weakened heart muscle that is unable to push blood forward; it backs up into the lungs and also causes swelling of the ankles, etc.

Heat cramps: painful muscle spasms due to excessive loss of fluid and salts by sweating.

Heat exhaustion: excessive sweating causing a loss of water and salts.

Heat stroke: A life-threatening emergency where the temperature regulation mechanism cannot cool the body, and the temperature is far above normal—also called hyperthermia or sunstroke

Heimlich manoeuvre: abdominal thrusts done to remove an airway obstruction.

History: information about the casualty's problem: symptoms, events leading up to the problem, applicable illnesses or medications, etc.

Hyperglycemia: abnormally elevated blood sugar.

Hypertension: high blood pressure.

Hyperthermia: too high body temperature.

Hyperventilation: too deep and rapid respirations.

Hypoglycemia: too low blood sugar levels.

Hypothermia: too low body temperature.

Hypoxia: too low levels of oxygen in the body tissues.

G

I

Impaled object: an object which remains embedded in a wound.

Immobilization: placing some type of restraint along a body part to prevent movement.

Incontinence: loss of bladder and bowel control.

Infarction: an area of tissue death due to lack of blood flow.

Infection: inflammation due to microbes.

Inflammation: a tissue reaction to irritation, illness or injury; shows as redness, heat, swelling, and pain.

Inhalation: breathing in; inspiration.

Insulin: hormone produced by the pancreas; important in the regulation of blood sugar levels.

Insulin coma/reaction/shock: hypoglycemia (too low blood sugar levels) due to excessive insulin.

Intrapleural space: a tiny space containing a negative pressure (vacuum) between the two pleural layers.

Involuntary muscle: muscles not under conscious control; heart, intestines etc.

Iris: coloured part of the eye; made of muscles which control light entering the eye.

Ischemic: lacking sufficient oxygen; as in ischemic heart disease.

J

Joint: a place where two or more bones meet.

Joint capsule: a tough covering over a joint.

K

Kidneys: a pair of organs which filter blood and produce urine.

L

Labour: the muscular contractions of the uterus which expel the fetus.

Laceration: a jagged wound from a rip or a tear.

Laryngectomy: removal of the larynx (voice-box); results in a neck-breather.

Lens: a part of the eye which focuses light rays on the retina.

Ligament: a tough cord of tissue which connects bone to bone.

Lipoproteins: substances floating in the blood; made of proteins and fats.

Lymph: a fluid similar to plasma that circulates in the lymphatic system.

Lymphatic system: a system of vessels, nodes and organs which collects strayed proteins leaked from blood vessels and cleanses the body of microbes and other foreign matter.

M

Mandible: the bone of the lower jaw.

Mechanism of injury: the force that causes an injury and the way it is applied to the body.

Medical alert: a means of identifying casualties (usually a bracelet, necklace) who have a condition that may alter first aid treatment.

Medical help: the treatment given by or under the supervision of a medical doctor, e.g. ambulance attendant.

Metacarpals: bones of the palm of the hand.

Metatarsals: bones of the arch of the foot; between the ankle and toes.

Micro-organisms: germs which can cause illness.

Miscarriage: the lay term for an abortion; the loss of the products of conception.

Mouth-to-mouth ventilation: artificial respiration by blowing air into the mouth of the casualty .

Mucous Membrane: thin, slick, transparent lining, covering tubes and cavities that open to the outside; the inner surface of the mouth, nose, eye, ear, rectum, etc.

Musculoskeletal system: all of the bones, muscles, and connecting tissues which allow locomotion (movement of the body).

Myocardial infarction: death of part of the cardiac (heart) muscle; heart attack.

N

Nail bed test: a method of assessing the adequacy of circulation to the extremities; gentle pressure is exerted on the nail bed until the tissue whitens; the return of colour to the area is assessed upon pressure release.

Negligence: failure to perform first aid at the level expected of someone with similar training and experience.

Nerve: a cord made up of fibres which carry nerve impulses to and from the brain.

Nervous system: the brain, spinal cord and nerves which control the body's activities.

Nitroglycerine: a drug used to ease the workload on the heart; often carried as a pill or spray by casualties with angina.

O

O₂: the chemical symbol for oxygen.

Obstructed airway: a blockage in the air passage-way to the lungs.

Oxygen: an odourless, colourless gas essential to life.

P

Pancreas: an organ located under the stomach; produces digestive enzymes and hormones which regulate blood sugar.

Paralysis: inability to move a part; loss of motor function.

Patella: the bone of the knee cap.

Phalanges: bones of the fingers and toes.

Pharynx: the back of the mouth and above the voice box (larynx); a passageway for both air and food.

Physiology: the study of functions of the body.

Placenta: an organ attached to the uterus which provides a fetus with nourishment.

Plasma: a pale yellow fluid containing blood cells, nutrients, gases and hormones.

Platelet: a small, cell-like blood element important in blood clotting.

Pleural membrane: a slick membrane covering the outside surface of the lungs and the inside surface of the chest cavity (thorax).

Pneumonia: inflammation of the lungs.

Pneumothorax: an accumulation of air in the pleural space. Normally the pleural space contains a negative pressure or a vacuum; the air mass (instead of a vacuum) collapes the lung under it.

Position of function: refers to the position an injured hand is placed in when bandaged and/or splinted; i.e. fingers are gently curved with palm slightly downwards.

Primary survey: a step of ESM—assessing the casualty for life-threatening injuries and giving appropriate first aid.

Proximal: refers to a part that is closest to the attachment of a leg/arm/finger/toe/intestine.

Pulmonary artery: the major artery emerging from the right ventricle; carries deoxygenated blood to the lungs.

Pulse: the rhythmic expansion and relaxation of the arteries caused by the contractile force of the heart; usually felt where the vessels cross a bone near the surface.

R

Radiate: the spreading of something; the pain of a heart attack in the chest radiates to the left arm.

Radius: the bone on the thumb side of the lower arm.

Red blood cells: the most numerous type of blood cells; carry oxygen.

Respiratory arrest: stopped breathing.

Retina: the covering at the back of the eyeball; changes light rays into nerve impulses.

Reye's Syndrome: A rare but serious disease in children and adolescents that is reported to be associated with taking ASA for a viral infection. Reye's Syndrome affects the brain, liver and blood. It can cause permanent brain damage or death.

R.I.C.E.: R=rest; I= ice; C= compression; E= elevation. First aid for certain bone and joint injuries.

Rule of Nines: a system of estimating the amount of skin surface burned.

S

Sacrum: a bone formed from five fused vertebra; forms the back of the pelvis.

Scapula: shoulder blade.

Scene survey: the initial step of ESM (emergency scene management) where the first aider takes control, assesses any hazards and makes the area safe, finds out what has happened, identifies self as a first aider, gains consent from the casualty, calls for help from bystanders and starts organizing them to get help for the casualty.

Sclera: the white of the eye; the tough, opaque layer of the eyeball.

Secondary survey: a step of ESM; assessing the casualty for non-life-threatening injuries and giving appropriate first aid.

S.I.D.S. (Sudden Infant Death Syndrome): death of an infant due to unexplainable causes.

Sign: objective evidence of disease or injury.

Sling: a support for an arm or shoulder, usually brought around the neck.

Spleen: an organ of the lymphatic system; functions to cleanse foreign matter from the blood; blood reservoir.

Spontanoeus pneumothorax: air in the pleural space due to an unexplained rupture of the underlying lung.

Splint: is a rigid and padded support used to prevent movement in a bone or joint injury.

Sprain: supporting tissues about a joint (such as ligaments) are stretched, partly or completely torn.

Sternum: the breastbone.

Stoma: an opening in the neck through which the person breathes.

Strain: a stretched or torn muscle.

Sucking chest wound: a wound in which air is pulled into the chest cavity through the chest wall; it can cause a collapse of the lung beneath.

Superficial: on the surface of the body; as opposed to deep.

Superior vena cava: one of the two largest veins; it drains the arms and head of deoxygenated blood and empties into the right atrium.

Symptom: an indication of illness or injury experienced by a casualty; cannot be detected by an observer without asking.

Syrup of ipecac: an emetic; used to cause vomiting.

T

Tendon: a tough cord of tissue that attaches muscles to bones or other tissues.

Tension pneumothorax: air in the pleural space presses on the heart and blood vessels and affects their function.

Tetanus: a type of bacteria in a wound; can cause severe muscle spasms.

TIA: Transient ischemic attack: a mini-stroke.

Tibia: the bone in the lower leg; on the large toe side; the shin bone.

Tonic phase: first stage of a convulsion where the muscles are rigid.

Tourniquet: a constricting band used to stop severe bleeding.

Trachea: a tube for air, kept open with cartilage rings; is located between the larynx (voice-box) and the bronchi.

Traction: gently but firmly pulling below a fracture to bring the limb into alignment.

Transient ischemic attack (TIA): temporary signs and symptoms of a stroke due to a lack of sufficient oxygen to the brain.

Trauma: any physical or psychological injury.

Triage: a system of placing priorities for first aid and/or transportation for multiple casualties.

U

Ulna: bone in the lower arm; on the little finger side.

Urethra: a tube which carries urine from the bladder to the outside.

Uterus: the muscular sac which holds, protects a fetus.

V

Vein: a blood vessel; carries blood to the heart.

Ventilation: supplying air to the lungs.

Ventricles: the muscular lower chambers of the heart which pump blood into the arteries.

Ventricular fibrillation: a quivering action of the heart muscles so that little blood is pumped.

Vital signs: the four signs that show the basic condition of the casualty: level of consciousness; breathing; pulse; skin condition and temperature (sources vary as to the components of vital signs).

W

White blood cells: blood cells which are involved in immunity and control of microbes.

X

Xiphoid process: the cartilage tip at the lower end of the breastbone.

G

Index

A

Abandonment of casualties 1-6, G-1
ABCs (Airway, Breathing, Circulation) 2-27, G-1
  primary survey, in 2-5 to 2-11, 2-31
  unresponsive casualties, first aider alone 1-18, 1-19
Abdominal injuries 6-23 to 6-24
Abdominal thrusts 3-15, G-1
  see also Heimlich manoeuvre
Abortions, spontaneous 12-2, 12-9, G-1
Abrasions 6-13, G-1
Acquired immunodeficiency syndrome (AIDS) 1-8 to 1-9, 13-6, G-1
Acute G-1
Adam's Apple 2-16, G-1
AIDS 1-8 to 1-9, 13-6, G-1
Air exchange 3-2
Airflow to lungs 3-2, 3-3, 11-7
Airway G-1
  artificial respiration 4-21, 4-22 to 4-23
  asthma attacks, in 11-7
  cardiopulmonary resuscitation 5-10 to 5-30
  head or spinal injuries 4-22, 5-12, 5-23, 5-27
  choking (*see* Choking)
  newborns, clearing in 12-7
  opening of 2-9, 2-31
    head or spinal injuries 2-9, 4-22
    head-tilt chin lift 2-9, 4-21, 4-26
    jaw thrust without chin lift 4-22
    oropharyngeal airways 7-16
    unconsciousness and 1-29
Alcohol-induced psychological emergencies 13-6
Allergens G-1
Allergic reactions (anaphylaxis) 4-13, 4-16 to 4-17, 8-11, G-1
  Ana-Kit® Anaphylaxis Kit 4-35
  EpiPen® Auto-Injector 4-34
  insect bites or stings 8-11
  medications for 4-34, 4-35
Alveoli (of lungs) 16-12, G-1
Ambulances 1-16, 1-21
Amniotic fluid 12-2, 12-3
Amniotic sac 12-2, G-1
Amputations 6-13, 6-20 to 6-22, G-1
  tourniquets 6-21
Ana-Kit® Anaphylaxis Emergency Treatment Kit 4-35
Anaphylaxis 4-13, 4-16 to 4-17, 8-11, G-1
  see also Allergic reactions
Anatomy 16-2 to 16-13, G-1
Angina pectoris 5-3, 5-5, 5-6, 5-7, G-1
Ankles 7-36, 16-6
Anterior (anatomical term) 16-2
Antihistamine tablets 4-35
Anxiety attacks 13-2, 13-4 to 13-5

Aorta (artery) 16-10, G-1
Aqueous humor (of eyes) 16-7, G-1
AR. *See* Artificial respiration
Arc-welders flashes, burns from 9-2, 9-13
Arteries 5-3, 5-5, 5-8, 16-10, G-1
Arterioles 16-10
Arteriosclerosis (hardening of arteries) 5-8, G-1
Artificial respiration (AR) 4-18 to 4-33
  assisted breathing 4-33
  direct methods 4-18 to 4-33
    gastric distention 4-28
    head or spinal injuries 4-22 to 4-23
    mouth-to-mouth, adult 4-20 to 4-24
    mouth-to-mouth, child 4-25 to 4-27
    mouth-to-mouth, infant 4-30 to 4-33
    mouth-to-nose 4-30
    mouth-to-stoma 4-29
  face masks or shields 1-9, 5-19, 8-4
  mouth-to-mouth contact, minimizing 1-9
  poisoning casualties 4-19, 8-6
  positioning casualties
    adults 4-21, 4-22 to 4-23
    children 4-22 to 4-23, 4-26
    head or spinal injuries 4-22, 4-23
    infants 4-22, 4-23, 4-31, 5-27
  vomiting 4-28
Assaults, psychological reactions to 13-5
Assisted breathing 4-33
Asthma, bronchial 4-13, 4-15, 11-7, G-1
  Ana-Kit® Anaphylaxis Kit 4-35
  EpiPen® Auto-Injector 4-34
  inhalers 4-36
  triggers 11-7
Atherosclerosis (narrowing of arteries) 5-3, G-1
Atrium (heart chamber) 16-10
Auras (in seizures) 11-4, G-1
Autonomic nervous system 16-7, G-1
Avulsions 6-13, G-1

B

Back blows 3-23, G-1
Back-pressure arm-lift (artificial respiration) 4-19, 4-34 to 4-37
Bacteria G-1
Baking soda 8-11, 8-13
Bandages 4-10, 6-3 to 6-9, 7-21, 7-26, 7-35, 7-36, G-1
Basic life support (BLS) G-1
Bile 16-8
Birth canal (vagina) 12-2, 12-3
Bites and stings, insect 8-11, 8-15, 11-7
Bites, animal or human 8-8 to 8-10, 8-15
Bladder 16-9
Blanket lifts 14-8
Blankets
  improvised stretchers 14-9
  use with stretchers 14-10, 14-11

Blast injuries 4-11
Bleeding 6-12 to 6-43
   amputations 6-20 to 6-22
   arterial 6-12
   circulation, checking 6-18
   controlling 6-16
   dressings, blood-soaked 6-17
   ear canals, bleeding from 6-31
   external 6-12, 6-14 to 6-17
   hands, palm of 6-34
   internal 6-12, 6-14 to 6-15, 6-19
   miscarriages 12-2, 12-9
   mouth or gums, bleeding from 6-33
   nosebleeds 6-32
   scalp, bleeding from 6-33
   shock 1-25, 16-11
   tourniquets 6-21
   vaginal 12-9
   varicose veins 6-35 to 6-36
   venous 6-12
Blood 16-9 to 16-11
   clots 5-5, 5-8, G-1
   pressure (BP) 5-2 to 5-3, 5-31, 9-5, 16-11, G-1
   vessels 16-10
   volume 16-11, G-1
"Bloody show" 12-3, G-1
BLS (Basic life support) G-1
Body mechanics (lifting casualties) 14-3
Bones 7-2 to 7-7, 7-31, 16-4 to 16-6
   dislocations 7-4, 7-5, 7-23 (*see also* Dislocations)
   fractures 7-2 to 7-3 (*see also* Fractures)
Bowels (intestines) 6-24, 16-8
BP (blood pressure) 5-2 to 5-3, 5-31, 9-5, 16-11
Brachial pulse (of upper arm) 2-16, 16-11, G-1
Brain 16-7
Breastbone (sternum) 4-9, 7-21, 16-5
Breathing 2-13, 2-15, 2-27, 4-2 to 4-4, 16-13
   assessing 2-15
   assisted 4-33
   depth 4-4
   difficulties (*see* Breathing emergencies)
   primary survey 2-9
   rates 2-15, 4-3
   respiratory system 16-13
   rhythms 4-4
   vital signs 2-13 to 2-15
Breathing emergencies 4-6 to 4-17
   allergic reactions (anaphylaxis) (*see* Allergic
      reactions)
   asthma (*see* Asthma, bronchial)
   blast injuries 4-11
   burns, in 9-5, 9-6
   chest injuries, in 4-6 to 4-10, 4-37, 7-21
   choking (*see* Choking)
   head or spinal injuries 4-8 (*see also* Head or
      spinal injuries)
   hyperventilation 4-17
   hypoxia 4-2
   illnesses, in 4-6, 4-13 to 4-17, 4-34, 4-35
   ineffective breathing 4-4

Breathing emergencies 4-6 to 4-17 *(continued)*
   inhalation injuries 4-12
   poisoning and 4-6
   severe breathing difficulties 4-4 to 4-5, 4-13
   sudden infant death syndrome (SIDS) 4-14
   unconsciousness 1-29
Breech births G-1
Bronchi 16-12, G-1
Bronchioles 16-12
Bronchospasms G-1
Bruises (contusions) 6-13, 6-30, 6-39, G-1
"Bumps on the head" 6-30
Burns 9-2 to 9-15
   area burned, estimating 9-4
   chemical burns 9-2, 9-4, 9-8 to 9-9, 9-15
   complications 9-5
   critical burns 9-4 to 9-5
   dressings 9-7
   electrical burns 9-2, 9-4, 9-10 to 9-11, 9-15, 10-14
   heat (thermal) burns 9-2, 9-7, 9-15
   light burns to eyes 9-13
   lightning strikes 10-14
   radiation burns 9-2, 9-12 to 9-13, 9-15
   "rule of nines" 9-4
   severity, estimating 9-3 to 9-5, 9-6
   thermal burns 9-2, 9-7, 9-15
Bystanders 1-12, 1-13, 1-17, 2-3

C

Canadian Injury Prevention Foundation 15-8
Capillaries 16-10, G-1
Capsule (of joint) 7-4, 16-4
Carbon dioxide (CO_2) 16-12, 16-13, G-2
Carbon monoxide (CO) 4-2, 4-12, 8-3, G-2
Cardiac arrests 5-4, 5-5, 5-10, 10-14, G-2
Cardiopulmonary resuscitation. *See* CPR
Cardiovascular diseases 5-2 to 5-10, G-2
   angina pectoris 5-3, 5-5, 5-6, 5-7
   cardiac arrests 5-10
   "chain of survival" 5-4
   congestive heart failure 4-2, 4-13, 5-7
   coronary artery disease 5-3
   heart attacks (myocardial infarctions)
      5-5 to 5-7
   high blood pressure (hypertension) 5-2, 5-3,
      5-31, 9-5
   narrowing of arteries (atherosclerosis) 5-3
   risk factors 5-31
   strokes (cerebrovascular accidents or CVAs)
      5-8 to 5-9, 10-4
   transient ischemic attacks (TIAs) 5-8
Carotid pulse (of neck) 2-16, 16-11
Carpals (wrist bones) 16-6, G-2
Carries, rescue 14-3 to 14-8, 14-9 to 14-14
Cars 14-14 to 14-15, 15-10 to 15-11
Cartilage 16-4, G-2
Casualties
   classification by age 1-3
   consent, right to refuse 1-5
   Good Samaritan principles 1-4 to 1-6, 1-16

Casualties (*continued*)
  moving (*see* Moving (casualties))
  multiple 2-26 to 2-28, 10-14
Central nervous system 16-6, G-2
Cerebrovascular accidents (CVAs or strokes) 5-8 to 5-9, 10-4, G-2
Cervical collars 7-15, 7-16, 14-15, G-2
Cervical vertebrae 7-13, 16-5
Cervix 12-2, 12-3, G-2
"Chain of survival" 5-4
Chest injuries
  closed chest wounds 4-6 to 4-7
  flail chests 4-7, 4-9 to 4-10
  open chest wounds 4-6
  penetrating chest wounds 4-7 to 4-9, 4-37
  pneumothorax 4-7, 4-9, 4-37, 7-21
  rib/breastbone injuries 7-21
  sucking chest wounds 4-7 to 4-9, 4-37
Chest thrusts 3-12, 3-13, 3-22 to 3-25, G-2
Child abuse 1-11
Child casualties, definition of 1-3
Childbirth, emergency 12-2 to 12-8
Childproofing a home 15-4
Children's Aid Society 1-11
Choking 3-2 to 3-29
  chest thrusts 3-12, 3-13, 3-23, 3-25
  first aid 3-4 to 3-28
    adult, conscious 3-4 to 3-8
    adult, obese 3-12, 3-13
    adult, pregnant 3-12, 3-13
    adult, self-help 3-13
    adult, unconscious 3-9 to 3-11
    adult, in wheelchair 3-14
    child, conscious 3-15 to 3-18
    child, unconscious 3-19 to 3-21
    infant, conscious 3-22 to 3-25
    infant, unconscious 3-26 to 3-28
  head or spinal injuries 3-9, 3-19, 3-26
  Heimlich manoeuvre 3-15 (*see also* Heimlich manoeuvre)
  ongoing casualty care 3-8
  swelling of airway (no foreign object) 3-4
Cholesterol 5-31, G-2
Chronic G-2
Chronic obstructive pulmonary disease (COPD) 4-2, 4-13, G-2
Cigarettes 5-31, 8-13
Circulation, blood 2-27, 16-9 to 16-11, G-2
  injuries, below 6-18
  primary survey 2-10, 2-31
  tourniquets 6-21
Classification of casualties by age 1-3
Clavicles (collarbones) 7-22, 16-6, G-2
"Clonic" phase (of seizures) 11-4, G-2
Closed wounds 6-12, G-2
Clotting of blood 16-11
Coccyx 7-13, 16-5
Collarbones (clavicles) 7-22, 16-6, G-2
Compression bandaging (in R.I.C.E.) 7-7
Compressions, chest. *See* CPR
Compressions (of skull) 7-11 to 7-12, G-2

Concussions 7-11 to 7-12, G-2
Congestive heart failure 4-2, 4-13, 5-7, G-2
Conjunctiva (of eye) 16-7, G-2
Consciousness, level of (LOC) 1-29 to 1-30
  assessing level 1-30, 2-13, 2-14
  breathing emergencies 1-29
  fainting 1-34, 1-35
  Glasgow Coma Scale 1-30, 2-14
  recovery position 1-27, 1-32, 1-33
  semi-conscious and unconscious 1-31
Consent (to first aid) 1-5
Contact dermatitis 8-7
Contact lenses 6-37, 9-9
Contamination (of wounds) 6-16, G-2
Contractions (in childbirth) 12-3, 12-4, 12-5, 12-6
Contractions (of muscles) 16-4, G-2
Contusions (bruises) 6-13, 6-30, 6-39
Convection of air 10-2, G-2
  see also Hypothermia
Convulsions 11-4 to 11-5
COPD (Chronic obstructive pulmonary disease) 4-2, 4-13, G-2
Cornea (of eye) 10-14, 16-7, G-2
Coronary arteries 5-3, 5-5, 16-10, G-2
Coronary disease. *See* Cardiovascular diseases
Corrosive chemicals 9-8 to 9-9
CPR (cardiopulmonary resuscitation) 5-10 to 5-30
  adult casualties 5-11 to 5-21
  chest compressions (*see below* cycles)
  child casualties 5-22 to 5-26
  courses 15-12
  cycles (compressions + ventilations)
    adults 5-14, 5-17, 5-19, 5-20, 5-21, 5-30
    children 5-25, 5-30
    infants 5-29, 5-30
    one-rescuer 5-14, 5-25, 5-29
    two-rescuer 5-17, 5-19, 5-21
  face masks or shields 1-9, 5-19
  hypothermic casualties 5-13
  infant casualties 5-26 to 5-30
  landmarking
    adults 5-13, 5-15, 5-19, 5-30
    children 5-24, 5-26, 5-30
    infants 5-28, 5-30
  one-rescuer 5-11 to 5-15, 5-22 to 5-26, 5-26 to 5-30
    taking over from 5-15
  two-rescuer 5-16 to 5-21
    switching positions 5-21
  ventilations (*see above* cycles)
Cranium (skull) 16-5, 16-6, G-2
Crepitus 7-3, G-2
Critical incident stress 2-25
Croup 3-2, G-2
Crowning (in childbirth) 12-4
Crush injuries 6-24 to 6-25
Crush syndrome 6-24 to 6-25
CVAs (cerebrovascular accidents or strokes) 5-8 to 5-9, 10-4

I

Cyanosis G-2
    allergic reactions 4-16
    asthma attacks 4-15
    choking 3-3
    inhalation injuries 4-12

D

Decapitation G-2
Defibrillation 5-4, G-2
Denial, in heart attacks 5-4
Deoxygenated blood 4-2, G-2
Dermatitis, contact 8-7
Dermis (skin layer) 9-3, 16-3, G-2
Diabetes 11-2, G-2
    burns and 9-5
    diabetic coma (hyperglycemia) 11-2 to 11-3
    insulin shock (hypoglycemia) 11-2 to 11-3
Diabetic coma (hyperglycemia) 11-2 to 11-3
Diaphragm 16-4, 16-12, G-2
Diarrhea 1-22, G-2
Digestive system 16-8
Direct methods of artificial respiration. *See*
    Artificial respiration
Direct pressure G-2
Discs (of vertebral column) 16-5
Dislocations (of joint) 7-4 to 7-6, 7-39, G-2
    elbow 7-25
    immobilization, general 7-23
    thumb/finger 7-30
Distal (anatomical term) 16-2, G-2
Dressings 6-2 to 6-3, G-3
    blood-soaked 6-17
    burn dressings 9-7
Drug abuse
    hypothermia, resemblance in 10-4
Drug-induced psychological emergencies 13-6
Drunkenness
    diabetic emergencies, resemblance in 11-3
    hypothermia, resemblance in 10-4
Dyspnea 4-5

E

Ears 6-31, 10-14
Elbows 6-6 to 6-7, 7-25
Elderly people
    burns and 9-4
    hypothermia, risk of 10-3
    safety precautions 15-5
Elevation (in R.I.C.E.) 7-7
Embedded objects in wound 6-26 to 6-29,
    6-39 to 6-40, G-3
Embolus 5-5, 5-8, G-3
Emergencies, priorities 2-23, 2-26 to 2-28
    multiple casualties 2-27, 10-14
    multiple injuries (one casualty) 2-23
Emergency Medical Services (EMS) 1-17
Emergency scene 1-12 to 1-14, 2-25

Emergency scene management (ESM)
    2-2 to 2-33
    critical incident stress 2-25
    handover of control 1-14, 2-25
    head or spinal injuries 2-4, 2-6 to 2-7
    lightning strikes 10-14
    multiple casualties 2-26 to 2-28, 10-14
    ongoing casualty care 2-24 to 2-25, 2-33
    power lines, downed 9-11
    primary survey 2-5 to 2-11, 2-31
    priorities 2-23, 2-26 to 2-28
    scene survey 2-2, 2-3 to 2-5, 2-30
    secondary survey 2-11 to 2-23, 2-32
        first aid 2-23
        head-to-toe examination 2-18 to 2-23, 2-32
        history of casualty (SAMPLE) 2-12, 2-32
        vital signs 2-13 to 2-18, 2-32
    summary of 2-30 to 2-33
    turning casualties face up 2-8
Emetic 8-5, G-3
Emphysema 4-13, G-3
EMS (Emergency Medical Services) 1-17, G-3
Energy and injuries 1-7, 1-20
Environmental emergencies
    cold (hypothermia) 10-2 to 10-10, 10-15
    heat 10-11 to 10-13
    lightning strikes 10-14
Epidermis (skin layer) 9-3, 16-3, G-3
Epiglottis 16-12, G-3
Epileptic seizures 11-4 to 11-5, G-3
EpiPen® Auto-Injector 4-34
ESM 2-2 to 2-33, G-3
    see also Emergency scene management
Evaporation. *See* Hypothermia
Examinations, head-to-toe 2-18 to 2-23, 2-32
Exhalation 4-3, G-3
Expansion waves (pulse) 16-10
Exposure. *See* Hypothermia
Extension (anatomical term) 16-2
Extinguishers, fire 15-3
Extrication (from car) 14-14 to 14-15, G-3
Eyelids 16-7
Eyes 16-7
    burns 9-9, 9-13, 9-15, 10-14
    embedded objects 6-39 to 6-40
    extruded eyeballs 6-41
    particles in 6-36 to 6-38
    wounds around 6-39

F

Face masks or shields 1-9, 5-19, 8-4
Falls, preventing 15-5
Femur (upper leg) 7-31 to 7-32, 16-6, G-3
Fetus 12-2
Fevers 11-6
Fibrillation G-3
Fibula (lower leg) 7-34 to 7-35, 16-6, G-3
Finger sweeps (in choking) 3-6, 3-10, 3-17, 3-20
Fingers 7-30, 16-6

Fire
 clothes on fire, extinguishing 9-14
 preparedness 15-3
Fire fighters 1-3, 1-13
 carries 14-6
 two-rescuer CPR 5-16
First aid 1-2 to 1-3, G-3
 alone, when first aider 1-18 to 1-19
 artificial respiration (see Artificial respiration)
 bandages 6-3 to 6-9
 courses 1-2, 1-3, 15-12
 CPR (see CPR)
 dressings 6-2, 6-3
 emergency scene, help at 1-12 to 1-14
 Good Samaritan principles 1-4 to 1-6, 1-16
 history of incident 1-23, 1-24, 2-4
 illnesses, guidelines for getting help 1-22
 injuries, background on 1-20 to 1-21
 kits 15-13
 legal duty to help 1-4 to 1-6
 medical help, getting 1-16 to 1-19
 moving casualties (see Moving casualties)
 priorities 2-23, 2-26 to 2-28
 recovery position 1-27, 1-32, 1-33
 report, sample of 2-29
 R.I.C.E. 7-7
 safety and first aid 1-7 to 1-11
 signs 1-23, 1-24
 slings 6-9 to 6-11, 6-34, 7-22, 7-23
 symptoms 1-23, 1-24
 syrup of ipecac 8-5
 vital signs 1-24, 2-13 to 2-18, 2-32
First aid, for specific injuries
 abdominal injuries 6-23 to 6-24
 alcohol-induced psychological emergencies 13-6
 allergic reactions 4-16 to 4-17, 4-34, 4-35
 amputations 6-20 to 6-22
 angina pectoris 5-6, 5-7
 anxiety attacks 13-5
 assaults 13-5
 asthma attacks 4-15, 4-34, 4-35, 4-36
 bites, animal and human 8-9
 bites or stings, insect 8-11
 blast injuries 4-11
 bleeding 6-15 to 6-17, 6-19
 bone or joint injuries 7-5 to 7-6 (see also
   Fractures;
   Dislocations; Sprains)
 breathing emergencies (see specific illnesses or
   injuries)
 breathing, ineffective 4-5 to 4-6
 bruises (contusions) 6-30
 "bumps on head" 6-30
 burns
   chemical 9-8
   dressings 9-7
   electrical 9-10 to 9-11
   eyes, to 9-9, 9-13
   heat 9-7
   radiation 9-12
   sunburns 9-12

First aid, for specific injuries (continued)
 cardiovascular emergencies 5-6, 5-7, 5-9
 cerebrovascular accidents (CVAs or strokes) 5-9
 choking (see Choking)
 compressions 7-12
 concussions 7-12
 congestive heart failure 5-7
 consciousness, level of 1-29, 1-30, 1-31, 2-14
 contusions (bruises) 6-30
 convulsions 11-5
 crush injuries 6-24 to 6-25
 diabetic emergencies 11-3
 drug-induced psychological emergencies 13-6
 ear canal, bleeding from 6-31
 embedded objects in wounds 6-26 to 6-29
 eye wounds 6-36 to 6-40
 eyeballs, extruded 6-41
 fainting 1-34 to 1-35
 fish hooks, embedded 6-29
 flail chests 4-10
 fractures (see Fractures)
 frostbite, superficial and deep 10-9, 10-10
 frostnip 10-9
 Glasgow Coma Scale 1-30, 2-14
 gunshot wounds 6-25 to 6-26
 hand injuries 6-34 to 6-35
 head injuries 7-9, 7-14 to 7-19
 heart attacks 5-6, 5-7
 heat cramps 10-11
 heat exhaustion 10-12
 heatstrokes 10-13
 hyperventilation 4-17
 hypothermia 10-5
 hysteria 13-4
 immobilization of bones or joints (see Fractures; Dislocations; Sprains)
 inhalation injuries 4-12, 8-6
 internal bleeding 6-19
 leeches 8-13
 miscarriages 12-9
 mouth or gums, bleeding 6-33
 moving casualties (see Moving (casualties))
 multiple casualties 2-26 to 2-28, 10-14
 nosebleeds 6-32
 penetrating chest wounds 4-7 to 4-9
 poisoning, general 8-4 to 8-8
 puncture wounds 6-25 to 6-26
 rewarming casualties 10-7
 rib or breastbone injuries 7-21
 scalp, bleeding from 6-33
 seizures 11-5
 shock 1-26 to 1-27
 smoke inhalation 4-12
 snakebites 8-9 to 8-10
 spinal injuries 7-14 to 7-19
 sprains 7-5 to 7-6, 7-36
 strains 7-5 to 7-6
 strokes (cerebrovascular accidents or CVAs) 5-9
 sunstroke 10-12 to 10-13
 tick bites 8-12
 transient ischemic attack (TIA) 5-9
 varicose veins, bleeding 6-36

First aiders 1-2, 1-3, 2-25
  emergency scene management 2-2 to 2-33
  emergency scene, on 1-12 to 1-14, 2-25
  getting help when alone 1-18, 1-19
First responders 1-13, 5-16, G-3
Fish hooks, embedded 6-29
"Five rights" (in giving medications) 8-14
Flail chests 4-7, 4-9 to 4-10, G-3
Flexion (anatomical term) 16-2, G-3
Flushing (for chemical burns) 9-8, 9-9
Flutter-type valves (in dressings) 4-8
Foot 6-7, 7-37, 16-6
Forearm (radius and ulna) 7-27 to 7-28, 16-6
Fractures 7-3, 7-5 to 7-7, 7-39, 10-14, G-3
  ankles 7-36
  burns and 9-4
  closed 7-2
  collarbones (clavicles) 7-22
  depression fractures (skull) 7-2
  elbows 7-25
  facial bones 7-8, 7-9 to 7-10
  fingers 7-30
  foot 7-37
  forearms (radius or ulna) 7-27 to 7-28
  hands 7-29
  hips 7-31 to 7-32
  jaw 7-8, 7-9 to 7-10
  knees 7-33
  lower legs (tibia or fibula) 7-34 to 7-35
  open 7-2, 7-34
  pelvis 7-20
  shock in 7-3
  shoulder blades (scapula) 7-22
  skull 7-8 to 7-9
  spinal 7-13 to 7-19
  thumbs 7-30
  toes 7-37
  traction 7-31
  types of 7-2
  upper arms (humerus) 7-24
  upper legs (femur) 7-31 to 7-32
  wrists 7-27 to 7-28
Frostbite 10-9 to 10-10, G-3
Frostnip 10-9

G

Gall bladder 16-8, G-3
Gas exchange 16-12
Gastric distention 4-28, G-3
Gauze G-3
"Gelled water" burn dressings 9-7
Glasgow Coma Scale 1-30, 2-14, G-3
Gloves 1-8, 1-10
"Golden hour" 1-15 to 1-16
Good Samaritan principles 1-4 to 1-6, 1-16
Guarding G-3
Gums, bleeding 6-33
Gunshot wounds 6-13, 6-25 to 6-26

H

Hands 7-29, 7-30, 16-6
  injuries 6-7, 6-34 to 6-35
  washing (precautions) 1-8
Hardening of arteries (arteriosclerosis) 5-8
Head 6-6, 16-6
Head or spinal injuries 1-28, 7-8 to 7-19
  airway, opening 2-9, 4-22
  artificial respiration and 4-22 to 4-23
  bleeding from mouth or gums 6-33
  breathing emergencies 4-8
  choking and 3-9, 3-19, 3-26
  compressions 7-11 to 7-12
  concussions 7-11 to 7-12
  CPR and 4-22, 4-23
  emergency scene management 2-4, 2-6 to 2-7
  extrication from car 14-14 to 14-15
  immobilization 7-14 to 7-19
  jaw-thrust without head-tilt manoeuvre 7-14
  lightning strikes and 10-14
  moving casualties 1-28, 2-4, 7-14 to 7-19
  ongoing casualty care 7-12, 7-19
  shock and 1-27, 7-13
  skull fractures 7-8 to 7-9
  spine boards 7-15, 7-17 to 7-19, 14-15
  turning casualties face up 2-8
Head-tilt chin-lift manoeuvre 2-9, 4-21, 4-26, G-3
Health professionals 1-14
Heart 16-9, 16-10, 16-12
Heart attacks (myocardial infarctions)
      5-4 to 5-7, 5-10, G-3
Heart failure 5-7, G-3
Heat cramps 10-11, G-3
Heat exhaustion 10-11, 10-12, G-3
Heat exposure 10-11 to 10-13
Heat loss. *See* Hypothermia
Heatstroke (sunstroke) 10-12 to 10-13, G-3
Heimlich manoeuvre 3-15, G-3
  adult, conscious 3-5
  adult, obese or pregnant 3-12
  adult, self-help 3-13
  adult, unconscious 3-7, 3-10
  child, conscious 3-16
  child, unconscious 3-18, 3-20
Hepatitis B 1-8, 13-6
HEROES™ program 15-8 to 15-9
High blood pressure (hypertension) 5-2, 5-3,
      5-31, 9-5
Hips, fractured 7-31 to 7-32
History (of casualty) 1-23, 2-12, 2-32, G-3
History (of situation) 1-23, 1-24, 2-4, G-3
Home safety 15-2 to 15-5
Human crutch (rescue carry) 14-5
Humerus (upper arm) 7-24, 16-6
Hydrogen sulphide (H_2S) 4-2
Hyperglycemia (diabetic coma) 11-2 to 11-3, G-3
Hypertension (high blood pressure) 5-2, 5-3,
      5-31, 9-5, G-3
Hyperthermia (heatstroke) 10-12 to 10-13, G-3

Hyperventilation 4-17, 13-3 to 13-5, 16-13, G-3
Hypoglycemia (insulin shock) 11-2 to 11-3, G-3
Hypothermia 10-2 to 10-10, 10-15, G-3
    frostbite 10-9 to 10-10
    frozen casualties 10-6
    pulse, taking 5-13, 10-5
    rewarming casualties 10-7
Hypoxia 4-2, 4-12, G-3
Hysteria 13-3 to 13-4

I

Ice, use of 6-42, 7-7, 7-23
Illnesses
    when to get medical help 1-22
    see also names of individual illnesses
Immobilization of casualties 7-5, 7-14 to 7-37, G-4
    cervical collars 7-15, 7-16, 14-15
    dislocations 7-23
    extrication, during 14-14 to 14-15
    fractures, other (*see* Fractures)
    head injuries 7-14 to 7-19
    pelvis, fractured 7-20
    spinal injuries 7-14 to 7-19
    splinting 7-26, 7-27, 7-32, 7-33, 7-35, 7-36
    traction 7-31
Impaled objects G-4
Implied consent 1-5
Improvisations
    dressings 6-3
    splints 7-26, 7-35, 7-36
    stretchers 14-9 to 14-10
Incisions 6-13
Incontinence G-4
Indirect methods. *See* Artificial respiration
Infant casualties, definition of 1-3
Infarctions 5-5, G-4
Infections G-4
    burns, complication of 9-5
    childbirth, prevention in 12-5
    universal precautions 1-8 to 9, 1-10
    wounds, in 6-12, 6-14, 6-16
Inferior (anatomical term) 16-2
Inflammation G-4
Inhalations 4-3, G-4
Inhalation injuries 4-12, 8-3, 8-6
    breathing emergencies 4-12
    burns and 9-6
    carbon monoxide 4-12, 8-3
    poisons, inhaled 8-3, 8-6
    smoke inhalation 4-12
Inhalers (for asthma) 4-36
Injuries 1-7, 1-20 to 1-22
    abdominal injuries 6-23 to 6-24
    dislocations (*see* Dislocations)
    fractures (*see* Fractures)
    head injuries 7-8 to 7-12
    immobilization (*see* Fractures; Immobilization of casualties)
    inhalation (*see* Inhalation injuries)

Injuries 1-7, 1-20 to 1-22 *(continued)*
    lightning strikes 10-14
    spinal injuries 7-13 to 7-19
    sprains (*see* Sprains)
    strains 7-38, 7-39, 10-14
Insect bites and stings 8-11, 8-15, 11-7
Insulin 11-2 to 11-3, 16-8, G-4
Insulin shock (hypoglycemia) 11-2 to 11-3, G-4
Intestines (bowels) 6-24, 16-8
Intrapleural spaces G-4
Involuntary muscles 16-4, G-4
Ipecac, syrup of 8-5
Iris (of eye) 16-7, G-4
Ischemic G-4

J

Jacket stretchers 14-10
Jaw thrust without head-tilt manoeuvre 4-22 to 4-23
Jaws (maxilla and mandible) 7-8, 7-9 to 7-10, 16-5, 16-6
Joints 7-3 to 7-4, 7-39, 16-4, G-4
    dislocations 7-4 to 7-7, 7-23, 7-25, 7-30
    fractures (*see* Fractures)
    lightning strikes and 10-14
    sprains 7-4, 7-5 to 7-7, 7-39
    see also names of individual joints

K

Kidneys 16-9, G-4
Knees 6-6 to 6-7, 7-33, 16-6

L

Labour, stages in childbirth 12-2 to 12-4, G-4
Lacerations 6-13, 6-39, G-4
    childbirth, after 12-8
Landmarking (in CPR) 5-13, 5-15, 5-19, 5-24, 5-26, 5-28, 5-30
Laryngectomy, artificial respiration and 4-29, G-4
Larynx 16-12
Lateral (anatomical term) 16-2
Leeches 8-13
Legal duty to help 1-4
Legal liabilities 1-4 to 1-6
Lens (of eye) 16-7, G-4
Level of consciousness (LOC). *See* Consciousness, level of
Lifting techniques 14-3 to 14-13
    casualties onto stretchers 14-11 to 14-12
    extrication, urgent 14-14 to 14-15
    head or spinal injuries 7-17 to 7-19
    rescue carries 14-3 to 14-8
Ligaments 16-4, G-4
Lightning injuries 10-14
Lipoproteins 4-31, G-4
Liver 16-8
Living alone 15-5

LOC. *See* Consciousness, level of
"Lockjaw" (tetanus) 6-16
"Logroll" 7-17, 7-18 to 7-19
Lower legs (tibia and fibula) 7-34 to 7-35, 16-6
Lubricating membrane (in joint) 16-4
Lumbar vertebrae 7-13, 16-5
Lungs 16-10, 16-12, 16-13
   pneumothorax 4-7 to 4-9, 4-37, 7-21
Lymph 16-12, G-4
Lymph nodes 16-12
Lymphatic system 16-12, G-4

M

Mandible (lower jaw) 7-8, 7-9 to 7-10, 16-5, 16-6,
   G-4
Material Safety Data Sheet (MSDS) 9-8, 15-7
Maxilla (upper jaw) 7-8, 7-9 to 7-10, 16-5
Mechanisms of injury 1-21, 4-11, 7-3, 7-38, 9-2, G-4
Medial (anatomical term) 16-2
Medical alert information 2-21, G-4
Medical help 1-15 to 1-19, 1-22, 7-37, G-4
   Emergency Medical Services (EMS) 1-17
Medications 8-14, 15-5
   allergic reactions 4-34, 4-35
   Ana-Kit Anaphylaxis Kit 4-35
   asthma 4-34, 4-35, 4-36
   EpiPen Auto-Injector 4-34
   inhalers 4-36
Mental illnesses 13-6 to 13-7
Metacarpals (bones in hand) 16-6, G-4
Metatarsals (bones in foot) 16-6, G-4
Microorganisms G-4
Miscarriages 12-2, 12-9, G-4
Motor nerves 16-7
Mouth, bleeding from 6-33
Mouth-to-mouth artificial respiration
   4-19 to 4-33, G-4
   see also Artificial respiration
Mouth-to-mouth contact 1-9
Moving (casualties) 14-2
   extrication, urgent 14-14 to 14-15
   head or spinal injuries 1-28, 2-4, 7-14 to 7-19
   lifting techniques 14-3
   "logroll" 7-17, 7-18 to 7-19
   rescue carries 14-3 to 14-8
   stretchers 14-9 to 14-14
   turning casualties face up 2-8
MSDS (Material Safety Data Sheet) 9-8, 15-7
Mucous membranes 8-2, G-4
Multiple casualty management (triage)
   2-26 to 2-28, 10-14
Muscles 16-3 to 16-4
   heat cramps 10-11
   strains 7-38, 7-39, 10-14
Musculoskeletal system 16-3 to 16-6, G-4
Myocardial infarctions (heart attacks) 5-4 to 5-7,
   5-10, G-4
   "chain of survival" 5-4

N

Nailbed test 6-18, G-4
Narrowing of arteries (atherosclerosis) 5-3
Natural gas, poisoning 8-3
"Natural" splints 7-26, 7-35
Neck injuries. *See* Head or spinal injuries
Negligence 1-5, 1-6, 1-16, G-4
Nerves 16-6 to 16-7, G-4
Nervous system 10-14, 16-6 to 16-7, G-5
Neutralizers, chemical 9-8
Newborns, care of 12-6 to 12-7
Nitrogen dioxide (silo gas) 4-2, 8-3, 8-6
Nitroglycerine G-5
Nosebleeds 6-32

O

O_2 (oxygen) 16-12, 16-13, G-5
Obese casualties 3-12, 3-13, 4-34
Obesity, risk factor 5-31
Obstructed airways G-5
Ongoing casualty care 2-24 to 2-25, 2-33
   choking 3-8
   head injuries 7-12, 7-19
OPAs (oropharyngeal airways) 7-16
Open fractures 7-2, 7-34
   see also Fractures
Optic nerves 10-14, 16-7
Organs 16-3, 16-8, 16-12
   see also names of individual organs
Oropharyngeal airways (OPAs) 7-16
Oxygen 16-12, 16-13, G-5

P

Padding (with splints) 7-26
Pancreas 16-8, G-5
Panic attacks 13-2, 13-4 to 13-5
Paradoxical chest movements 4-9, 4-10
Paralysis G-5
   hysteria, in 13-3
   spinal injuries 7-13
   strokes, determining in 5-8, 5-9
Patella (kneecap) 7-33, 16-6, G-5
Pelvis 7-20, 16-6
Peripheral nerves 16-7
Personal safety 15-2
Phalanges (bones in fingers and toes) 16-6, G-5
Pharynx 16-12, G-5
Physiology 16-2 to 16-11, G-5
Placenta 12-2, 12-3, 12-8, G-5
Plasma (blood component) 16-8, 16-11, G-5
Platelets (blood component) 16-11, G-5
Pleura 16-13
Pleural membranes 16-13, G-5
Pleural spaces 4-37
Pneumonia 4-2, 4-13, G-5
Pneumothorax 4-7 to 4-9, 4-37, 7-21, G-5
Poison Information Centre 8-2 to 8-3, 8-4
Poison ivy 8-7

Poisoning 8-2 to 8-8, 8-14
  artificial respiration 4-19, 4-34, 8-6
  breathing emergencies and 4-6
  Poison Information Centre 8-2 to 8-3, 8-4
  syrup of ipecac 8-5
Position of function 7-29, G-5
Positioning (casualties)
  artificial respiration 4-21, 4-22, 4-23, 4-26,
    4-31, 4-34, 5-27
  CPR 5-12, 5-13, 5-23, 5-27
  facial or jaw fractures 7-9 to 7-10
  head or spinal injuries (*see* Head or spinal
    injuries)
  pregnant casualties 3-12
  recovery position 1-27, 1-32, 1-33
  seizures or convulsions 11-5
  shock, in 1-27
  turning casualties face up 2-8
Posterior (anatomical term) 16-2
Post-traumatic acute renal failure 6-24
Power lines, downed 9-11
Pregnant casualties
  artificial respiration and 4-34
  childbirth, emergency 12-2 to 12-8
  choking and 3-12, 3-13
Preparedness. *See* Safety
Prevention of injuries
  bites and stings 8-15
  bleeding 6-43
  bone/joint/muscle injuries 7-39
  burns 9-15
  choking 3-29
  cold injuries 10-15
  infection 1-8 to 1-10
  poisoning, prevention 8-14
  wounds 6-43
Primary survey (emergency scene management)
    2-5 to 2-11, 2-31, G-5
Priorities in first aid 2-23, 2-26 to 2-28
  lightning strikes 10-14
  multiple casualties 2-27
Proximal (anatomical term) 16-2, G-5
Psychological emergencies 13-2 to 13-7
Pulmonary artery 16-10, G-5
Pulmonary circulation 16-11
Pulse 2-13, 2-16, 5-13, 10-5, 16-10, 16-11, G-5
Puncture wounds 6-13, 6-25 to 6-26
Pupil (of eye) 16-7

Q

Quebec, legal duty to help 1-4

R

Rabies 8-8
Radial (wrist) pulse 2-16, 16-11
Radiate G-5
Radioactive material 9-12
Radius (bone in forearm) 7-27 to 7-28, 16-6, G-5
"Reasonable skill and care" 1-5, 1-6

Recovery position 1-27, 1-32, 1-33
Recreational safety 15-8 to 15-9
Rectum 16-8
Red blood cells 16-11, G-5
Reef knots 6-5
Renal failure, post-traumatic acute 6-24
Repetitive strain injury (RSI) 7-39
Report, first aid 2-29
Reproductive system, female 12-2
Rescue carries 14-3 to 14-8
  stretchers, using 14-9 to 14-14
Respiratory arrests 4-4, G-5
Respiratory distress 4-4
Respiratory system 16-12 to 16-13
Responsiveness, assessing 2-4
Rest (in R.I.C.E.) 7-7
Retina (of eye) 16-7, G-5
Rewarming casualties (hypothermic) 10-7
Ribs 7-21, 16-5
R.I.C.E. 7-7, G-5
Ring pads 6-5, 6-27, 6-40
Risk factors (cardiovascular disease) 5-31
RSI (repetitive strain injury) 7-39
"Rule of nines" 9-4

S

Sacrum 7-13, 16-5, 16-6, G-5
Safety
  children, emergency skills 15-4
  driving a car 15-10 to 15-11
  elderly people 15-5
  fires 15-3
  first aid courses 1-2, 1-3, 15-12
  first aid kits 15-13
  HEROES program 15-8 to 15-9
  home, at 15-2 to 15-5
  personal 15-2
  recreation, during 15-8 to 15-9
  work, at 15-6 to 15-7
Safety for the first aider 1-7 to 1-11
  assessing emergency scene 2-3
  infection prevention 1-8 to 1-9, 1-10
  lifting techniques 14-3, 14-11 to 14-12
  violent situations 1-9, 1-11
SAMPLE (history of casualties) 2-12, 2-32
Scalds 9-2, 9-7, 9-15
Scalp, bleeding from 6-33
Scapula (shoulder blade) 7-22, 16-6, G-5
Scene survey (emergency scene management)
    2-2, 2-3 to 2-5, 2-30, G-5
Sclera (of eye) 16-7, G-5
Scrapes 6-13
Seatbelts, in car 15-11
Secondary survey (emergency scene manage-
    ment) 2-11 to 2-23, 2-32, G-5
Seizures 11-4 to 11-5
  burns and 9-5
Semi-consciousness 1-29, 1-30
Sensory nerves 16-7
Sexual assaults, psychological reactions to 13-5

Shivering (in hypothermia) 10-3
Shock 1-25 to 1-27, 6-12
    burns, in 9-5
    fractures, following 7-3, 7-29
    heat exhaustion, and 10-11
    insulin shock 11-2 to 11-3
    miscarriages, and 12-9
    pelvic injuries, and 7-20
    skin condition 2-17
    spinal injuries 7-13
Shoulder blades (scapula) 7-22, 16-6
Shoulder joints 7-23, 16-6
SIDS (Sudden infant death syndrome) 4-14, G-5
Signs and/or symptoms 1-23, 1-24, G-5, G-6
    allergic reactions (anaphylaxis) 4-16
    angina pectoris 5-3, 5-5
    anxiety attacks 13-4
    assaults, psychological reaction to 13-5
    asthma attacks 4-15
    bleeding, internal 6-14 to 6-15
    breathing problems 4-3, 4-4, 4-5
    burns 9-5, 9-6, 9-13
    cerebrovascular accidents (CVAs or strokes) 5-8
    choking 3-3, 3-22
    collarbone fractures 7-22
    compressions 7-11 to 7-12
    concussions 7-11 to 7-12
    congestive heart failure 5-7
    convulsions 11-4
    diabetic emergencies 11-2
    dislocations 7-5
    elbow fractures 7-25
    fainting 1-34
    flail chests 4-10
    fractures, in general 7-3
    frostbite 10-9
    head injuries 7-8
    heart attacks 5-5
    heat cramps 10-11
    heat exhaustion 10-11
    heatstrokes (sunstrokes) 10-12 to 10-13
    hip fractures 7-31
    hyperventilation 4-17
    hypothermia 10-4, 10-6, 10-7, 10-8
    hypoxia 4-12
    hysteria 13-3
    inhalation injuries 4-12
    insect bites or stings 8-11
    miscarriages 12-9
    muscle strains 7-38
    pelvic injuries 7-20
    poisoning 8-3
    rib/breastbone injuries 7-21
    seizures 11-4
    shock 1-26
    shoulder blade fractures 7-22
    smoke inhalation 4-12
    snowblindness 9-13
    spinal injuries, and 7-13
    sprains 7-4
    strokes (cerebrovascular accidents or CVAs) 5-8

Signs and/or symptoms 1-23, 1-24, G-5, G-6
(continued)
    transient ischemic attacks (TIAs) 5-8
    upper leg (femur) fractures 7-31
    vital signs 1-24, 2-13 to 2-18, 2-32
Silent killer (high blood pressure) 5-3
Silo gas (nitrogen dioxide) 4-2, 8-6
Skeleton 16-4 to 16-6
Skin 2-13, 2-17, 16-3
Skull 7-8 to 7-9, 16-5, 16-6
Slings 6-9 to 6-11, 6-34, 7-22, 7-23, G-5
Smoke detectors 15-3
Smoke-filled room, exiting 9-14
Smoke inhalation 4-12, 9-14
Snakebites 8-9 to 8-10, 8-15
Snowblindness 9-13
Spinal injuries 7-13, 7-14 to 7-19
    see also Head or spinal injuries
Spine 7-13, 16-5
Spine boards 7-15, 7-17 to 7-19, 14-15
Spleen 16-12, G-6
Splints 7-26, 7-27, 7-32, 7-33, 7-35, 7-36, G-6
Spontaneous pneumothorax 4-9, 4-37, G-6
Sprains 7-4, 7-5 to 7-6, 7-39, G-6
    ankles 7-36
    elbows 7-25
    foot or toes 7-37
    thumbs or fingers 7-30
    wrists 7-27 to 7-28
St. John Ambulance 1-2, 1-3, 15-12 to 15-13
Sternum 4-9, 4-10, 7-21, 16-5, G-6
Stoma (from laryngectomy) 4-29, G-6
Stomach 16-8
Strains (of muscles) 7-38, 7-39, 10-14, G-6
Stress
    critical incident 2-25
    risk factor 5-31
Stretchers 14-9 to 14-14
    carrying 14-13 to 14-14
    improvised 14-9 to 14-10
    placing casualties on 14-11 to 14-12
Strokes (cerebrovascular accidents or CVAs)
        5-8 to 5-9, 10-4
Subcutaneous tissue (skin layer) 16-3
Sucking chest wounds 4-7 to 4-9, 4-37, G-6
Sudden infant death syndrome (SIDS) 4-14
Suicide gestures 13-7
Sunburns 9-12, 9-15
Sunstrokes (heatstrokes) 10-12 to 10-13
Superficial G-6
Superior (anatomical term) 16-2
Superior vena cava 16-10, G-6
Swelling, in burns 9-5
Symptoms. See Signs and/or symptoms
Syrup of ipecac 8-5, G-6
Systemic circulation 16-11
Systems, body 16-3 to 16-13

T

Tarsals (ankle and foot bones) 16-6
Temperature, body 11-6
Tendons 16-4, G-6
Tension pneumothorax 4-9, 4-37, 7-21, G-6
Tetanus 6-16, G-6
Thigh bone (femur) 7-31 to 7-32, 16-6
Thorax 7-13, 16-5
Thumb injuries 7-30
TIAs (transient ischemic attacks) 5-8, 5-9, G-6
Tibia (lower leg bone) 7-34 to 7-35, 16-6, G-6
Ticks 8-12
Toes 7-37, 16-6
"Tonic" phase (of seizure) 11-4
Tooth, knocked-out 6-22
Tourniquets 6-21, G-6
Trachea 16-12, G-6
Traction in first aid 7-31, G-6
Transient ischemic attacks (TIAs) 5-8, 5-9, G-6
Transportation. *See* Moving (casualties)
Trauma G-6
Tremors, in hysteria 13-3
Triage (prioritizing casualties) 2-26 to 2-28, G-6
Triggers (of asthma attacks) 11-7
Two-rescuer CPR. *See* CPR (cardiopulmonary resuscitation)

U

Ulna (bone of forearm) 7-27 to 7-28, 16-6, G-6
Umbilical cord 12-2, 12-3, 12-8
Unconsciousness 1-29
    Glasgow Coma Scale 1-30, 2-14
Universal precautions 1-8 to 1-9, 1-10
Upper arms (humerus) 7-24, 16-6
Upper legs (femur) 7-31 to 7-32, 16-6
Ureters 16-9
Urethra 16-9, G-6
Urinary system 16-9
Urine 16-9
Uterus (womb) 12-2, G-6

V

Vagina 12-2, 12-3
Valves
    flutter-type, in dressings 4-8
    one-way, in face mask 1-9
Veins 6-35, 6-36, 16-10, G-6
    varicose veins, bleeding 6-35 to 6-36
Vena cava, superior 16-10
Ventilations G-6
    see also CPR
Ventricles (of heart) 16-10, G-6
Ventricular fibrillation G-6
Venules 16-10
Vertebral columns 16-5
Violent situations 1-9, 1-11

Vital signs 1-24, 2-13 to 2-18, 2-32, G-6
    Glasgow Coma Scale 1-30, 2-14
    psychological emergencies 13-2
Vitreous humor (of eye) 16-7
Voluntary muscles 16-4
Voluntary nervous system 16-7
Vomiting 4-28, 8-5, 8-6

W

"Waters breaking" (in childbirth) 12-3
White blood cells 16-11, G-6
Wind chill 10-2
WHMIS labelling 15-7
Womb (uterus) 12-2
Workplace Hazardous Materials Information
    System (WHMIS) 15-7
Workplace, safety in 9-8, 15-6 to 15-7
Wounds 6-12, 6-13, 6-20 to 6-43
    bandages 6-3 to 6-9
    bleeding, internal 6-12 to 6-19
    contamination prevention 6-16
    dressings 6-2 to 6-3
    types of wounds 6-13
        see also names of areas injured
Wrists 7-27 to 7-28, 16-6

X

Xiphoid process (sternum) 16-5, G-6